Baillière's
CLINICAL OBSTETRICS AND GYNAECOLOGY

INTERNATIONAL PRACTICE AND RESEARCH

Baillière's

CLINICAL OBSTETRICS AND GYNAECOLOGY

INTERNATIONAL PRACTICE AND RESEARCH

Volume 4/Number 3
September 1990

Induction of Ovulation

P. G. CROSIGNANI MD
Guest Editor

Baillière Tindall
London Philadelphia Sydney Tokyo Toronto

This book is printed on acid-free paper. ∞

Baillière Tindall   24–28 Oval Road,
W.B. Saunders   London NW1 7DX

The Curtis Center, Independence Square West,
Philadelphia, PA 19106–3399, USA

55 Horner Avenue
Toronto, Ontario M8Z 4X6, Canada

Harcourt Brace Jovanovich Group (Australia) Pty Ltd,
30–52 Smidmore Street, Marrickville, NSW 2204, Australia

Harcourt Brace Jovanovich Japan, Inc,
Ichibancho Central Building,
22-1 Ichibancho, Chiyoda-ku, Tokyo 102, Japan

ISSN 0950–3552

ISBN 0–7020–1478–8 (single copy)

Baillière's Clinical Obstetrics and Gynaecology is published four times each year by Baillière Tindall. Annual subscription prices are:

TERRITORY	ANNUAL SUBSCRIPTION	SINGLE ISSUE
1. UK	£49.00 post free	£22.50 post free
2. Europe	£57.00 post free	£22.50 post free
3. All other countries	Consult your local Harcourt Brace Jovanovich office for dollar price	

The editor of this publication is Margaret Macdonald, Baillière Tindall, 24–28 Oval Road, London NW1 7DX.

Baillière's Clinical Obstetrics and Gynaecology was published from 1983 to 1986 as *Clinics in Obstetrics and Gynaecology*.

Typeset by Phoenix Photosetting, Chatham.
Printed and bound in Great Britain by Mackays of Chatham PLC, Chatham, Kent.

Contributors to this issue

J. M. ANTOINE MD, Department of Obstetrics and Gynaecology, Hôpital Tenon, 4 rue de la Chine, 75020 Paris, France.

F. ARNAL, Biologist, Laboratoire de Fécondation in Vitro Maternite, 13 Avenue du Professeur Grasset, 34059 Montpellier Cédex, France.

F. AUDIBERT MD, Gynécologue Obstétricien, Faculté de Medecine Montpellier-Nimes, Services de Gynécologie-Obstétrique—Maternité, 13 Avenue du Professeur Grasset, 34059 Montpellier Cédex, France.

C. AYALA ADN, Research Coordinator, Texas Foundation for Research in Reproductive Medicine, 7800 Fannin Suite 502, Houston, TX 77054, USA.

DAVID T. BAIRD DSc, FRCOG, FRCP, MRC Clinical Research Professor, Department of Obstetrics and Gynaecology, University of Edinburgh, Centre for Reproductive Biology, 37 Chalmers Street, Edinburgh EH3 9EW, UK.

PAUL BENOS MD, Gynécologue Obstetricien Faculté de Medecine Montpellier-Nimes, Services de Gynécologie-Obstétrique—Maternité, 13 Avenue du Professeur Grasset, 34059 Montpellier Cédex, France.

GERHARD BETTENDORF, Prof Dr Med, Division of Endocrinology, Center for Reproductive Medicine, Univers. Franenklinik, Martinistr. 52, D-2000 Hamburg 20, FRG.

P. BOULOT MD, Gynécologue Obstétricien, Services de Gynécologie-Obstétrique—Maternité, 13 Avenue du Professeur Grasset, 34059 Montpellier Cédex, France.

J. BRINGER, Professeur d'Endocrinologie, Faculte de Médicine Montpellier-Nimes, Services d'Endocrinologie—Hopital Lapeyionie, Rte de Gauges, 34059 Montpellier Cédex, France.

PIERGIORGIO CROSIGNANI MD, Professor and Chairman, III Department of Obstetrics and Gynecology, University of Milan, Via M. Melloni 52, 20129 Milan, Italy.

CARLO FERRARI MD, Associate Professor, II Specialty School of Endocrinology, University of Milan; Senior Registrar, Responsible for the Endocrine Unit, Fatebenefratelli Hospital, Milan; Hospital, Corso di Porta Nuova 23, 20121 Milan, Italy.

STEPHEN FRANKS MD, FRCP, Professor of Reproductive Endocrinology, St Mary's Hospital Medical School, Norfolk Place, London W2 1PG, UK.

ROSE E. FRISCH BA, MA, PhD, Associate Professor of Population Sciences, Harvard Center for Population Studies, 9 Bow Street; School of Public Health, Cambridge, MA 02138, USA.

R. FRYDMAN, MD, Professor of the University of Paris, Hopital Antoine Beclere, 157 rue de la Porte de Trivaux, 923140 Clamart, France.

ANNA F. GLASIER BSc, MD, MB ChB, MRCOG, Clinical Research Scientist, Medical Research Council, Centre for Reproductive Biology, 37 Chalmers Street, Edinburgh EH3 9EW, UK.

LARS HAMBERGER, Professor, Department of Obstetrics & Gynaecology, University of Göteborg, S-71375 Göteborg, Sweden.

DIANA HAMILTON-FAIRLEY MRCOG, Research Fellow, Department of Obstetrics & Gynaecology, St Mary's Hospital Medical School, Norfolk Place, London W2 1PG, UK.

B. HEDON, Professeur Gynécologue Obstétricien, Faculté de Medecine Montpellier-Nimes, Services de Gynécologie-Obstetrique—Maternité, 13 Avenue du Professeur Grasset, 34059 Montpellier Cédex, France.

GARY D. HODGEN PhD, Scientific Director, The Jones Institute for Reproductive Medicine, Department of Obstetrics and Gynecology, Eastern Virginia Medical School, 855 W. Brambleton Avenue, Suite B, Norfolk, VA 23510, USA.

ROY HOMBURG MB BS, Senior Lecturer in Obstetrics & Gynaecology, Sackler School of Medicine, University of Tel Aviv, Israel; Previously, Clinical Research Fellow, Middlesex Hospital, Mortimer Street, London W1N 8AA, UK.

C. HUMEAU, Professeur de Biologie de la Reproduction, Faculté de Médecine Montpellier-Nimes, Laboratoire de Fécondation in Vitro Maternité, 13 Avenue du Professeur Grasset, 34059 Montpellier Cédex, France.

VACLAV INSLER MD, FRCOG, Director, Department of Ob/Gyn, Kaplan Hospital, Rehovot (affiliated to the Hebrew University Hadassah Medical School, Jerusalem); Professor of Obstetrics and Gynaecology, Ben Gurion University of the Neveg, Beer Sheba, Israel.

HOWARD S. JACOBS MD, FRCP, Professor of Reproductive Endocrinology, Middlesex Hospital, Mortimer Street, London W1N 8AA, UK.

F. LAFFARGUE, Professeur Gynécologue Obstétricien, Faculté de Médecine Montpellier-Nimes, Services de Gynécologie-Obstétrique—Maternité, 13 Avenue du Professeur Grasset, 34059 Montpellier Cédex, France.

WILLIAM L. LEDGER BA, MA, BM, BCh, MRCOG, Lecturer, Reproductive Medicine, Department of Obstetrics & Gynaecology, University of Edinburgh, Centre for Reproductive Biology, 37 Chalmers Street, Edinburgh EH3 9EW, UK.

BRUNO LUNENFELD MD, FRCOG, Director, Institute of Endocrinology, Sheba Medical Center, Tel-Hashomer, Ramat Gan 52621; Professor of Endocrinology, University of Bar Ilan, Ramat Gan, Israel.

P. MARES, Professeur Gynécologue Obstetricien, Services de Gynécologie Obstetrique, Hopital Carémeau, rue du Professeur Debré, 30006 Nimes, France.

SYLVIE NEVEU MD, Gynécologue Obstetricien, Faculté de Gynécologie-Obstetrique, Hopital Carémeau, 30006 Nimes, France.

LARS B. E. NILSSON MD, PhD, Assistant Professor, Department of Obstetrics & Gynecology, University of Göteborg, Sahlgren Hospital, S-41345 Göteborg, Sweden.

SERGIO OEHNINGER MD, The Jones Institute for Reproductive Medicine, Department of Obstetrics & Gynecology, Eastern Virginia Medical School, 855 West Brambleton Avenue, Suite B, Norfolk, VA 23510, USA.

STEVEN MICHAEL PETAK MD, Adjunct Assistant Professor, Department of Pharmacology, University of Texas Medical School, Houston and Texas Institute of Reproductive Medicine and Endocrinology, PO Box 20708, Houston, TX 77030, USA.

LUIS J. RODRIGUEZ-RIGAU MD, Clinical Associate Professor of Endocrinology, University of Texas Medical School at Houston, Texas, USA.

J. SALAT-BAROUX, Department of Obstetrics and Gynaecology, Hôpital Tenon, 4 rue de la Chine, 75020 Paris, France.

ZEEV SHOHAM MD, Lecturer in Obstetrics and Gynaecology, Kaplan Hospital, Rehovot, Israel; Present address: Clinical Research Fellow, Middlesex Hospital, Mortimer Street, London W1N 8AA, UK.

KEITH D. SMITH MD, Clinical Professor, Dept of Internal Medicine (Endocrinology), University of Texas Medical School at Houston, PO Box 20708, Houston TX 77030; Mailing address: 7800 Fannin St, Houston, TX 77054, USA.

EMIL STEINBERGER MSc, MD, Clinical Professor, University of Texas Medical School of Houston, 6431 Fannin, Houston, TX 77030, USA.

J. L. VIALA, Professeur Gynécologue Obstétricien, Faculté de Médecine Montpellier-Nimes, Services de Gynécologie-Obstetrique—Maternité, 13 Avenue du Professeur Grasset, 34059 Montpellier Cédex, France.

E. R. WEIDMAN MD, Texas Institute for Reproductive Medicine and Endocrinology, 7800 Fannin Suite 500, Houston, TX 77054; Clinical Assistant Professor, Dept of Medicine, University of Texas Medical School, Houston, PO Box 20708, TX 77030, USA.

Table of contents

PREVIOUS ISSUES

FORTHCOMING ISSUE

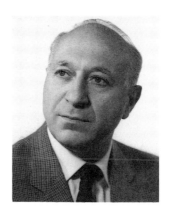

Foreword

Ovulation is still a mysterious phenomenon: its regulatory mechanism is poorly understood and its occurrence is difficult to detect. It is crucial for fertility and also has definite links to a woman's health. A lack of or defective ovulation is one of the commonest causes of sterility in humans.

Sometimes this is due to unfavourable conditions such as low body weight, excess prolactin or androgen, and once the problem has been corrected regular ovulatory cycles start again. Abnormal prolactin secretion is, for instance, a well-known cause of chronic anovulation and can be easily treated with dopaminergic drugs, with a remarkable 80–90% rate of success.

However, the pathophysiology that underlies most anovulations is still unknown and therefore no specific treatment can be prescribed for these patients. Nevertheless, the great advances in the study of ovarian physiology and the availability of powerful drugs allow an effective treatment today for the vast majority of anovulatory women.

Induction of ovulation through a mediated ovarian stimulation was made possible for the first time with the anti-oestrogens, and the industrial preparation of human gonadotrophins, introduced 30 years ago by P. Donini, has given clinicians the only direct ovarian stimulator. Today, pulsatile administration of hypothalamic LHRH is the new strategy for anovulation due to a variety of hypothalamic defects.

Thanks to these strategies, thousands of births have been enjoyed by infertile couples in the last 2–3 decades; however, the results are not ideal. Pharmacological stimulation of the ovary leads to a multiple follicular development that is quite different from monoovulation elicited by the pituitary gland. This is why the pregnancies achieved are associated with increased rates of abortion and twins.

In the recent past, the extensive use of the strategies of assisted procreation has spread the pharmacological induction of superovulation even to normally ovulating women to increase the pregnancy rate, but again, the effectiveness in achieving pregnancies is still paid for, with early and late complications of those gestations.

This comprehensive book, the collaborative work of a group of outstanding scientists, covers the past history and the present practice of ovulation induction, showing its possibilities and limitations to date.

ix

There is some indication, however, that we are just at the beginning of a long and fascinating story.

P. G. CROSIGNANI

1

The right weight: body fat, menarche and ovulation

ROSE E. FRISCH

Women who are underweight, or too lean, because of injudicious dieting or excessive athletic activity or both, experience disruption of their reproductive ability (Frisch and McArthur, 1974; Frisch et al, 1980, 1981b; Green et al, 1988). It is now well documented that moderate weight loss, in the range of 10–15% of normal weight for height, unassociated with anorexia nervosa (where weight loss is in the range of 30% below ideal weight) results in amenorrhoea due to hypothalamic dysfunction (Vigersky et al, 1977; Nillius, 1983). Weight loss in this moderate range is equivalent to a loss of one third of body fat (Frisch and McArthur, 1974). If the excessive leanness occurs before menarche, menarche may be delayed until as late as 19 or 20 years of age (Frisch et al, 1980, 1981b). Under special medical circumstances, normal menarche and ovulatory cycles can be delayed until after 30 years of age (Feigelman et al, 1987).

In addition to these disruptive effects of weight loss and athletic activity on the menstrual cycle, women who exercise moderately or who are regaining weight into the normal range may have a menstrual cycle which appears to be normal, but which actually has a shortened luteal phase or is anovulatory (Cumming et al, 1985; Prior, 1985). All of these partial or total disruptions of reproductive ability are usually reversible, after varying periods of time, following weight gain, decreased athletic training, or both (McArthur et al, 1976; Frisch et al, 1981).

Excessive fatness is also associated with infertility in women (Hartz et al, 1979; Pasquali et al, 1989) as was observed for animals almost a century ago by Marshall and Peel (1908). Loss of weight restores fertility of the women and of the animals.

Too little or too much fat are thus both associated with infertility. I have hypothesized that these associations are causal, and that the high percentage of body fat, 26–28% in women after completion of growth, is necessary for and may influence reproduction directly (Frisch, 1974, 1984, 1985, 1988). The hypothesis led to the prediction of minimum or threshold weights for height for the onset and maintenance of regular ovulatory menstrual cycles (Frisch and McArthur, 1974), as will be described below. These weights have been found to be useful clinically as target weights for the restoration of ovulatory cycles in cases of amenorrhoea due to weight loss (Nillius, 1983;

Baillière's Clinical Obstetrics and Gynaecology—
Vol. 4, No. 3, September 1990
ISBN 0–7020–1478–8

Speroff et al, 1983). I have hypothesized that both the absolute and relative amounts of fat are important, since the lean mass and the fat must be in a particular absolute range, as well as relative range, i.e., the female must be big enough to reproduce successfully (Frisch, 1985).

WHY FAT? CALORIC COST OF REPRODUCTION

A human pregnancy and lactation each have a high caloric cost: a pregnancy requires about 50 000 calories over and above normal metabolic require-ments (Emerson et al, 1972). Lactation requires about 1000 calories a day (FAO, 1957). In premodern times lactation was an essential part of repro-duction.

While the reproductive system is slowly maturing during growth, the body changes in composition as well as in size and proportions. Direct measurements of body water of girls from birth to completion of growth at ages 16–18 years show a continuous decline in the proportion of body water, because girls have a large relative increase in body fat (Friis-Hansen, 1956) (Figure 1). This decrease is particularly rapid during the adolescent growth spurt in height and weight which precedes menarche (Frisch, 1974).

At the completion of growth, between ages 16 and 18 years, the body of a well-nourished woman contains about 26–28% fat and about 52% water, whereas the body of a man at completion of growth contains about 14% fat and 61% water (Edelman et al, 1952; Moore et al, 1963). A young girl and boy of the same height and weight, as shown in Table 1, differ markedly in the percentages of body water and fat (Frisch, 1981). The main function of

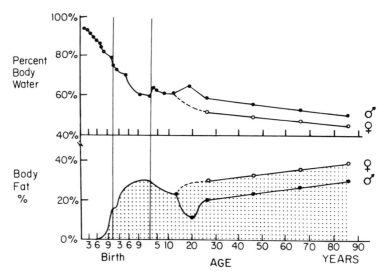

Figure 1. Changes in body water as a percentage of body weight throughout the life-span, and corresponding changes in the percentage of body fat. Adapted from Friis-Hansen (1965) with permission.

Table 1. Total water/body weight percentage as an index of fatness: comparison of a girl aged 18 and a boy aged 15 years of same height and weight.

	Girl aged 18 years	Boy aged 15 years
Height (cm)	165.0	165.0
Weight (kg)	57.0	57.0
Total body water (TW) (litres)	29.5	36.0
Lean body weight (LBW) (kg; TW/0.72)	41.0	50.0
Fat (kg)	16.0	7.0
(Fat/body weight) %	28.0	12.0
(Total body water/body weight) %	51.8	63.0

(Fat/body weight) % = 100 − [(TW/BW%)/0.72].
From Frisch (1981).

the 16 kg of stored female fat, which is equivalent to 144 000 calories, may be to provide energy for a pregnancy and for about 3 months' lactation. In prehistoric times when the food supply was scarce, or fluctuated seasonally, stored fat would have been necessary for successful reproduction. Fat is the most labile component of body weight. Body fat therefore would reflect environmental changes in food supplies more rapidly than other tissues (Frisch, 1984).

BODY WEIGHT AND INFANT SURVIVAL

Infant survival is correlated with birth weight, and birth weight is correlated with the prepregnancy weight of the mother and, independently, her weight gain during pregnancy (Eastman and Jackson, 1968). From a teleological and evolutionary view, it is economical to hypothesize that the physical ability to deliver a viable infant and the hypothalamic control of reproduction are synchronized. Adipose tissue may be the synchronizer.

HOW ADIPOSE TISSUE MAY REGULATE FEMALE REPRODUCTION

There are at least four mechanisms already known by which adipose tissue may directly affect ovulation and the menstrual cycle, and hence fertility:

1. Adipose tissue is a significant extragonadal source of oestrogen (Siiteri and MacDonald, 1973; Siiteri, 1981). Conversion of androgen to oestrogen takes place in adipose tissue of the breast and abdomen (Nimrod and Ryan, 1975), the omentum (Perel and Killinger, 1979), and the fatty marrow of the long bones (Frisch et al, 1975). This conversion accounts for roughly a third of the circulating oestrogen of premenopausal women. It is the main source of oestrogen in postmenopausal women. Men also convert androgen into oestrogen in body fat (Siiteri and MacDonald, 1973).

2. Body weight, and hence fatness, influences the direction of oestrogen metabolism to more potent or less potent forms (Fishman et al, 1975).

Very thin women have an increase in the 2-hydroxylated form of oestrogen, which is relatively inactive and has little affinity for the oestrogen receptor. Lean women athletes also have an increase in the 2-hydroxylated form of oestrogen (Snow et al, 1989). In contrast, obese women metabolize less of the 2-hydroxylated form and have a relative increase in the 16-hydroxylated form, which has potent oestrogenic activity (Schneider et al, 1983).

3. Obese women (Siiteri, 1981) and young girls who are relatively fatter (Apter et al, 1984) have a diminished capacity for oestrogen to bind to serum sex-hormone-binding globulin (SHBG); this results in an elevated percentage of free serum oestradiol. Since SHBG regulates the availability of oestradiol to the brain and other target tissues, the changes in the proportion of body fat to lean mass may influence reproductive performance through the intermediate effects of SHBG.

4. Adipose tissue of obese women stores steroid hormones (Kaku, 1969).

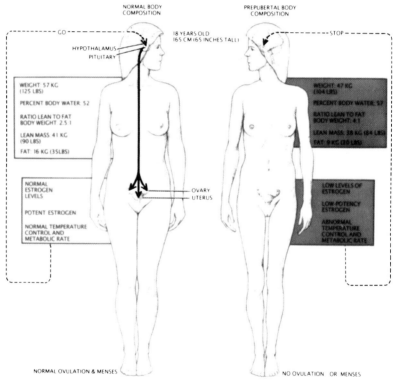

Figure 2. Women with moderate weight loss, in the range 10–15% of body weight, become amenorrhoeic due to hypothalamic dysfunction. Weight loss in this range is mainly loss of fat; the body reverts to a prepubertal body composition of lean mass to fat (4:1). How the hypothalamus perceives the fat loss is not known. Hypothalamic control of reproduction may be disrupted by decreases in the concentration and potency of circulating oestrogen and by signals of disturbed temperature control and abnormal metabolic rate. From Frisch (1988) with permission.

Changes in relative fatness might also affect reproductive ability indirectly through disturbance of the regulation of body temperature and energy balance by the hypothalamus (Figure 2). Very lean women, both anorectic and non-anorectic, display abnormalities of temperature regulation, in addition to delayed response or lack of response to exogenous luteinizing hormone-releasing hormone (Vigersky et al, 1977).

HYPOTHALAMIC DYSFUNCTION, GONADOTROPHIN SECRETION AND WEIGHT LOSS

It is now known that the amenorrhoea of underweight and excessively lean women is due to hypothalamic dysfunction (Vigersky et al, 1977; Nillius, 1983). Hypothalamic dysfunction has been implicated also in the amenorrhoea of athletes (Cumming et al, 1985). Consistent with the view that this type of amenorrhoea is adaptive, the pituitary–ovarian axis is apparently intact, and functions when exogenous gonadotrophin-releasing hormone (GnRH) is given in pulsatile form (Nillius, 1983) (Figure 3) or in a bolus (Vigersky et al, 1977).

Women with this type of hypothalamic amenorrhoea have both quantitative and qualitative changes in the secretion of the gonadotrophins luteinizing hormone (LH) and follicle-stimulating hormone (FSH), and of oestrogen:

1. LH, FSH, and oestradiol levels are low.
2. The secretion of LH and the response to gonadotrophin-releasing hormone (GnRH) are reduced in direct correlation with the amount of weight loss (Warren et al, 1975; Vigersky et al, 1977).
3. Underweight patients respond to exogenous GnRH with a pattern of secretion similar to that of prepubertal children; the FSH response is greater than the LH response. The return of LH responsiveness is correlated with weight gain (Warren et al, 1975; Nillius and Wide, 1977).
4. The maturity of the 24-h LH secretory pattern and body weight are related; weight loss results in an age-inappropriate secretory pattern resembling that of prepubertal or early pubertal children. Weight gain restores the postmenarcheal secretory pattern (Boyar et al, 1974).
5. A reduced response or absence of response to clomiphene is correlated with the degree of the loss of body weight and, hence, fat. A normal response occurs after weight gain to the normal range (Marshall and Fraser, 1971).

Supportive, also, of the view that this type of hypothalamic amenorrhoea is adaptive are the findings of van der Spuy et al (1988) that women in whom ovulation had been induced had a higher risk of babies who were small for dates, and this risk was greatest (54%) in those who were underweight. These authors conclude that the most suitable treatment for infertility secondary to weight-related amenorrhoea is dietary rather than induction of ovulation.

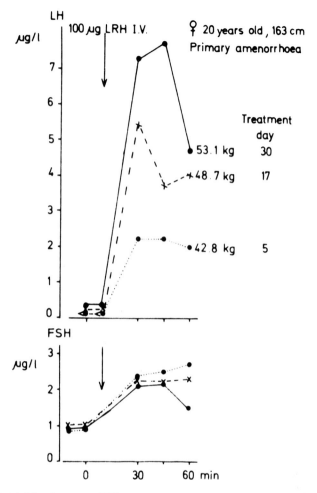

Figure 3. Luteinizing hormone (LH) and follicle-stimulating hormone (FSH) responses to luteinizing-releasing hormone (LRH) during refeeding of an anorectic woman, age 20 years, height 163 cm, with rapid weight gain (11 kg in 30 days), showing normalization of the LH responsiveness and change from a prepubertal to a mature gonadotrophic secretory pattern after LRH administration. From Nillius (1983) with permission.

THE PHYSIOLOGICAL BASIS OF REPRODUCTIVE ABILITY: WEIGHT AT MENARCHE

The idea that relative fatness is important for female reproductive ability followed from the findings that the events of the adolescent growth spurt, particularly menarche in girls, were closely related to an *average* critical body weight (Frisch and Revelle, 1971). This result was unexpected for human beings, although it was well known for monkeys (van Wagenen, 1949) and rats (Kennedy and Mitra, 1963) that puberty (defined by vaginal opening or, more precisely, by first oestrus) was more closely related to body weight than to chronological age.

The mean weight at menarche for United States girls was 47.8 ± 0.5 kg, at the mean height of 158.5 ± 0.5 cm at the mean age of 12.9 ± 0.1 years. This mean age included girls from Denver, who had a slightly later age of menarche than the sea-level populations because of the slowing effect of altitude on prenatal and postnatal weight growth (Frisch and Revelle, 1971).

THE SECULAR TREND TOWARD AN EARLIER AGE OF MENARCHE

Even before analysing the meaning of the critical weight for an *individual* girl, the idea that menarche is associated with a critical weight for a population provided a simple explanation for many observations associated with early or late menarche. Observations of earlier menarche are associated with attaining the critical weight more quickly. The most important example is the secular (long-term) trend to an earlier menarche of about 3 or 4 months per decade in Europe in the last 100 years (Wyshak and Frisch, 1982) (Figure 4). Our explanation is that children now are bigger sooner; therefore, girls on average reach 46–47 kg, the mean weight at menarche of

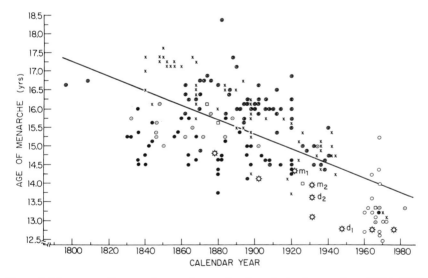

Figure 4. Mean or median age of menarche as a function of calendar year from 1790 to 1980. The symbols refer to England (○); France (●); Germany (⊗); Holland (□); Scandinavia (Denmark, Finland, Norway, and Sweden) (×); Belgium, Czechoslovakia, Hungary, Italy, Poland (rural), Romania (urban and rural), Russia (15.2 years at an altitude of 2500 m and 14.4 years at 700 m), Spain and Switzerland (all labelled ○); and the United States (✿) (data not included in the regression line). Twenty-seven points were identical and do not appear on the graph. The regression line of course cannot be extended indefinitely. The age of menarche has already levelled off in some European countries, as it has in the United States (see text). From Wyshak and Frisch (1982) with permission.

the United States and many European populations, more quickly. According to our hypothesis also, the secular trend should end when the weight of children of successive cohorts remains the same because of the attainment of maximum nutrition and child care; this has now happened in the United States (Frisch and Revelle, 1971).

Conversely, a late menarche is associated with body weight growth that is slower prenatally, postnatally, or both, so that the average critical weight is reached at a later age. Malnutrition delays menarche (Tanner, 1962), twins have later menarche than do singletons of the same population, and high altitude delays menarche (Frisch and Revelle, 1971).

COMPONENTS OF WEIGHT AT MENARCHE

Individual girls have menarche at various weights and heights (Frisch and Revelle, 1971). In order to make the notion of a critical weight meaningful for an individual girl at menarche, we analysed the components of body weight at menarche (Frisch et al, 1973). We investigated body composition at menarche because total body water (TW) and lean body weight (LBW, TW/0.72) are more closely correlated with metabolic rate than is body weight, since they represent the metabolic mass as a first approximation. Metabolic rate was considered an important clue, since Kennedy hypothesized a food intake–lipostat–metabolic signal to explain his elegant findings on weight and puberty in the rat (Kennedy and Mitra, 1963; Kennedy, 1969).

The greatest change in estimated body composition of both early- and late-maturing girls during the adolescent growth spurt was a large increase in body fat, from about 5 kg to 11 kg, a 120% increase, compared to a 44% increase in lean body weight. There was thus a change in the ratio of lean body weight to fat from 5:1 at initiation of the spurt to 3:1 at menarche. The shortest, lightest girls at menarche have a smaller absolute amount of fat, 8.9 ± 0.4 kg, compared to that of the tallest, heaviest girls, 12.3 ± 0.6 kg (the mean of all subjects is 11.5 ± 0.3 kg). However, both extreme groups have about 22% of their body weight as fat at menarche as do all subjects, and the ratio of lean body weight to fat of both groups is in the range of 3:1, as it is in all subjects (Frisch et al, 1973).

Since adipose tissue can convert androgens to oestrogens (Siiteri and MacDonald, 1973) the relative degree of fatness can be directly related to the quantity of circulating oestrogen. The biological effectiveness of the oestrogen is also related to body weight (Fishman et al, 1975). Rate of fat gain is therefore a neat mechanism for relating rate of growth, nutrition, and physical work to the energy requirements for reproduction.

FATNESS AS A DETERMINANT OF MINIMAL WEIGHTS FOR MENSTRUAL CYCLES

As shown in Table 1 and Figure 1, total water/body weight per cent is an

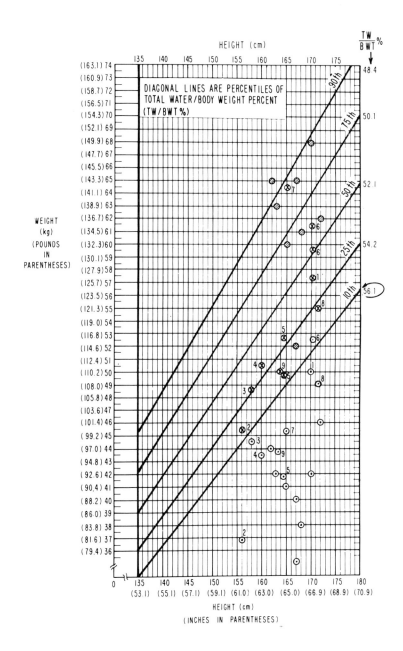

Figure 5. The minimal weight necessary for a particular height for restoration of menstrual cycles is indicated on the weight scale by the 10th percentile diagonal line of total water/body weight per cent, 56.1%, as it crosses the vertical height line. For example, a 20-year-old woman whose height is 165 cm (65 in) should weigh at least 49 kg (108 lb) before menstrual cycles would be expected to resume. From Frisch and McArthur (1974) with permission.

index of fatness (Friis-Hansen, 1956). The total water/body weight per cent data of each of the same 181 girls followed from menarche to the completion of growth at ages 16–18 years provided a method of determining a minimal weight for height necessary for menarche in primary amenorrhoea and for the resumption of normal ovulatory cycles in cases of secondary amenorrhoea, when the amenorrhoea is due to undernutrition and/or intensive exercise (Frisch and McArthur, 1974). These weights have been found useful in the evaluation and treatment of patients with primary or secondary amenorrhoea due to weight loss (Nillius, 1983).

Percentiles of total body water/body weight per cent, which are percentiles of fatness, were made at menarche and for the same 181 girls at age 18 years, the age at which body composition was stabilized (Frisch, 1976). Patients with amenorrhoea due to weight loss, other possible causes having been excluded, were studied in relation to the weights indicated by the diagonal percentile lines of total water/body weight per cent in Figure 5. We found that 56.1% of total water/body weight, the 10th percentile at age 18 years, which is equivalent to about 22% fat of body weight, indicated a minimal weight for height necessary for the restoration and maintenance of menstrual cycles. For example, a 20-year-old woman whose height is 165 cm (65 in) should weigh at least 49 kg (108 lb) before menstrual cycles would be expected to resume (Figure 5).

The weights at which menstrual cycles ceased or resumed in postmenarcheal patients age 16 years and older were about 10% heavier than the minimal weights for the same height observed at menarche (Frisch and McArthur, 1974) (Figure 6).

The explanation was that both early- and late-maturing girls gain an average of 4.5 kg of fat from menarche to age 18 years. Almost all this gain is achieved by age 16 years, when mean fat is 15.7 ± 0.3 kg, 27% of body weight. At age 18 years mean fat is 16.0 ± 0.3 kg, 28% of the mean body weight of 57.1 ± 0.6 kg. Reflecting this increase in fatness, the total water/body weight per cent decreases from $55.1 \pm 0.2\%$ of menarche (12.9 ± 0.1 years in our sample) to $52.1 \pm 0.2\%$ (SD 3.0) at age 18 years (Frisch, 1976).

Because girls are less fat at menarche than when they achieve stable reproductive ability, the minimal weight for onset of menstrual cycles in cases of primary amenorrhoea due to undernutrition or exercise is indicated by the 10th percentile of fractional body water at menarche, 59.8%, which is equivalent to about 17% of body weight as fat. For example, a 15-year-old girl whose completed height is 165 cm (65 in) should weigh at least 43.6 kg (96 lb) before menstrual cycles can be expected to begin (Figure 6).

The minimum weights indicated in Figure 6 would also be used for girls who become amenorrhoeic as a result of weight loss shortly after menarche, as is often found in cases of anorexia nervosa in adolescent girls (Crisp, 1970).

The absolute and relative increase in fatness from menarche to ages 16–18 years coincides with the period of adolescent subfecundity (Montague, 1979). During this time there is still rapid growth of the uterus, the ovaries, and the oviducts (Scammon, 1930).

Other factors, such as emotional stress, affect the maintenance or onset of menstrual cycles. Therefore, menstrual cycles may cease without weight loss and may not resume in some subjects even though the minimum weight for height has been achieved. Also, our standards apply as yet only to Caucasian United States females and European females; different races have different critical weights at menarche, and it is not yet known whether the different

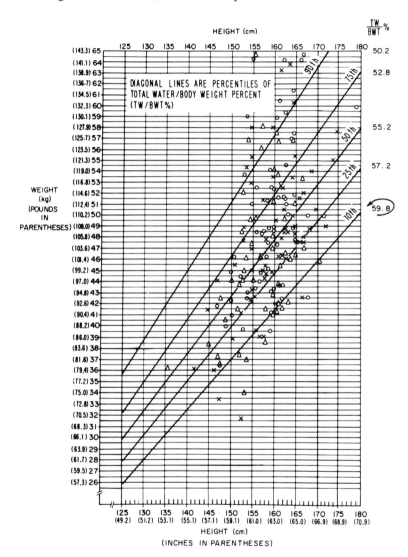

Figure 6. The minimal weight necessary for a particular height for onset of menstrual cycles is indicated on the weight scale by the 10th percentile diagonal line of total water/body weight per cent, 59.8%, as it crosses the vertical height lines. Height growth of girls must be completed, or approaching completion. For example, a 15-year-old girl whose completed height is 165 cm (65 in) should weigh at least 43.6 kg (96 lb) before menstrual cycles can be expected to start. From Frisch and McArthur (1974) with permission.

critical weights represent the same critical body composition of fatness (Frisch and McArthur, 1974).

Since the prediction of the minimum weights for height is from TW/BW% (not fat/BW%), I have hypothesized that the successful prediction is related to a lean mass:fat ratio, which is normally about 3:1 at menarche and 2.5:1 at the completion of growth at age 18 years. No prediction can as yet be made above the threshold weight for a particular height.

PHYSICAL EXERCISE, DELAYED MENARCHE AND AMENORRHOEA

Does intense exercise cause delayed menarche and amenorrhoea of athletes, or do late maturers choose to be athletes and dancers? Frisch et al (1980) found that the mean age of menarche of 38 college swimmers and runners was 13.9 ± 0.3 years, significantly later ($P < 0.001$) than that of the general population, 12.8 ± 0.05 years, in accord with other reports (Malina et al, 1978). However, the mean menarcheal age of the 18 athletes whose training began *before* menarche was 15.1 ± 0.5 years, whereas the mean menarcheal age of the 20 athletes whose training began after their menarche was 12.8 ± 0.2 years ($P < 0.001$). The latter mean age was similar to that of the college controls, 12.7 ± 0.4 years, and the general population. Therefore, training, not preselection, is the delaying factor. Each year of premenarcheal training delayed menarche by 5 months (0.4 year). This suggests that one constructive way to reduce the incidence of teenage pregnancy would be to have girls join teams at ages 8–9 years and maintain regular moderate exercise. Such a programme may also reduce the risk of the serious diseases of women in later life, as I will present below.

The training also directly affected the regularity of the menstrual cycles during the training year. Of the premenarche trained athletes, only 17% had regular cycles; 61% were irregular and 22% were amenorrhoeic. In contrast, 60% of the postmenarcheal trained athletes were regular, 40% were irregular, and none were amenorrhoeic. However, during intense training, the incidence of oligomenorrhoea and amenorrhoea increased in both groups.

As other workers have found (Dale et al, 1979; Schwartz et al, 1981) plasma gonadotrophins and oestrogen levels were in the low–normal range for the athletes with irregular cycles or amenorrhoea. Progesterone was at follicular phase level. Thyroid hormones, however, were in the normal range (Frisch et al, 1981a). These athletes had increased muscularity and decreased adiposity compared to non-athletes. The explanation of their menstrual disturbances may therefore be the same as for dieting, non-athletic women: too little fat in relation to the lean mass. Some of the swimmers and track and field athletes were above average weight for height. A raised lean/fat ratio may nevertheless have caused their menstrual problems, because their body weight undoubtedly represented a greater amount of muscle and less adipose tissue than the same weight of a non-athletic woman. Behnke et al (1942) found, over 4 decades ago, that physically fit male football players, who had been misclassified as overweight, in fact had little adipose tissue and a great deal of muscle.

PSYCHOLOGICAL STRESS AND CHANGES IN WEIGHT

The psychological stress of competition, which may increase the secretion of adrenal corticosteroids and catecholamines, thus affecting the hypothalamic control of gonadotrophins (Reichlin, 1982), may also be involved; however, stress does not seem to be the main factor in many individuals. For example, a top-ranked 17.5-year-old swimmer who had a high tension score on the Profile Moods State test had not had a menstrual period in 5 months. She was very lean: her height was 169.2 cm (66.6 in) and her weight was 48.9 kg (108 lb), which is 82.5% of ideal weight and 2.1 kg below the critical weight for her height found necessary for regular cycles (Frisch and MacArthur, 1974). After 2 months of training and no menses, this swimmer suddenly reported a 4-day period. On inquiry she reported she had gained 5 lb (2.3 kg) 'on purpose, by eating a lot of carbohydrate', to see if she would have a cycle. She lost the 5 lb by the next month and had no more cycles. What this small change in weight represents physiologically or endocrinologically is an intriguing question.

In contrast to the lean swimmer, a woman swimmer of the English channel (9 hr 20 min), who was studied during the training and after the swim, had an ample supply of body fat (about 30%) which preswim tests showed was necessary for maintenance of her body temperature. The reproductive changes during training included a shortened luteal phase, absence of ovulation and increased LH secretion relative to FSH. However, this swimmer did not become amenorrhoeic, even after the swim, although the metabolic and hormonal (except cortisol) data after the swim reflected the severe physiological stress, and presumably there was also psychological stress (Frisch et al, 1984).

DOUBLE-MUSCLED CATTLE AND OTHER ANIMAL DATA

That loss of fat and extreme leanness, not weight loss per se, is the important factor in infertility, can be deduced from the relative infertility of the breed of double-muscled Charolais cattle. As described by Vissac et al (1974): 'Female cattle with muscular hypertrophy have evident physiological troubles with their puberty, their fertility, and their sexuality in general' (translation from French). Cows of this breed produce insufficient milk to nourish their calves by the second month of lactation. The Charolais bulls also are not very fertile. It may be relevant that these very lean cattle are more subject to heat stress than normal breeds; the lean bulls have a greater increase in rectal temperature as the ambient temperature rises (Halipré, 1973).

EXPERIMENTAL EVIDENCE

Rats fed a high-fat diet, the fat being substituted isocalorically for carbohydrate, had oestrus significantly earlier ($P<0.001$) than did rats fed a low-fat diet (Frisch et al, 1975). Confirming and extending Kennedy's findings, we found that the caloric intake per 100 g body weight of the high-fat-diet (HFD) and low-fat-diet (LFD) rats did not differ at vaginal opening or at first oestrus, whereas the two groups differed significantly at both events in age, absolute food intake, relative food intake, and absolute caloric intake.

Direct carcass analysis data showed that the HFD and LFD rats had similar body compositions at oestrus, although the HFD rats had oestrus at a lighter body weight than the LFD rats (Frisch et al, 1977). The means ($\pm$ SEM) of total water as percentage of wet weight were $66.2 \pm 0.3\%$ for the HFD rats and $66.4 \pm 0.3\%$ for the LFD rats, whereas the mean absolute total body water for the two diet groups was 69.7 ± 2.2 g and 81.1 ± 2.4 g, respectively ($P<0.01$).

FOOD INTAKE, OVULATION AND 'FLUSHING'

'Flushing' is the increase in the rate of twinning in sheep resulting from short-term (e.g. a week) high-caloric feeding before mating to the ram (Coop, 1966). The well-nourished human female fortunately does not normally superovulate in response to a high caloric intake, like a large steak dinner, although, interestingly, there is evidence for some residual flushing effect even in human beings. The rate of human dizygotic twinning, but not monozygotic twinning, fell during wartime restrictions of nutrition in Holland and the rate returned to normal after the return of a normal food supply (Bulmer, 1970).

NUTRITION AND MALE REPRODUCTION

Undernutrition delays the onset of sexual maturation in boys (Tanner, 1962) similar to the delaying effect of undernutrition on menarche. Undernutrition and weight loss in men also affects their reproductive ability. The sequence of effects, however, is different from that in the female. In men loss of libido is the first effect of a decrease in caloric intake and subsequent weight loss. Continued caloric reduction and weight loss results in a loss of prostate fluid, and decreases of sperm motility and sperm longevity, in that order. Sperm production ceases when weight loss is in the range of 25% of normal body weight. Refeeding results in a restoration of function in the reverse order of loss (Keys et al, 1950).

EFFECTS OF EXERCISE ON MALES

Men marathon runners have recently been shown to have decreased hypothalamic gonadotrophin-releasing hormone secretion (MacConnie et al, 1986). Also reported are changes in serum testosterone levels with weight loss in wrestlers (Strauss et al, 1985), a reduction in serum testosterone and prolactin levels in male distance runners (Wheeler et al, 1984), and changes in reproductive function and development in relation to physical activity (Wall and Cumming, 1985).

NUTRITION, PHYSICAL WORK AND NATURAL FERTILITY: HUMAN REPRODUCTION RECONSIDERED?

The effects of hard physical work and nutrition on reproductive ability, set forth above, suggested that differences in the fertility of populations, historically and today, may be explained by a direct pathway from food intake to fertility (Frisch, 1975, 1978) (Figure 7), in addition to the classic Malthusian pathway through mortality. Charles Darwin (1859, 1894) described this commonsense direct relationship between food supplies and fertility, observing that: (1) domestic animals, which have regular, plentiful food without working to get it, are more fertile than the corresponding wild animals; (2) 'hard living retards the period at which animals conceive'; (3) the amount of food affects the fertility of the same individual; and (4) it is difficult to fatten a cow which is lactating. All of Darwin's dicta apply to human beings (Frisch, 1978).

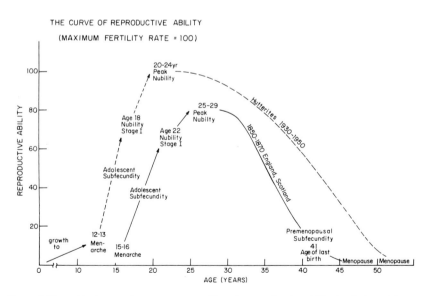

Figure 7. The mid-nineteenth-century curve of female reproductive ability (variation of the rate of childbearing with age) compared to that of the well-nourished, non-contracepting, modern Hutterites. The Hutterite fertility curve results in an average of 10–12 children, the 1850–1870 fertility curve in about six to eight children. From Frisch (1978) with permission.

THE PARADOX OF RAPID POPULATION GROWTH IN UNDERNOURISHED POPULATIONS

In many historical populations with slow population growth, poor couples living together to the end of their reproductive lives had only six to seven living births. Most poor couples in many developing countries today also only have six to seven living births during their reproductive life-span. This total fertility rate is far below the human maximum of 11 to 12 children observed among well-nourished, non-contracepting peoples such as the Hutterites. However, six children per couple today in developing countries results in a very rapid rate of population growth because of decreased mortality rates resulting from the necessary introduction of modern public health procedures. The difference between the birth rate/1000 and the death rate/1000 (which gives the growth rate [%]), is now as high as 2%, 3%, and 4%. Populations growing at these rates double in 35 years, 23 years, and 18 years, respectively.

British mid-19th-century data on growth rates, food intake, age-specific fertility, sterility, and ages of menarche and menopause show that females who grew relatively slowly to maturity, completing height growth at ages 20–21 years (instead of 16–18 years as in well-nourished contemporary populations), also differ from well-nourished females in each event of the reproductive span: menarche is later, for example 15.0–16.0 years compared to 12.8 years; adolescent sterility is longer, the age of peak nubility is later; the levels of specific fertility are lower; pregnancy wastage is higher; the duration of lactational amenorrhoea is longer; the birth interval is therefore longer; and the age of menopause is earlier, preceded by a more rapid period of perimenopausal decline (Figure 7) (additional references in Frisch, 1978, 1983).

Thus, the slower, submaximum growth of women to maturity is subsequently associated with a shortened and less efficient reproductive span. The differences in the rate of physical growth of women and men result not only in a displacement of the age-specific fertility curve in time, but in a difference in the ultimate level: the faster the growth of the females and males, the earlier and more efficient the reproductive ability (Frisch, 1983).

Recent endocrinological data show that undernourished women have a longer lactational amenorrhoea than do well-nourished women (Lunn et al, 1984). The amount of suckling is not the only factor, as has been suggested in explaining reduced natural fertility. In addition, age of menarche and the other events of the reproductive span, which are known to be affected by the nutritional state, are pertinent to overall fertility (Frisch, 1978).

LONG-TERM REGULAR EXERCISE LOWERS THE RISK OF SEX-HORMONE-SENSITIVE CANCERS

The amenorrhoea and delayed menarche of athletes raised the question: are there differences in the long-term reproductive health of athletes with moderate training compared to non-athletes?

A study of 5398 college alumnae aged 20–80 years, 2622 of whom were former athletes and 2776 were non-athletes, showed that the former athletes had a significantly lower life-time occurrence of breast cancer and cancers of the reproductive system compared to non-athletes. Over 82.4% of the former college athletes began their training in high school or earlier, compared to 24.9% of the non-athletes. The analysis controlled for potential confounding factors, including age, age of menarche, age of first birth, smoking, cancer family history, etc. (Frisch et al, 1985). The relative risk (RR) for non-athletes/athletes for cancers of the reproductive system was 2.53, 95% confidence limits (CL) (1.17, 5.47). The RR for breast cancer was 1.86, 95% CL (1.00, 3.47). The former college athletes were leaner in every age group compared to the non-athletes.

Although one can only speculate at present as to the reasons for the lower risk, the most likely explanation is that in the long term, the former athletes had lower levels of oestrogen because they were leaner, and more of the oestrogen was metabolized to the non-potent catechol oestrogens (Frisch et al, 1985; Hershcopf and Bradlow, 1987). Also, the former athletes may have consumed diets lower in fat and saturated fat (Frisch et al, 1981b). Such diets shift the pattern of oestrogen metabolism toward the less active catechol oestrogens (Longcope et al, 1987).

The lower risk of breast cancer observed among the former college athletes is in accord with the hypothesis of Henderson et al (1985) that regular, ovulatory menstrual cycles would be expected to *increase* the risk of breast cancer. The former college athletes also had a lower life-time occurrence (prevalence) of benign tumours of the breast and reproductive system (Wyshak et al, 1986), a lower prevalence of diabetes, particularly after age 40, compared to the non-athletes (Frisch et al, 1986) and no greater risk of bone fractures, including risk of wrist and hip fractures, in the menopausal period compared to non-athletes (Wyshak et al, 1987).

These data indicate that long-term exercise, which was not Olympic or marathon level but moderate and regular, reduces the risk of sex-hormone-sensitive cancers, and the risk of diabetes, for women later in life. Recent data showing that moderate exercise also reduces the risk of non-reproductive system cancers (Blair et al, 1989; Frisch et al, 1989) suggest that other factors, such as changes in immunosurveillance, may also be involved.

SUMMARY

Women with moderate weight loss (10–15% of ideal weight), as well as women with the severe weight loss of anorexia nervosa (30% of ideal weight), have secondary or primary amenorrhoea. A high proportion of well-trained dancers and athletes also have amenorrhoea, though weight may be in the normal range, since muscles are heavy (80% water, compared to 5–10% water in adipose tissue). The amenorrhoea is usually reversible with weight gain, decreased exercise or both. The amenorrhoea is due to hypothalamic dysfunction; the pituitary–ovary axis is intact, suggesting that this type of amenorrhoea is adaptive, preventing an unsuccessful pregnancy outcome. Evidence is presented that the high percentage of body fat (26–28%) in mature women is necessary for regular ovulatory cycles. Target weights for height are given for the evaluation and treatment of primary and secondary amenorrhoea due to weight loss. The high percentage of body fat in women may influence reproductive ability directly: (1) as an extragonadal source of oestrogen by aromatization of androgen to oestrogen; (2) by influencing the direction of oestrogen metabolism to more potent or less potent forms; or (3) by changes in the binding properties of sex-hormone-binding globulin. Indirect signals may be of abnormal control of temperature and changes in energy metabolism, which accompany excessive leanness.

Acknowledgements

The research on athletes reported here was in part under the auspices of the Advanced Medical Research Foundation, Boston, and in part funded by a grant from the National Science Foundation (No. BNS 85–20614). I thank Dan Holzner for the preparation of the manuscript.

REFERENCES

Apter D, Bolton NJ, Hammond GL et al (1984) Serum sex hormone-binding globulin during puberty in girls and in different types of adolescent menstrual cycles. *Acta Endocrinologica* **107**: 413–419.

Behnke AR, Feen GB & Welham WC (1942) The specific gravity of healthy men. Body weight:volume as an index of obesity. *Journal of the American Medical Association* **118**: 495–498.

Blair SN, Kohl HW III, Paffenbarger RS et al (1989) Physical fitness and all-cause mortality. *Journal of the American Medical Association* **262**: 2395–2401.

Boyar RM, Katz J, Finkelstein JW et al (1974) Anorexia nervosa: immaturity of the 24-hour luteinizing hormone secretory pattern. *New England Journal of Medicine* **291**: 861–865.

Bulmer MG (1970) *The Biology of Twinning in Man.* Oxford: Oxford University Press.

Coop IE (1966) Effect of flushing on reproductive performance of ewes. *Journal of Agricultural Science* **67**: 305–323.

Crisp AH (1970) Anorexia nervosa: 'feeding disorder', 'nervous malnutrition', or 'weight phobia'? *World Review of Nutrition and Diet* **12**: 452–504.

Cumming DC, Vickovic MM, Wall SR et al (1985) Defects in pulsatile LH release in normally menstruating runners. *Journal of Clinical Endocrinology and Metabolism* **6**: 810–812.

Dale D, Gerlach DH & Wilhite AL (1979) Menstrual dysfunction in distance runners. *Obstetrics and Gynecology* **54**: 47–53.

Darwin C (1859) *Origin of Species* (first edition facsimile, 1975), p 147. Cambridge, Massachusetts: Harvard University Press.

Darwin C (1894) *The Variation of Animals and Plants Under Domestication*, Volume 2, 2nd edn, pp 88–99. New York: Appleton.

Eastman NJ & Jackson E (1968) Weight relationships in pregnancy. I: The bearing of maternal weight gain and pre-pregnancy weight on birth weight in full term pregnancies. *Obstetrical and Gynecological Survey* **23**: 1003–1025.

Edelman IS, Haley HB, Scholerb PR et al (1952) Further observations on total body water. I. Normal values throughout the life span. *Surgery Gynecology and Obstetrics* **95**: 1–12.

Emerson K Jr, Saxena BN & Poindexter EL (1972) Caloric cost of normal pregnancy. *Obstetrics and Gynecology* **40**: 786–794.

FAO (1957) *Calorie Requirements*. Rome: Food and Agriculture Organization of the United Nations (FAO).
Feigelman T, Frisch RE, Wilmore D et al (1987) Sexual maturation in third and fourth decades, after nutritional rehabilitation by internal feeding. *Journal of Pediatrics* **111:** 620–623.
Fishman J, Boyar RM & Hellman L (1975) Influence of body weight on estradiol metabolism in young women. *Journal of Clinical Endocrinology and Metabolism* **41:** 989–991.
Friis-Hansen BJ (1956) Changes in body water compartments during growth. *Acta Paediatrica* **110 (supplement):** 1–67.
Friis-Hansen B (1965) Hydrometry of growth and aging. In Brözek J (ed.) *Human Body Composition*. Symposia of the Society for the Study of Human Biology. Volume VII, pp 191–209. Oxford: Pergamon.
Frisch RE (1974) Critical weight at menarche, initiation of the adolescent growth spurt, and control of puberty. In Grumbach M, Grave D & Meyer FE (eds) *Control of the Onset of Puberty*, pp 403–423. New York: John Wiley.
Frisch RE (1975) Demographic implication of the biological determinants of female fecundity. *Social Biology* **22:** 17–22.
Frisch RE (1976) Fatness of girls from menarche to age 18 years, with a nomogram. *Human Biology* **48:** 353–359.
Frisch RE (1978) Population, food intake and fertility. *Science* **199:** 22–30.
Frisch RE (1981) What's below the surface? *New England Journal of Medicine* **305:** 1019–1020.
Frisch RE (1983) Population, nutrition and fecundity. In Dupaquier J (ed.) *Malthus Past and Present*, pp 393–404. London: Academic Press.
Frisch RE (1984) Body fat, puberty and fertility. *Biological Reviews* **59:** 161–188.
Frisch RE (1985) Fatness, menarche and female fertility. *Perspectives in Biology and Medicine* **28:** 611–633.
Frisch RE (1988) Fatness and fertility. *Scientific American* **258:** 88–95.
Frisch RE & McArthur JW (1974) Menstrual cycles: fatness as a determinant of minimum weight for height necessary for their maintenance or onset. *Science* **185:** 949–951.
Frisch RE & Revelle R (1971) Height and weight at menarche and a hypothesis of menarche. *Archives of Diseases in Childhood* **46:** 695–701.
Frisch RE, Revelle R & Cook S (1973) Components of weight at menarche and the initiation of the adolescent growth spurt in girls: estimated total water, lean body weight and fat. *Human Biology* **45:** 469–483.
Frisch RE, Hegsted DM & Yoshinaga K (1975) Body weight and food intake at early estrus of rats on high fat diet. *Proceedings of the National Academy of Sciences USA* **72:** 4172–4176.
Frisch RE, Hegsted DM & Yoshinaga K (1977) Carcass components at first estrus of rats on high fat and low fat diets: body water, protein, and fat. *Proceedings of the National Academy of Sciences* **74:** 379–383.
Frisch RE, Canick JA & Tulchinsky D (1980) Human fatty marrow aromatizes androgen to estrogen. *Journal of Clinical Endocrinology and Metabolism* **51:** 394–396.
Frisch RE, Wyshak G & Vincent L (1980) Delayed menarche and amenorrhea of ballet dancers. *New England Journal of Medicine* **303:** 17–19.
Frisch RE, von Gotz-Welbergen A, McArthur JW et al (1981a) Abstract no 147. *Program, Annual Meeting of the Endocrine Society*, Cincinnati, p 119.
Frisch RE, von Gotz-Welbergen A, McArthur JW et al (1981b) Delayed menarche and amenorrhea of college athletes in relation to age of onset of training. *Journal of the American Medical Association* **246:** 1559–1563.
Frisch RE, Hall G, Aoki TT et al (1984) Metabolic, endocrine and reproductive changes of a woman channel swimmer. *Metabolism* **33:** 1106–1111.
Frisch RE, Wyshak G, Albright NL et al (1985) Lower prevalence of breast cancer and cancers of the reproductive system among former college athletes compared to non-athletes. *British Journal of Cancer* **52:** 885–981.
Frisch RE, Wyshak G, Albright TE et al (1986) Lower prevalence of diabetes in female former college athletes compared with nonathletes. *Diabetes* **35:** 1101–1105.
Frisch RE, Wyshak G, Albright NL et al (1989) Lower prevalence of non-reproductive system cancers among female former college athletes. *Medicine and Science in Sports and Exercise* **21:** 250–253.
Green BB, Weiss NS & Daling JR (1988) Risk of ovulatory infertility in relation to body weight. *Fertility and Sterility* **50:** 721–725.

Halipré A (1973) Étude du caractère culard X. Sensibilité des bovins culards au stress thémique. *Annales de Génétique et de Sélection Animale* **5(A):** 441–449.

Hartz AJ, Barboriak PN, Wong A et al (1979) The association of obesity with infertility and related menstrual abnormalities in women. *International Journal of Obesity* **3:** 57–73.

Henderson BE, Ross RK, Judd HL et al (1985) Do regular ovulatory cycles increase breast cancer risk? *Cancer* **56:** 1206–1208.

Hershcopf RJ & Bradlow HL (1987) Obesity, diet, endogenous estrogens, and the risk of hormone-sensitive cancer. *American Journal of Clinical Nutrition* **45:** 283–289.

Kaku M (1969) Disturbance of sexual function and adipose tissue of obese females. *Sanfujinka No Jissai* (Tokyo) **18:** 212–218.

Kennedy GC (1969) Interactions between feeding behavior and hormones during growth. *Annals of the New York Academy of Sciences* **157:** 1049–1061.

Kennedy GC & Mitra J (1963) Body weight and food intake as initiation factors for puberty in the rat. *Journal of Physiology* **166:** 408–418.

Keys A, Brŏzek J, Henschel A et al (1950) *The Biology of Human Starvation*, Volume I, pp 753–763, Volume II, pp 839–840, 850–851. Minneapolis: University of Minnesota Press.

Longcope C, Gorbach S, Goldin B et al (1987) The effect of a low fat diet on estrogen metabolism. *Journal of Endocrinology and Metabolism* **64:** 1246–1250.

Lunn PG, Austin S, Prentice AM et al (1984) The effect of improved nutrition on plasma prolactin concentrations and postpartum infertility in lactating Gambian women. *American Journal of Clinical Nutrition* **39:** 227–235.

MacConnie SE, Barkan A, Lampman RM et al (1986) Decreased hypothalamic gonadotropin-releasing hormone secretion in male marathon runners. *New England Journal of Medicine* **315:** 411–417.

Malina RM, Spirduso WW, Tate C et al (1978) Age at menarche and selected menstrual characteristics in athletes at different competitive levels and in different sports. *Medicine and Science in Sports and Exercise* **10:** 218–222.

Marshall JC & Fraser TR (1971) Amenorrhea and loss of weight. *British Journal of Obstetrics and Gynaecology* **84:** 801–807.

Marshall FHA & Peel WR (1908) 'Fatness' as a cause of sterility. *Journal of Agricultural Science* **3:** 383–389.

McArthur JW, O'Loughlin KM, Beitins IZ et al (1976) Endocrine studies during the refeeding of young women with nutritional amenorrhea and infertility. *Mayo Clinic Proceedings* **51:** 607–615.

Montagu A (1979) *The Reproductive Development of the Female: A Study in the Comparative Physiology of the Adolescent Organism.* Littleton, Massachusetts: PSG Publishing.

Moore FK, Olesen H, McMurrey JD et al (1963) *The Body Cell Mass and Its Supporting Environment.* Philadelphia: W.B. Saunders.

Nillius SJ (1983) Weight and the menstrual cycle. In *Understanding Anorexia Nervosa and Bulimia, Report of the Fourth Ross Conference on Medical Research*, pp 77–81. Columbus, Ohio: Ross Laboratories.

Nillius SJ & Wide L (1977) The pituitary responsiveness to acute and chronic administration of gonadotropin releasing hormone in acute and recovery stages of anorexia nervosa. In Vigersky RA (ed.) *Anorexia Nervosa*, pp 225–241. New York: Raven Press.

Nimrod A & Ryan KJ (1975) Aromatization of androgens by human abdominal and breast fat tissue. *Journal of Clinical Endocrinology and Metabolism* **40:** 367–372.

Pasquali R, Antenucci D, Casimirri F et al (1989) Clinical and hormonal characteristics of obese amenorrheic hyperandrogenic women before and after weight loss. *Journal of Clinical Endocrinology and Metabolism* **68:** 173–179.

Perel E & Killinger DW (1979) The interconversion and aromatization of androgens by human adipose tissue. *Journal of Steroid Biochemistry* **10:** 623–626.

Prior JC (1985) Luteal phase defects and anovulation: adaptive alterations occurring with conditioning exercise. *Seminars in Reproductive Endocrinology* **3:** 27–33.

Reichlin S (1982) Neuroendocrinology. In Williams RH (ed.) *Textbook of Endocrinology*, 6th edn, pp 588–645. Philadelphia: W.B. Saunders.

Scammon RE (1930) The measurement of the body in childhood. In Harris AJ, Jackson CM & Paterson DG (eds) *The Measurement of Man*, pp 174–215. Minneapolis: University of Minnesota Press.

Schneider J, Bradlow HL, Strain G et al (1983) Effects of obesity on estradiol metabolism: decreased formation of nonuterotropic metabolites. *Journal of Clinical Endocrinology and Metabolism* **56:** 973–978.

Schwartz B, Cumming DC, Riordan E et al (1981) Exercise-associated amenorrhea: a distinct entity? *American Journal of Obstetrics and Gynecology* **141:** 662–670.

Siiteri PK (1981) Extraglandular oestrogen formation and serum binding of estradiol: relationship to cancer. *Journal of Endocrinology* **89:** 119P–129P.

Siiteri PK & MacDonald PC (1973) Role of extraglandular estrogen in human endocrinology. In Geiger SR, Astwood EB & Greep RO (eds) *Handbook of Physiology*, Section 7, Volume 2, part I, pp 615–629. New York: American Physiology Society.

Snow RC, Barbieri RL & Frisch RE (1989) Estrogen 2-hydroxylase oxidation and menstrual function among elite oarswomen. *Journal of Clinical Endocrinology and Metabolism* **69:** 369–376.

Speroff L, Glass RH & Kase NG (1983) *Clinical, Gynecologic Endocrinology and Infertility*, 3rd edn, pp 175–178. Baltimore: Williams and Wilkins.

Strauss RH, Lanese RR & Malarkey WB (1985) Weight loss in amateur wrestlers and its effect on serum testosterone levels. *Journal of the American Medical Association* **254:** 3337–3338.

Tanner JW (1962) *Growth at Adolescence*, 2nd edn. Oxford: Blackwell.

van der Spuy ZM, Steer PJ, McCusken M et al (1988) Outcome of pregnancy in underweight women after spontaneous and induced ovulation. *British Medical Journal* **296:** 962–965.

van Wagenen G (1949) Accelerated growth with sexual precocity in female monkeys receiving testosterone propionate. *Endocrinology* **45:** 544–546.

Vigersky RA, Andersen AE, Thompson RH et al (1977) Hypothalamic dysfunction in secondary amenorrhea associated with simple weight loss. *New England Journal of Medicine* **297:** 1141–1145.

Vissac B, Perreau B, Mauleon P et al (1974) Étude du caractère culard: IX: Fertilité des femelles et aptitude maternelle. *Annales de Génétique et de Sélection Animale* **6:** 35–48.

Wall SR & Cumming DC (1985) Effects of physical activity on reproductive function and development in males. *Seminars in Reproductive Endocrinology* **3:** 65–80.

Warren M (1980) The effects of exercise on pubertal progression and reproductive function in girls. *Journal of Clinical Endocrinology and Metabolism* **51:** 1050–1057.

Warren MP, Jewelewicz R, Dyrenfurth I et al (1975) The significance of weight loss in the evaluation of pituitary response to LHRH in women with secondary amenorrhea. *Journal of Clinical Endocrinology and Metabolism* **40:** 601–611.

Wheeler GD, Wall SR, Belcastro AN et al (1984) Reduced serum testosterone and prolactin levels in male distance runners. *Journal of the American Medical Association* **252:** 514–516.

Wyshak G & Frisch RE (1982) Evidence for a secular trend in age of menarche. *New England Journal of Medicine* **306:** 1033–1035.

Wyshak G, Frisch RE, Albright NL et al (1986) Lower prevalence of benign diseases of the breast and benign tumors of the reproductive system among former college athletes compared to non-athletes. *British Journal of Cancer* **54:** 841–845.

Wyshak G, Frisch RE, Albright TE et al (1987) Bone fractures among former college athletes compared with non-athletes in the menopausal and postmenopausal years. *Obstetrics and Gynecology* **69:** 121–126.

2

Dopaminergic treatments for hyperprolactinaemia

P. G. CROSIGNANI
C. FERRARI

INCIDENCE OF HYPERPROLACTINAEMIA IN WOMEN

Hyperprolactinaemia is by far the most common disorder of the hypothalamic–pituitary axis. Estimates of the frequency of hyperprolactinaemia have been obtained by measuring serum prolactin (PRL) levels in population studies or by searching for prolactinomas at autopsy (Table 1). A Japanese study of 10 550 people found evidence of pathological hyperprolactinaemia in 0.07% of men and 0.5% of women (Miyai et al, 1986). On the other hand, postmortem studies found pituitary adenomas (99.9% of which were microadenomas) in 1.5–27% of subjects not suspected while alive of having pituitary disease, with a frequency of 11% in a total of 10 123 pituitaries examined (Molitch et al, 1986 for review; Abd El-Hamid et al, 1988); 45% of the tumours studied by immunohistochemistry stained positively for PRL as true prolactinomas. These studies mean that approximately 5% of the adult population bear microprolactinoma that usually go unrecognized due to lack of symptoms, as indicated by a recent study in which the clinical case notes of 57 subjects with pituitary microadenomas

Table 1. Prevalence of microprolactinoma or hyperprolactinaemia in various populations (Miyai et al, 1986; Molitch, 1986; Abd El-Hamid et al, 1988).

Population	Method of assessment	Prevalence (%)
Unselected (male and female)	Autopsy: pituitary microadenoma	11
Unselected (male and female)	Autopsy: microprolactinoma	≈ 5
Unselected women	Prolactin measurement	0.5*
Amenorrhoeic women	Prolactin measurement	15
Women with galactorrhoea	Prolactin measurement	28
Women with oligo–amenorrhoea and galactorrhoea	Prolactin measurement	75
Infertile women	Prolactin measurement	33
Hirsute women	Prolactin measurement	13

* After having excluded iatrogenic and pregnancy-related hyperprolactinaemia.

Baillière's Clinical Obstetrics and Gynaecology—
Vol. 4, No. 3, September 1990
ISBN 0–7020–1478–8

found at autopsy were reviewed, and the overall fertility rate was found to be over 50% (Abd El-Hamid et al, 1988).

The frequency of clinical diagnosis of pituitary adenoma during life is much lower. A population study in Minnesota found a mean annual incidence of this diagnosis of 8.2 per 100000 women over 15 years of age (Annegers et al, 1978); even assuming an additional 30 years of life during which the diagnosis of pituitary tumour could be made, only 0.25% of women will have the tumour diagnosed.

Hyperprolactinaemia is usually associated with hypogonadism and/or galactorrhoea. Among women with reproductive disturbances the prevalence of hyperprolactinaemia has been found to be high: approximately 15% of women with amenorrhoea (usually secondary but sometimes primary) or oligomenorrhoea, 28% of women with galactorrhoea, 75% of those with oligo–amenorrhoea and galactorrhoea and 33% of infertile women in many large series (Molitch, 1986 for review). Women with hirsutism are also often hyperprolactinaemic (13% of hirsute patients with normal menses, 26% of those with associated oligo–amenorrhoea, and 33% of those with oligo–amenorrhoea and the polycystic ovary syndrome). The existence of hyperprolactinaemia in women with polycystic ovaries has been known for many years, but in almost all instances it is mild and is only a consequence of increased oestrogen secretion; cases of polycystic ovary syndrome associated with primary idiopathic hyperprolactinaemia or prolactinoma have, however, been reported (Futterweit, 1983; Franks, 1989).

CLINICAL PRESENTATION OF HYPERPROLACTINAEMIC ANOVULATION

Although slightly to moderately elevated PRL levels are found in many subjects who have no major clinical disturbances (Crosignani et al, 1985), hyperprolactinaemia is frequently associated with menstrual irregularities (amenorrhoea, oligomenorrhoea, irregular bleeding) and/or sterility due to either chronic anovulation or defective luteal phase (Kredenster et al, 1981; Archer, 1987). Approximately 50% of these patients show evidence of pituitary adenoma (Keye et al, 1980) while many others do not show abnormalities even in high-resolution computed tomography (CT) or nuclear magnetic resonance (NMR) scans of the pituitary fossa. In some of these subjects a slightly elevated PRL level can be found preferentially in the supposed luteal phase; they are classified as patients having variable hyperprolactinaemia (Coutts et al, 1978; Archer, 1987).

Several studies of the natural history of untreated hyperprolactinaemic patients with either idiopathic disease or microprolactinoma have shown no progression or only slow progression of the disease over several years of follow-up (Johnston et al, 1983; Koppelman et al, 1984; Martin et al, 1985), while some studies have reported a frequent worsening of the disease (Weiss et al, 1983; Pontiroli and Falsetti, 1984). Other investigators have found reduced or even normalized PRL levels at follow-up in several patients (Martin et al, 1985; Sisam et al, 1987; Corenblum and Taylor, 1988;

Schlechte et al, 1989), and this was particularly common after pregnancy for women who had conceived spontaneously (Crosignani et al, 1985).

SPONTANEOUSLY OCCURRING PREGNANCY IN HYPERPROLACTINAEMIC WOMEN

Hyperprolactinaemia does not preclude fertility in women, and the occurrence of presumptive ovulation and in some cases pregnancy has been reported for small series of untreated hyperprolactinaemic women (Magyar and Marshall, 1978; Crosignani et al, 1981). Crosignani et al (1985) reported 29 pregnancies occurring spontaneously in 28 women with mild to moderate hyperprolactinaemia (PRL levels up to 100 ng/ml). Only four of them showed tomographic evidence of microprolactinoma; one of the prolactinoma patients experienced a visual field defect at week 30, which was quickly controlled by bromocriptine treatment. Pregnancy in the rest of the patients was uneventful. Normal values were found in nine of 22 women in whom PRL levels were re-evaluated at least 1 month after delivery and/or lactation.

A practical consequence of these observations is that hyperprolactinaemia of moderate degree does not protect against pregnancy (in that series five accidental conceptions occurred). The possibility of prolactinoma suprasellar enlargement suggests the need for close monitoring of the subjects during pregnancy. Consistent lowering of PRL levels or even their normalization after delivery or lactation have also been observed after induced pregnancies, but is particularly frequent in those women who conceived spontaneously, probably because the hyperprolactinaemia was mild to begin with.

DIAGNOSTIC WORK-UP

The causes of pathological hyperprolactinaemia are numerous (Table 2). The commonest are microprolactinoma (about 50% of cases) and idiopathic disease (i.e., hyperprolactinaemia in the absence of recognizable causes, about 30% of cases). Macroprolactinomas are less frequent but tend to invade the suprasellar region, with eventual visual disturbances, and other parasellar structures. Other pituitary tumours which do not secrete PRL, primary empty sella syndrome and hypothalamic or parasellar tumours may frequently cause hyperprolactinaemia, typically mild to moderate, due to interference of the tumour mass with the delivery of hypothalamic dopamine to the lactotrophs (Ferrari et al, 1982b).

Differential diagnosis between the different aetiologies relies primarily on basal serum PRL levels and neuroradiological evaluation by either CT or NMR (Ferrari and Crosignani, 1985). PRL levels >100 µg/litre are almost always due to prolactinomas: very high levels (>500–1000 µg/litre) are only found in macroprolactinomas; PRL levels <50–100 µg/litre in the presence of pituitary or parapituitary macrotumours indicate that the lesion is not a

Table 2. Causes of pathological hyperprolactinaemia.

Pituitary disorders
    Prolactinoma (PRL cell adenoma, micro or macro)
    Plurihormonal pituitary tumours
    Non-PRL-secreting pituitary tumours causing hypothalamopituitary disconnection
       (acromegaly, Cushing's disease, Nelson's syndrome)
    Non-secreting pituitary tumours
    Pituitary cysts
    Granulomatous hypophysitis
    Autoimmune hypophysitis
    Stalk section
    Empty sella syndrome
Multiple endocrine neoplasia type I
Hypothalamic disorders
    Tumours (craniopharyngioma, meningioma, glioma, neuroblastoma, ependymoma,
       pinealoma, germinoma, metastatic carcinoma)
    Granulomatous diseases (sarcoidosis, histiocytosis X)
    Vascular disorders (aneurysms)
    Postirradiation
    Post-traumatic
Idiopathic hyperprolactinaemia
Primary hypothyroidism
Polycystic ovary disease
Oestrogen-secreting tumours
Chronic renal failure
Liver cirrhosis
Lesions of the chest wall
Pseudocyesis

PRL, prolactin.

prolactinoma ('pseudoprolactinoma'). Many PRL stimulation and suppression tests have been devised, but none of them has proved to be able to differentiate tumoral from idiopathic hyperprolactinaemia (Crosignani et al, 1984a). On the other hand, probably many patients with idiopathic disease have microprolactinomas too small to be detected radiologically; this may account for the difficulty in discriminating between these two entities (Crosignani et al, 1981). Nevertheless, a thyrotrophin-releasing hormone test may be of value to more fully evaluate thyroid function in hyperprolactinaemic patients (and, concomitantly, the presence or absence of PRL response). Obviously in patients with evidence or suspicion of other endocrine abnormalities or with large pituitary tumours or suprasellar lesions, a complete endocrine work-up is needed.

The essential examinations to be performed for all hyperprolactinaemic

Table 3. Hyperprolactinaemic anovulation: diagnostic work-up.

1. Women with menses: measure PRL and progesterone in the supposed luteal phase
   (during at least two cycles)
2. Women with oligo–amenorrhoea: measure FSH and PRL on two different occasions
3. If PRL ↑ CT or NMR can be considered
4. Measure TSH, T_3 and T_4 (to exclude hypothyroidism)

PRL, prolactin; FSH, follicle-stimulating hormone; CT, computed tomography; NMR, nuclear magnetic resonance; TSH, thyroid-stimulating (thyrotrophic) hormone; T_3, tri-iodothyronine; T_4, thyroxine.

women are outlined in Table 3. Determination of serum follicle-stimulating hormone (FSH) is of utmost importance to exclude ovarian failure in subjects seeking pregnancy.

TREATMENT OPTIONS

The decision to treat a hyperprolactinaemic woman because of amenorrhoea, infertility, severe menstrual irregularities, spontaneous galactorrhoea, or because of the presence of a large pituitary or parasellar tumour is obvious, but many subjects with mild to moderate hyperprolactinaemia have no major clinical disturbances. Lack of symptoms despite hyperprolactinaemia may be due either to only mild PRL excess (usually serum PRL levels <50 μg/litre) or to high concentrations of high-molecular-weight PRL forms (big PRL and big big PRL) or glycosylated forms that, though immunoreactive, have low biological activity (Malarkey, 1986; Pellegrini et al, 1988; Fraser et al, 1989; Larrea et al, 1989; Lewis et al, 1989). Many asymptomatic patients with mild to moderate hyperprolactinaemia or with 'macroprolactinaemia' do not show abnormalities in high-resolution CT or NMR imaging of the pituitary fossa; furthermore, as discussed above, patients with either idiopathic disease or microprolactinoma only infrequently show progression of the disease over several years of follow-up. Thus, there is a subset of hyperprolactinaemic patients for whom the indication to treat is still debatable, particularly since knowledge about the possible hazards of chronic hyperprolactinaemia (impaired libido, osteoporosis, breast disorders, impaired glucose and lipid metabolism) is presently insufficient (Ferrari and Crosignani, 1986).

Clearly, if the woman is complaining of anovulation or infertility and has hyperprolactinaemia, the best treatment is to lower the serum PRL levels. Several therapeutic modalities are available: ergoline derivatives, surgery and radiotherapy. Medical treatment may be an option for all causes of pathological hyperprolactinaemia and will be discussed in detail in the next section, while surgical and radiation treatments may only be considered for cases with pituitary or parasellar tumours.

Pituitary adenomectomy or hypophysectomy by the trans-sphenoidal or, for large adenomas, the transcranial route is a well-established form of treatment for prolactinomas (reviews in Arafah et al, 1986; Melmed et al, 1986; Post, 1986; Schlechte et al, 1986; Bevan et al, 1987, Molitch, 1989). Normalization of PRL levels has been reported for approximately 75% of patients with preoperative PRL values <200 μg/litre but only for 35% of those with higher values. Similarly, 'cure' of prolactinoma has been obtained for 70–85% of microadenomas but only for 10–40% of macroadenomas. The recurrence rates within 5 years after surgery are also high: 5–50% (usually about 20%) in patients with microprolactinomas and 16–80% in those with macroprolactinomas. Furthermore, surgical therapy results in hypopituitarism in many cases, particularly those with large adenomas, and has a major morbidity rate of 0.4% in microprolactinomas and 5.5% in macroprolactinomas (Laws, 1987). Treatment with bromocriptine for more than 6 weeks before surgery induces fibrosis in some tumours, either micro or macro, and thus resulted in worse surgical outcomes in some series but not others (review in Molitch, 1989). Taken together, and considering the excellent results of medical treatment (see below), available data do not suggest that surgery is the primary therapy for prolactinomas, either small or large. However, it has an important role in the management of the uncommon patient who is intolerant of or resistant to drug treatment or, when there is a large prolactinoma, to decrease the tumour mass before pregnancy and increase the response to drug and radiation therapy (Murphy et al, 1987). On the other hand, surgery is the treatment of choice for patients with hyperprolactinaemia due to non-secreting pituitary adenomas or parasellar tumours (Ferrari and Crosignani, 1985; Bevan et al, 1987) who, despite normalization of PRL levels and possible improvement of visual field defects during drug treatment (D'Emden and Harrison, 1986) do not show any considerable tumour shrinkage (Gasser et al, 1987; Bevan et al, 1987).

Conventional or heavy-particle radiotherapy results in gradual lowering of PRL levels in prolactinoma patients over several (1–15) years, with eventual normalization in many cases, but drug treatment is needed for years while awaiting the benefits of radiation therapy, which, furthermore, induces hypopituitarism over years in most cases (Johnston et al, 1986; Mehta et al, 1987). Thus radiotherapy may be considered only for macroprolactinomas and for non-secreting pituitary adenomas or parasellar tumours as adjunctive treatment to dopamine agonists and/or surgery.

DOPAMINERGIC TREATMENT

The effectiveness of ergoline dopaminergic drugs for treatment of hyperprolactinaemic disorders has been established for many years, and world-wide clinical experience indicates that they are the treatment of first choice for either idiopathic disease or prolactinoma. Bromocriptine is by far the most widely used drug, and given in daily doses of 1.25–20 mg (usually 5–7.5 mg) divided into two or three administrations normalizes serum PRL levels in about 80% of patients with microprolactinoma or idiopathic disease, together with restoration of ovarian function in approximately 85% of cases (Vance et al, 1984; Ferrari and Crosignani, 1986) and a pregnancy rate of 80% in women with hyperprolactinaemic infertility who wish to conceive, provided there are no other infertility factors (Weil, 1986). In patients with macroprolactinoma, PRL levels become normal in about 65% of cases, with restoration of gonadal function in over 50%, and an additional benefit is a decrease in tumour size, reported in approximately 70% of cases (Robbins, 1986; Murphy et al, 1987). Tumour shrinkage is due to a number of actions of the drug: decreased nuclear and nucleolar volume associated with inhibition of PRL gene transcription; reduction of the rough endoplasmic reticulum membranes, of the ribosomes and the Golgi cisternae, with resulting decrease in cytoplasmic volume (within days of treatment); and perivascular fibrosis and partial cell necrosis (after long-term treatment)

(Landolt et al, 1987; Duffy et al, 1988).

Resistance to bromocriptine or other dopamine agonists is usually partial, i.e., PRL levels decrease under treatment (but not to normal or near-normal levels); however, resistance is complete in occasional patients and seems to be due to a decrease in D2 dopamine receptors within the prolactinoma, although postreceptor defects may also contribute (Bevan and Burke, 1989; Pellegrini et al, 1989).

Bromocriptine therapy should to be initiated with low doses (1.25 mg with dinner), to be gradually increased up to 2.5 mg twice daily with food over 1–2 weeks to minimize side-effects; subsequently the drug dose should be increased if PRL values do not become normal or near-normal and ovarian function is not restored. Drug treatment must be continued up to the occurrence of pregnancy or, when this is not the case, for at least 1 year; serum PRL and progesterone levels during presumed luteal phases should be monitored periodically to check effectiveness of treatment, and if progesterone does not rise in the luteal phase despite lowered PRL, the cyclic use of an anti-oestrogen to stimulate the ovary can be advised. After drug withdrawal, PRL levels usually rebound to pretreatment values within a few weeks (Ferrari and Crosignani, 1986); however, some patients may have persistently normal or only slightly elevated PRL levels for at least several months and occasionally for years. The percentage of such cases seems higher after more prolonged (2–4 years) drug therapy (Faglia et al, 1987; Rasmussen et al, 1987; Wang et al, 1987). Furthermore, many patients continue to menstruate and frequently to have ovulatory menses for several months despite recurrence of hyperprolactinaemia (Ferrari et al, 1982a; Rasmussen et al, 1987). Bromocriptine has a high incidence (69%) of side-effects, though usually mild to moderate and transient, nausea, headache, dizziness and fatigue being the most frequent; however, only approximately 5% of patients have to discontinue treatment because of intolerance (Physician's Desk Reference, 1989). Many other dopamine agonists, including metergoline, lisuride, pergolide, terguride, dihydroergocristine, dihydroergokryptine, cabergoline and the non-ergoline drug CV 205-502 have been shown to be effective treatment for hyperprolactinaemia, but only cabergoline and CV 205-502 may offer advantages over bromocriptine in effectiveness, safety and convenient administration schedules.

Cabergoline, presently under clinical investigation, will probably represent a major breakthrough for treatment of hyperprolactinaemia. This drug has an exceptionally long duration of action, being able to lower serum PRL levels significantly for up to 7–14 days after oral administration of single 0.3–0.6 mg doses to hyperprolactinaemic patients (Ferrari et al, 1986; Mattei et al, 1988). As chronic treatment, cabergoline was given to 70 hyperprolactinaemic patients (68 women and two men) for 3–34 months, at doses from 0.2–3 mg per week, administered one to three times weekly (Ferrari et al, 1989; Ferrari, 1989). Serum PRL levels declined to normal in 62 (89%) and to nearly normal values in six; resumption of menses occurred in 36 of 38 women with amenorrhoea, with presumptive evidence of ovulation in most cases and pregnancy in four; and tumour shrinkage seen in control CT or NMR scans in 10 of 11 patients with macroprolactinoma after

3 months of therapy and in 9 of 12 with microprolactinoma re-evaluated after 12 months of therapy. Side-effects (including weakness, dizziness, postural hypotension and nausea), all mild and transient, occurred in only seven patients and vanished despite continued cabergoline treatment at the same or reduced, but still effective, doses. The experience of another group was similar (Ciccarelli et al, 1989), with PRL normalized in 22 of 26 hyperprolactinaemic women (85%) treated with 0.5–2 mg once weekly for 6–12 months; side-effects occurred in 13 patients, but only three had to discontinue treatment. An interesting point was that seven of 20 patients in this series who had been previously intolerant to bromocriptine tolerated this medication, a significantly higher number than the three who did not tolerate cabergoline. Thus, the excellent efficacy and tolerability results together with the very simple administration schedule of cabergoline (once or twice weekly for almost all patients) may make it the drug of choice for treatment of hyperprolactinaemia.

The compound CV 205-502 is also interesting because it is administered once daily like pergolide, but appears to have lesser side-effects. To date, four subchronic or chronic studies with this drug have been reported (Rasmussen et al, 1988; Newman et al, 1989; Vance et al, 1989; van der Heijden et al, 1989), showing that once daily administration of doses from 0.025 to 0.175 mg could normalize PRL levels in 64 of 99 patients. Adverse reactions to CV 205-502 were mild to moderate, included headache, nausea, dizziness, tiredness, light-headedness and nasal congestion, and were reported by 34 patients, of whom only three, however, had to discontinue treatment. It is noteworthy that only one of 14 patients who had not previously tolerated bromocriptine also had to discontinue CV 205-502.

A new formulation of bromocriptine to be injected intramuscularly at monthly intervals at the dose of 50–100 mg also deserves attention because of its simple schedule (although it must be injected by a nurse) and its reported safety. However, experience at present is nearly limited to a single injection, which normalized or reduced serum PRL levels for up to 6 weeks in most patients with prolactinoma and rapidly shrank macroadenomas in many cases (Grossman et al, 1986; Montini et al, 1986; Ciccarelli et al, 1987). Nausea, vomiting and postural hypotension are not uncommon in the first 24 h, but are minimal thereafter. Recently, a repeatable preparation of long-acting bromocriptine has been reported to have normalized PRL levels in three of five patients with macroprolactinomas and to have shrunk the tumours in all (van't Verlaat et al, 1988). However, adverse reactions were noticed in four cases, including nausea and vomiting for several days in one and severe postural hypotension in another patient. A modified-release bromocriptine capsule that causes fewer side-effects than the marketed oral formulation and that might be used as once daily treatment of hyperprolactinaemia is also under investigation (Drewe et al, 1988).

THE RESULTING PREGNANCY

The data for large series of dopaminergic treatment-induced pregnancies

(Krupp and Turkalj, 1984; Weil, 1986) do not show increased rates of spontaneous abortion (11%), multiple pregnancies (2%) or congenital abnormalities (3–4%). All of these figures compare favourably with those quoted for pregnancies achieved after treatment with anti-oestrogens, pulsatile gonadotrophin-releasing hormone (GnRH) and human menopausal gonadotrophin (hMG), both for abortion and for the multiple pregnancy rates. Interestingly, there is no indication that, on discontinuing the bromocriptine treatment at an early stage of pregnancy, the rise in plasma PRL induces a rise in the abortion rate.

On the other hand, despite the clear experimental evidence that not only an excess but also a deficit in PRL can impair progesterone secretion by the corpus luteum (Wyss et al, 1977), the marked hypoprolactinaemia induced by dopaminergic treatments does not affect the spontaneous abortion rate. Similarly, for the few women treated continuously throughout gestation, it does not appear that the inhibition of PRL secretion had any effect on placental function that might adversely influence the course of pregnancy, the subsequent breast feeding (Ho Yuen et al, 1980; Miyakawa et al, 1982) or the postnatal development of the children (Weil, 1986).

EFFECT OF PREGNANCY ON HYPERPROLACTINAEMIA

For many years pregnancy was thought to be a specific risk for hyperprolactinaemic patients (especially those with prolactinoma) because of the effects of oestrogen stimulation on the pituitary (Shupnik et al, 1979). However, since the introduction of bromocriptine, pregnancy has become a normal situation because anovulatory infertility due to hyperprolactinaemia can be treated successfully with drugs, even in patients with pituitary adenomas. Early reports (Magyar and Marshall, 1978; Gemzell and Wang, 1979) indicated considerable risk of complications developing during pregnancy in the patients with pituitary prolactinoma. However, many subsequent reports on larger series of cases divided on the basis of the initial presence of tumour and of its size clearly showed that the risk of clinically significant adenoma growth during pregnancy is indeed small, except in women with macroadenoma. Thus, in the Molitch review (1985) symptomatic enlargement occurred in only four and asymptomatic enlargement in 11 of 246 pregnancies in women with microprolactinomas and no prior operation or irradiation, and in no case was surgical intervention necessary. The figures were seven symptomatic and four asymptomatic enlargements for 45 pregnancies in women with macroadenomas not previously treated by surgery or radiotherapy, and in four cases surgical treatment was required during pregnancy, while only two of 46 such patients who had been operated on or irradiated before pregnancy had symptomatic tumour enlargement. In addition, it is possible to quickly suppress the symptomatic suprasellar growth of a prolactinoma during pregnancy with bromocriptine (Corenblum, 1979; Konopka et al, 1983; Bergh et al, 1984; Crosignani et al, 1984b; Holmgren et al, 1986). This is the reason for close monitoring of the pregnancy. Plasma PRL changes are usually not a reliable index unless the subject shows a very sharp increase (Andersen et al, 1983). Visual field evaluation is a good indicator of possible suprasellar tumour growth and should be performed regularly in the second part of the pregnancy.

Many reports have also shown that pregnancy may be beneficial to hyperprolactinaemic women, since in some patients (usually with idiopathic disease or microprolactinoma) postpartum PRL levels are actually lower than before pregnancy (Mornex et al, 1978; Bergh et al, 1981; Crosignani et al, 1981; Andersen et al, 1983; Daya et al, 1984; Crosignani et al, 1985).

There are few reports of the long-term effects of pregnancy on PRL hypersecretion (Molitch, 1985; Rasmussen et al, 1985; Bergh, 1987). In a recent series (Crosignani et al, 1989) of 64 pregnancies in 54 women with functional hyperprolactinaemia or microprolactinoma, the PRL concentrations were lower 12 months after delivery or at the end of lactation (median values, 43 ng/ml versus 67.5 ng/ml). Figure 1 shows the PRL levels before and after pregnancy for those women. Pregnancy by itself normalized plasma PRL in 11 patients (17%). It is worth noting that five of 11 PRL normalizations occurred in women with radiological evidence of microadenomas. PRL concentrations were substantially lowered (at least halved) in 15 additional patients, six with prolactinoma. In addition, menstrual cyclicity started in five of the 28 previously amenorrhoeic patients (18%). Enlargement of the pituitary gland during normal pregnancy has been documented by serial NMR imaging (Gonzales et al, 1988). Whether the improvement of the hyperprolactinaemic disorder that may follow pregnancy is due to autoinfarction of the adenoma (Daya et al, 1984) or some other mechanism(s) related to the pregnant state is not certain. There is a suspicion that partial infarction of the gland could possibly explain it. However, the effects of pregnancy on patients without evidence of adenoma and the absence of signs of hypopituitarism after pregnancy speak against this infarction theory. In fact, infarction would be more likely in the ade-

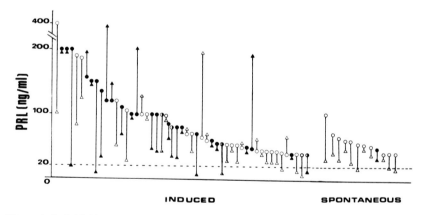

Figure 1. Individual serum prolactin (PRL) values before and after gestation for 12 spontaneous pregnancies (12 patients) and 52 induced pregnancies (46 patients). Circles: PRL before pregnancy; triangles; PRL after pregnancy. The presence of adenoma is indicated by black symbols. ◐, adenoma previously treated by surgery. From Crosignani et al (1989).

noma patients, and if there were general infarction of the gland, one would expect subsequent impairment of at least the more fragile pituitary functions, such as gonadotrophin secretion. Interestingly, a recent report showed significantly lower PRL values in parous than in nulliparous normoprolactinaemic women (Musey et al, 1987) and the same group of normal subjects showed blunted PRL responses to perphenazine after pregnancy, as compared to their prepregnancy tests.

SUMMARY

Hyperprolactinaemia is a frequent cause of anovulatory sterility, although spontaneous pregnancy may occur occasionally. Dopaminergic treatment is highly effective for the treatment of both idiopathic and tumoral hyperprolactinaemia. If the only cause of infertility is chronic anovulation due to hyperprolactinaemia, an 80% pregnancy rate can be anticipated.

Because of these results, surgical treatment is still needed only rarely. Pregnancy, either spontaneous or drug-related, is usually uneventful for the mother and is not associated with any increase in abortion, twins or malformations.

Pregnancy-related tumour growth occurs rarely and can be treated successfully with dopaminergic drugs. On the contrary, there is more frequently improvement after pregnancy of the biochemical and clinical disorders associated with hyperprolactinaemia.

REFERENCES

Abd El-Hamid MW, Joplin GF & Lewis PD (1988) Incidentally found small pituitary adenomas may have no effect on fertility. *Acta Endocrinologica* **117:** 361–364.

Andersen AN, Starup J, Tabor A, Jensen HK & Westergaard JG (1983) The possible prognostic value of serum prolactin increment during pregnancy in hyperprolactinaemic patients. *Acta Endocrinologica* **102:** 1–5.

Annegers JF, Coulam CB, Abboud CF, Laws ER & Kurland LT (1978) Pituitary adenoma in Olmstead County, Minnesota, 1935–1977. A report of an increasing incidence of diagnosis in women of childbearing age. *Mayo Clinical Proceedings* **53:** 661–643.

Arafah BM, Brodkey JS & Pearson OH (1986) Gradual recovery of lactotroph responsiveness to dynamic stimulation following surgical removal of prolactinomas: long-term follow-up studies. *Metabolism* **35:** 905–912.

Archer DF (1987) Prolactin response to thyrotropin-releasing hormone in women with infertility and/or randomly elevated serum prolactin levels. *Fertility and Sterility* **47:** 559–564.

Bergh T, Nillius SJ, Larsson S-G & Wide L (1981) Effects of bromocriptine-induced pregnancy on prolactin-secreting pituitary tumours. *Acta Endocrinologica* **98:** 333–338.

Bergh T, Nillius SJ & Wide L (1982) Menstrual function and serum prolactin levels after long-term bromocriptine treatment of hyperprolactinemic amenorrhea. *Clinical Endocrinology* **16:** 587–592.

Bergh T, Nillius SJ, Enoksson P & Wide L (1984) Bromocriptine-induced regression of a suprasellar extending prolactinoma during pregnancy. *Journal of Endocrinological Investigation* **7:** 133–136.

Bevan JS & Burke CW (1989) Perifusion studies of bromocriptine-treated and untreated macroprolactinomas: effects of dopamine, bromocriptine and TRH. *Clinical Endocrinology* **30:** 667–680.

Bevan JS, Adams CBT, Burke CW et al (1987) Factors in the outcome of transsphenoidal surgery for prolactinoma and non-functioning pituitary tumours, including preoperative bromocriptine therapy. *Clinical Endocrinology* **26:** 541–556.

Ciccarelli E, Ghigo E, Mazza E et al (1987) Effects of a new long-acting form of bromocriptine on tumorous hyperprolactinemia. *Journal of Endocrinological Investigation* **10:** 179–182.

Ciccarelli E, Giusti M, Miola C et al (1989) Effectiveness and tolerability of long-term treatment with cabergoline, a new long-lasting ergoline derivative, in hyperprolactinemic patients. *Journal of Clinical Endocrinology and Metabolism* **69:** 725–728.

Corenblum B (1979) Successful outcome of ergocryptine-induced pregnancies in twenty-one women with prolactin secreting pituitary adenomas. *Fertility and Sterility* **32:** 183–187.

Corenblum B & Taylor PJ (1988) Idiopathic hyperprolactinaemia may include a distinct entity with a natural history different from that of prolactin adenomas. *Fertility and Sterility* **49:** 544–546.

Coutts JRT (1978) The defective luteal phase. In Jacobs HS (ed.) *Advances in Gynaecological Endocrinology*, pp 65–91. London: The Royal College of Obstetricians and Gynaecologists.

Crosignani PG, Ferrari C, Scarduelli C et al (1981) Spontaneous and induced pregnancies in hyperprolactinemic women. *Obstetrics and Gynecology* **58:** 708–713.

Crosignani PG, Ferrari C, Scarduelli C et al (1984a) Dynamic functional testing in hyperprolactinemic disorders. In Camanni F & Muller EE (eds) *Pituitary Hyperfunction: Physiopathology and Clinical Aspects*, pp 321–331. New York: Raven Press.

Crosignani PG, Ferrari C & Mattei AM (1984b) Visual field defects and reduced visual acuity during pregnancy in two patients with prolactinoma: rapid regression of symptoms under bromocriptine. Case reports. *British Journal of Obstetrics and Gynaecology* **91:** 821–823.

Crosignani PG, Scarduelli C, Brambilla G, Cavioni V & Ferrari C (1985) Spontaneous pregnancies in hyperprolactinemic women. *Gynecologic and Obstetric Investigation* **19:** 17–20.

Crosignani PG, Mattei AM, Scarduelli C, Cavioni V & Boracchi P (1989) Is pregnancy the best treatment for hyperprolactinaemia? *Human Reproduction* **4:** 910–912.

Daya S, Shewchuk AB & Brycelond N (1984) The effect of multiparity on intrasellar prolactinomas. *American Journal of Obstetrics and Gynecology* **148:** 512–515.

D'Emden MC & Harrison LC (1986) Rapid improvement of visual field defects following bromocriptine treatment of patients with non-functioning pituitary adenomas. *Clinical Endocrinology* **25:** 697–702.

Drewe J, Mazer N, Abisch E, Krummen K & Keck M (1988) Differential effects of food on kinetics of bromocriptine in a modified release capsule and a conventional formulation. *European Journal of Clinical Pharmacology* **35:** 535–541.

Duffy AE, Asa SL & Kovacs K (1988) Effect of bromocriptine on secretion and morphology of human prolactin cell adenomas in vitro. *Hormone Research* **30:** 32–38.

Faglia G, Conti A, Muratori M et al (1987) Dihydroergocriptine in management of microprolactinomas. *Journal of Clinical Endocrinology and Metabolism* **65:** 779–784.

Ferrari C (1989) New dopamine agonists in the treatment of hyperprolactinemia. In Casanueva FF & Dieguez C (eds) *Recent Advances in Basic and Clinical Neuroendocrinology*, pp 333–339. Amsterdam: Elsevier.

Ferrari C & Crosignani PG (1985) Hypothalamic disease presenting as amenorrhoea: value of computed tomography. *British Journal of Obstetrics and Gynaecology* **92:** 1251–1257.

Ferrari C & Crosignani PG (1986) Review. Medical treatment of hyperprolactinaemic disorders. *Human Reproduction* **1:** 507–514.

Ferrari C, Mattei A, Rampini P et al (1982a) Long-term effects of drug treatment on hyperprolactinemic disorders: a study after discontinuation of bromocriptine and metergoline. In Molinatti GM (ed.) *A Clinical Problem. Microprolactinoma. Diagnosis and Treatment*, pp 141–147. Amsterdam: Excerpta Medica.

Ferrari C, Rampini P, Benco R et al (1982b) Functional characterization of hypothalamic hyperprolactinemia. *Journal of Clinical Endocrinology and Metabolism* **55:** 897–901.

Ferrari C, Barbieri C, Caldara R et al (1986) Long-lasting prolactin-lowering effect of cabergoline, a new dopamine agonist, in hyperprolactinemic patients. *Journal of Clinical Endocrinology and Metabolism* **63:** 941–945.

Ferrari C, Mattei A, Melis GB et al (1989) Cabergoline: long-acting oral treatment of hyperprolactinemic disorders. *Journal of Clinical Endocrinology and Metabolism* **68:** 1201–1206.

Franks S (1989) Polycystic ovary syndrome: a changing perspective. *Clinical Endocrinology* **31:** 87–120.

Fraser IS, Guang Lun Z, Ping Zhon J et al (1989) Detailed assessment of big big prolactin in women with hyperprolactinemia and normal ovarian function. *Journal of Clinical Endocrinology and Metabolism* **69:** 585–592.

Futterweit W (1983) Pituitary tumors and polycistic ovarian disease. *Obstetrics and Gynecology* **62:** 74S–79S.

Gasser RW, Mueller-Holzner E, Skrabal F et al (1987) Macroprolactinomas and functionless pituitary tumours. Immunostaining and effect of dopamine agonist therapy. *Acta Endocrinologica* **116:** 253–259.

Gemzell C & Wang CF (1979) Outcome of pregnancy in women with pituitary adenoma. *Fertility and Sterility* **31:** 363–372.

Gonzales JG, Elizondo G, Saldivar D et al (1988) Pituitary gland growth during normal pregnancy: an in vivo study using magnetic resonance imaging. *American Journal of Medicine* **85:** 217–220.

Grossman A, Ross R, Wass JAH & Besser GM (1986) Depot-bromocriptine treatment for prolactinomas and acromegaly. *Clinical Endocrinology* **24:** 231–238.

Holmgren U, Bergstrand G, Hagenfeldt K & Werner S (1986) Women with prolactinoma— effect of pregnancy and lactation on serum prolactin and on tumour growth. *Acta Endocrinologica* **111:** 452–459.

Ho Yuen B, Cannon W, Lewis J, Sy L & Wooley S (1980) A possible role for prolactin in the control of human chorionic gonadotropin and estrogen secretion by the fetoplacental unit. *American Journal of Obstetrics and Gynecology* **136:** 286–291.

Johnston DG, Prescott RWG, Kendall-Taylor P et al (1983) Hyperprolactinemia: long-term effects of bromocriptine. *American Journal of Medicine* **75:** 868–874.

Johnston DG, Hall K, Kendall-Taylor P et al (1986) The long-term effects of megavoltage radiotherapy as sole or combined therapy for large prolactinomas: studies with high definition computerized tomography. *Clinical Endocrinology* **24:** 675–685.

Keye WR Jr, Chang RJ, Wilson CB & Jaffe RB (1980) Prolactin-secreting pituitary adenomas in women, III. Frequency and diagnosis in amenorrhea–galactorrhea. *Journal of the American Medical Association* **244:** 1329–1333.

Konopka P, Raymond JP, Merceron RE & Seneze J (1983) Continuous administration of bromocriptine in the prevention of neurological complications in pregnant women with prolactinomas. *American Journal of Obstetrics and Gynecology* **146:** 935–938.

Koppelman MCS, Jaffe MJ, Rieth KG, Caruso RC & Loriaux DL (1984) Hyperprolactinemia, amenorrhea, and galactorrhea: a retrospective assessment of twenty-five cases. *Annals of Internal Medicine* **100:** 115–121.

Kredenster JV, Hoskins CF & Scott JZ (1981) Hyperprolactinemia: a significant factor in female infertility. *American Journal of Obstetrics and Gynecology* **139:** 264–267.

Krupp P & Turkalj I (1984) Surveillance of Parlodel (bromocriptine) in pregnancy and offspring. In Jacobs HS (ed.) *Prolactinomas and Pregnancy*, pp 45–50. Lancaster: MTP Press.

Landolt AM, Osterwalder V & Landolt TA (1987) Storage and release of secretory granules in human prolactinomas: modification by bromocriptine. *Journal of Endocrinology* **113:** 495–499.

Larrea F, Escorza A, Valero A et al (1989) Heterogenicity of serum prolactin throughout the menstrual cycle and pregnancy in hyperprolactinemic women with normal ovarian function. *Journal of Clinical Endocrinology and Metabolism* **68:** 982–987.

Laws ER Jr (1987) Pituitary surgery. *Endocrinology and Metabolism Clinics of North America* **16:** 647–665.

Lewis UJ, Singh RNP & Lewis LJ (1989) Two forms of glycosylated human prolactin have different pigeon crop sac-stimulating activities. *Endocrinology* **124:** 1558–1563.

Magyar DM & Marshall JR (1978) Pituitary tumors and pregnancy. *American Journal of Obstetrics and Gynecology* **132:** 739–751.

Malarkey WB (1986) Effects of hyperprolactinemia on other endocrine systems. In Olefsky JM & Robbins RJ (eds) *Prolactinomas*, pp 21–41. New York: Churchill Livingstone.

Martin TL, Kim M & Malarkey WB (1985) The natural history of idiopathic hyperprolactinaemia. *Journal of Clinical Endocrinology and Metabolism* **60:** 855–858.

Mattei AM, Ferrari C, Baroldi P et al (1988) Prolactin-lowering effect of acute and once weekly repetitive oral administration of cabergoline at two dose levels in hyperprolactinemic patients. *Journal of Clinical Endocrinology and Metabolism* **66:** 193–198.

Mehta AE, Reyes FI & Faiman C (1987) Primary radiotherapy of prolactinomas. Eight- to 15-year follow-up. *American Journal of Medicine* **83:** 49–58.

Melmed S, Braunstein GS, Chang RJ & Becker DP (1986) Pituitary tumours secreting growth hormone and prolactin. *Annals of Internal Medicine* **105:** 238–253.

Miyai K, Ichihara K, Kondo K & Mori S (1986) Asymptomatic hyperprolactinaemia and prolactinoma in the general population—mass screening by paired assays of serum prolactin. *Clinical Endocrinology* **25:** 249–554.

Miyakawa I, Taniyama K, Koike H et al (1982) Successful pregnancy in an acromegalic patient during 2-Br-a-ergocryptine (CB-154) therapy. *Acta Endocrinologica* **101:** 333–338.

Molitch ME (1985) Pregnancy and the hyperprolactinemic woman. *New England Journal of Medicine* **312:** 1364–1370.

Molitch ME (1986) Manifestations, epidemiology and pathogenesis of prolactinomas in women. In Olefsky JM & Robbins RJ (eds) *Prolactinomas*, pp 67–95. New York: Churchill Livingstone.

Molitch ME (1989) Management of prolactinomas. *Annual Review of Medicine* **40:** 225–232.

Montini M, Pagani G, Gianola D et al (1986) Long-lasting suppression of prolactin secretion and rapid shrinkage of prolactinomas after a long-acting injectable form of bromocriptine. *Journal of Clinical Endocrinology and Metabolism* **63:** 266–268.

Mornex R, Orgiazzi J, Hugues B, Gagnaire JC & Claustrat B (1978) Normal pregnancies after treatment of hyperprolactinemia with bromoergocryptine, despite suspected pituitary tumors. *Journal of Clinical Endocrinology and Metabolism* **47:** 290–295.

Murphy FY, Vesely DL, Jerdan RM, Flanigan S & Kohler PO (1987) Giant invasive prolactinomas. *American Journal of Medicine* **83:** 995–1002.

Musey VC, Collina DC, Musey PI, Martino-Saltzman D & Preedy JRK (1987) Long-term effect of a first pregnancy on the secretion of prolactin. *New England Journal of Medicine* **316:** 229–234.

Newman CB, Hurley AM & Kleinberg DL (1989) Effect of CV 205-502 in hyperprolactinaemic patients intolerant of bromocriptine. *Clinical Endocrinology* **31:** 391–400.

Pellegrini I, Gunz G, Ronin C et al (1988) Polymorphism of prolactin secreted by human prolactinoma cells: immunological, receptor binding, and biological properties of the glycosylated and nonglycosylated forms. *Endocrinology* **122:** 2667–2674.

Pellegrini I, Rasolonjanahary R, Gunz G et al (1989) Resistance to bromocriptine in prolactinomas. *Journal of Clinical Endocrinology and Metabolism* **69:** 500–509.

Physician's Desk Reference (1989) Parlodel Sandoz, 43rd edition, pp 1888–1890. New York: Medical Economics.

Pontiroli AE & Falsetti L (1984) Development of pituitary adenoma in women with hyperprolactinaemia: clinical, endocrine and radiological characteristics. *British Medical Journal* **288:** 515–518.

Post KD (1986) Surgical approaches to the treatment of prolactinomas. In Olefsky JM & Robbins RJ (eds) *Prolactinomas*, pp 159–194. New York: Churchill Livingstone.

Rasmussen C, Bergh T, Nillius SJ & Wide L (1985) Return to menstruation and normalization of prolactin in hyperprolactinemic women with bromocriptine-induced pregnancy. *Fertility and Sterility* **44:** 31–34.

Rasmussen C, Bergh T & Wide L (1987) Prolactin secretion and menstrual function after long-term bromocriptine treatment. *Fertility and Sterility* **48:** 550–554.

Rasmussen C, Bergh T, Wide L & Brownell J (1988) Long-term treatment with a new non-ergot long-acting dopamine agonist, CV 205-502, in women with hyperprolactinemia. *Clinical Endocrinology* **29:** 271–279.

Robbins RJ (1986) Medical management of prolactinomas. In Olefsky JM & Robbins RJ (eds) *Prolactinomas*, pp 97–114. New York: Churchill Livingstone.

Schlechte JA, Sherman BM, Chapler FK & van Gilder J (1986) Long-term follow-up of women with surgically treated prolactin secreting pituitary tumours. *Journal of Clinical Endocrinology and Metabolism* **62:** 1296–1301.

Schlechte J, Dolan K, Sherman B, Chapter F & Luciano A (1989) The natural history of untreated hyperprolactinemia: a prospective analysis. *Journal of Clinical Endocrinology and Metabolism* **68:** 412–418.

Shupnik MA, Baxter LA, French LR & Gorski J (1979) In vivo effects of estrogen on ovine pituitaries: prolactin and growth hormone biosynthesis and messenger ribonucleic acid translation. *Endocrinology* **104:** 729–735.

Sisam DA, Saheehan JP & Sheeler LR (1987) The natural history of untreated microprolactinomas. *Fertility and Sterility* **48:** 67–71.

Vance ML, Evans WS & Thorner MO (1984) Bromocriptine. *Annals of Internal Medicine* **100:** 78–91.

Vance ML, Cragun JR, Reimnitz C et al (1989) CV 205-502 treatment of hyperprolactinemia. *Journal of Clinical Endocrinology and Metabolism* **68:** 336–339.

van der Heijden PFM, Lappöhn RE, Corbey RS et al (1989) The effectiveness, safety, and tolerability of CV 205-502 in hyperprolactinemic women: a 12-month study. *Fertility and Sterility* **52:** 574–579.

van't Verlaat JW, Lancranjan I, Hendriks MJ & Croughs RJM (1988) Primary treatment of macroprolactinomas with Parlodel LAR. *Acta Endocrinologica* **119:** 51–55.

Wang C, Lam KSL, Ma JTC et al (1987) Long-term treatment of hyperprolactinaemia with bromocriptine: effect of drug withdrawal. *Clinical Endocrinology* **27:** 363–371.

Weil C (1986) The safety of bromocriptine in hyperprolactinaemic female infertility: a literature review. *Current Medical Research and Opinion* **10:** 172–195.

Weiss MH, Teal J, Gott P et al (1983) Natural history of microprolactinomas: six-year follow-up. *Neurosurgery* **12:** 180.

Wyss HI, del Pozo E, Huber P et al (1977) Corpus luteum-induffizienz bei Hyperprolaktinämie. *Gynäkologie* **10:** 109–112.

3

Glucocorticoid therapy in hyperandrogenism

EMIL STEINBERGER
LUIS J. RODRIGUEZ-RIGAU
STEVEN M. PETAK
E. RUSSELL WEIDMAN
KEITH D. SMITH
CARMA AYALA

The first case in which a glucocorticoid, specifically cortisone, was used for therapy of hyperandrogenism was reported in 1950 by Wilkins et al. Bartter et al (1951) clearly demonstrated that in patients with adrenogenital syndrome the adrenal gland produced an excess of androgens, and that this increase in adrenal androgen production could be prevented by administration of cortisone. They also showed that the suppression of adrenal androgens in these patients was due not to direct action of cortisone on the adrenal gland, but to a negative feedback inhibition of adrenocorticotrophic hormone (ACTH) production. These fundamental studies laid the groundwork for all subsequent investigations of pathophysiology and glucocorticoid therapy in hyperandrogenism. Following the publication of these two reports, the concept of 'mild adrenal dysfunction' in patients with ovulatory dysfunction was introduced (Jones et al, 1953). Later, the association of 'mild adrenal dysfunction' with hirsutism (Greenblatt, 1953) and infertility (Greenblatt et al, 1956) was demonstrated. It should be emphasized that in the 1950s the diagnosis of hyperandrogenism in patients with 'mild adrenal dysfunction' was based primarily on clinical signs and symptoms, since the only laboratory technique available was measurement of urinary 17-ketosteroids, a highly non-specific and insensitive technique for detecting mild elevations of androgens. A beneficial effect of cortisone treatment in patients with ovulatory dysfunction was reported (Jones et al, 1953) and a 30% incidence of pregnancy was observed (Greenblatt et al, 1956). With respect to hirsutism, the first report (Greenblatt, 1953) noted that this treatment only slows its progression, an observation that is still valid.

In 1959, Perloff and Channick introduced the use of prednisone for treatment of ovulatory dysfunction in clinically hyperandrogenic females. In 1965, Perloff et al demonstrated the effectiveness of prednisone therapy in a large group of patients with infertility and clinical signs of hyperandrogenism. In the same year, Smith et al reported beneficial effects of prednisone therapy in a large group of patients with polycystic ovarian disease (PCO). The development of sensitive and precise techniques for measurement of blood levels of androgens in the late 1960s allowed the clinician to objectively diagnose hyperandrogenaemia. Elevated plasma levels of androgens in women with various 'hyperandrogenic syndromes' were reported by Bardin et al (1968) and in women with PCO by Horton and Neisler (1968). During the 1970s the emphasis of investigations into the various androgen disorders was primarily directed towards establishment of a laboratory marker for diagnosis of hyperandrogenism (Wright et al, 1978). This included measurement of various androgens in blood and urine, as well as investigation of production, distribution, transport, metabolism and excretion of androgens. By the early 1980s it became clear that determination of plasma levels of total testosterone, when using a highly specific and sensitive radio-immunoassay technique, provided a good quantitative tool for diagnosing hyperandrogenism and for follow-up of hyperandrogenic patients on suppressive therapy (Steinberger et al, 1981a). This finding offered an opportunity for investigation of specific clinical conditions associated with hyperandrogenaemia and for assessment of the effectiveness of therapy. Thus, efficacy of glucocorticoid treatment in ovulatory dysfunction (Rodriguez-Rigau et al, 1979a), infertility (Steinberger et al, 1979) and acne (Nader et al, 1984) was shown. While the clinical usefulness of glucocorticoid therapy was demonstrated, questions remained concerning duration of treatment, recurrence of hyperandrogenaemia after discontinuation of therapy and the occurrence of adverse side-effects. This report will address these issues and review the current status of glucocorticoid treatment of hyperandrogenism.

HYPERANDROGENISM

Since hair follicles and sebaceous glands are androgen-dependent structures (Hay and Hodgins, 1978), the physical manifestations of hyperandrogenism include hirsutism (male-pattern excessive hair growth), acne, and increased sebaceous gland secretion (oily skin, oily hair). In severe forms of hyperandrogenism virilization may also develop (i.e. clitoromegaly, deepening of the voice male-pattern alopecia, etc.). Clinical hyperandrogenism may result from either increased sensitivity of target cells to normal circulating androgen levels or from hyperandrogenaemia. The relative frequency of these two mechanisms has been a subject of controversy for many years. Prior to the advent of specific and sensitive assays for measurement of circulating androgen levels, the literature suggested that most cases of hirsutism were due to end-organ hypersensitivity to androgens (Lorenzo, 1970) and that hyperandrogenaemia was infrequent in women with acne (Kligman, 1974). The current consensus is that circulating androgen levels are elevated in a majority of patients with hirsutism and/or acne (Rosenfield, 1975; Paulson et al, 1977; Steinberger et al, 1981b; Marynick et al, 1983; Reingold and Rosenfield, 1987). Some patients with hirsutism have normal circulating androgen levels and it has been suggested that they have increased target cell sensitivity due to increased receptor affinity for androgens (Biffignandi et al, 1981; Mowszowicz et al, 1981) or elevated 5α-reductase activity (Biffignandi et al, 1984).

Hyperandrogenaemia may result from hypersecretion of androgens by the adrenal glands or the ovaries, from abnormality in plasma protein transport, and from increased peripheral conversion of precursors to biologically active androgens. The classic example of the latter is obesity. Increased production rates of testosterone and dihydrotestosterone have been reported in obesity, presumably from increased peripheral conversion of androstenedione to testosterone. However, increased blood production rates of dehydroepiandrosterone (DHEA), DHEA sulphate and androstenedione have also been reported in obesity. In addition, levels of sex-hormone-binding globulin (SHBG) are decreased in obesity, leading to increased free testosterone levels (Parker, 1989). Decreased SHBG and elevated free testosterone levels are common findings in hyperandrogenic women (Paulson et al, 1977; Rosenfield and Moll, 1983). Excepting obesity, iatrogenic and rare genetic causes, it appears that in most cases of hyperandrogenism excessive androgen secretion is responsible for the decrease in SHBG levels. This is supported by reports of excellent correlations between circulating total and free testosterone levels in hyperandrogenic women (Steinberger et al, 1981a). Thus, for the vast majority of patients measurement of total testosterone suffices.

Increased adrenal secretion of androgenic steroids may be the result of benign or malignant adrenal neoplasias, Cushing's syndrome, congenital and acquired adrenal hyperplasias due to enzyme deficiencies, or may be 'idiopathic'. It appears that the latter is the most common (Rodriguez-Rigau et al, 1979a; Steinberger et al, 1981a, 1984; Rodriguez-Rigau et al, 1989). A number of theories were proposed to explain the pathophysiology of this idiopathic glucocorticoid-suppressible hyperandrogenism (IGSH): 'cryptic' or 'subclinical' adrenal enzyme deficiencies, excessive pituitary secretion of the putative corticoadrenal androgen-stimulating hormone (CASH), 'exaggerated' or 'persistent' adrenarche, 'stress', etc.

Purely ovarian hypersecretion of androgens may occur as a result of neoplasias (arrhenoblastoma, Sertoli–Leydig cell tumour, hilus-cell tumour, lipid-cell tumour, cystadenoma, cystadenocarcinoma, etc.), in ovarian hyperthecosis, and in some cases of polycystic ovarian disease. Combined adrenal–ovarian androgen hypersecretion is found in most cases of polycystic ovarian disease (Lobo, 1984).

In summary, hyperandrogenaemia is found in a majority of women with clinical signs of hyperandrogenism. Development of specific and sensitive assays for serum testosterone determination and precise establishment of the normal range for serum testosterone levels in women led to the conclusion that increased serum testosterone concentrations are found in most women showing clinical signs of hyperandrogenism. Determinations of free testosterone levels and other androgens are useful when serum testosterone levels are normal. In a majority of hyperandrogenic women adrenal overproduction of androgens is responsible, at least in part, for the hyperandrogenic state.

CLINICAL CONSEQUENCES OF HYPERANDROGENISM

The clinical manifestations of hyperandrogenism consist of readily apparent effects on the skin and more subtle effects on ovulatory function. In the skin, both hair follicles and sebaceous glands are androgen-dependent structures (Hay and Hodgins, 1978). An increase in circulating androgen levels stimulates androgen-dependent hair growth. This effect is mediated by androgen receptors. The stimulation of sebaceous glands by androgens is also mediated by androgen receptors. This explains why the cutaneous manifestations of hyperandrogenism are less pronounced in the Oriental female with a limited number of androgen receptors than in a woman of Mediterranean ethnic origin with more androgen receptors. Increase in sebaceous gland activity results in enlargement of the pores in the skin, excessively oily skin, excessively oily hair and acne. Androgen stimulation of the hair follicles results in hirsutism, a clinical finding that is sometimes difficult to quantify. Most clinicians employ the scale of Ferriman and Gallwey (1961) or its modification to quantify hirsutism.

Hyperandrogenism is associated with varying degrees of ovulatory dysfunction and infertility. As plasma androgen levels increase, the length of the follicular phase of the menstrual cycle increases and the length of the luteal phase decreases, sometimes without any change in the overall length of the cycle (Smith et al, 1979a). Hyperandrogenism has been associated with a decrease in progesterone production by the corpus luteum (Rodriguez-Rigau et al, 1979b). As progesterone levels decline, a multitude of luteal phase symptoms may occur (e.g. mastodynia, cyclic oedema, premenstrual syndrome). The luteal phase deficiency may be severe enough to prevent conception or be associated with an increased incidence of spontaneous

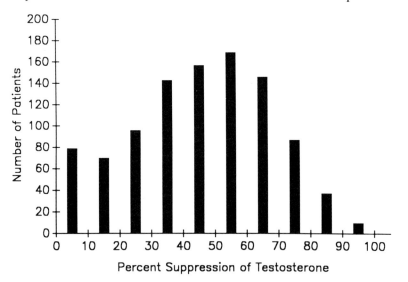

Figure 1. Per cent suppression of serum testosterone levels in 994 hyperandrogenic women following a dexamethasone suppression test (0.5 mg four times daily for 2 days).

abortions. As androgen levels become higher, the disturbance of the menstrual cycle progresses to anovulation and ultimately to amenorrhoea (Smith et al, 1979a; Steinberger et al, 1981a). This sequence of events relating degree of androgen elevation to severity of disturbance of ovulatory function has been experimentally demonstrated to occur after administration of progressively increasing doses of testosterone to normally ovulating females (Rodriguez-Rigau et al, 1986). Indeed, one observes first prolongation of the follicular phase and shortening of the luteal phase, then anovulatory cycles, and finally amenorrhoea. Interestingly enough, the ratio of circulating luteinizing hormone (LH) to follicle-stimulating hormone (FSH) levels first increases and, once amenorrhoea ensues, the levels of both gonadotrophins drop.

Another consequence of hyperandrogenaemia is formation of ovarian cysts of varying sizes. These cysts represent the end result of disturbed follicular development and rupture (Yen, 1980). Increased serum LH levels with normal or suppressed FSH levels are also a consequence of hyperandrogenaemia (Yen, 1980; Steinberger et al, 1981a; Karpas et al, 1984; Rodriguez-Rigau et al, 1986). In turn, increased LH levels stimulate androgen-producing cells in the ovaries. This results in the development of the so-called polycystic ovarian syndrome (Yen, 1980).

THERAPY OF HYPERANDROGENISM

In a majority of hyperandrogenic women androgen levels can be suppressed, at least in part, with low-dose glucocorticoid treatment (Rodriguez-Rigau et al, 1979a; Steinberger et al, 1979). We have recently studied a large population of women with clinical signs of hyperandrogenism ($n = 994$). The suppressibility of testosterone levels by glucocorticoids was investigated utilizing a dexamethasone suppression test (Figure 1). Testosterone levels failed to suppress more than 20% in only 15.2% of cases. It has been shown previously that such patients do not benefit from chronic glucocorticoid therapy (Steinberger et al, 1984).

Management of glucocorticoid-resistant hyperandrogenism (GRH)

Failure of circulating androgen levels to suppress after glucocorticoid administration indicates the need for a diagnostic work-up to exclude androgen-producing tumours, Cushing's syndrome and purely ovarian forms of hyperandrogenism. The management of patients with glucocorticoid-resistant hyperandrogenism or patients in whom glucocorticoid treatment is contraindicated is based on individual circumstances and particularly on the goals of the treatment. If the patient is obese, weight loss is the preferred therapeutic approach. If the primary goal of the treatment is amelioration of the cutaneous manifestations of hyperandrogenism and pregnancy is not desired, ovarian suppression with oestrogens or gonadotrophin-releasing hormone analogues or therapy with antiandrogens like cyproterone acetate can be considered. Although these treatments may be effective in achieving reduction of hirsutism and acne, they do not correct the ovarian dysfunction and can be associated with significant side-effects. Spironolactone treatment also appears to be effective in some cases of hyperandrogenism (Koksal et al, 1987). However, at high doses spironolactone is associated with a significant incidence of metrorrhagia (Helfer et al, 1988). Cimetidine has been proposed for treatment of hyperandrogenism, but its effectiveness is marginal at best (Lardinois and Mazzaferri, 1985). Ketoconazole has been proposed (Martikainen et al, 1988) as a therapeutic modality, but it has potentially serious side-effects and thus is rarely used.

In glucocorticoid-resistant hyperandrogenic patients desiring pregnancy, treatment with anti-oestrogens (e.g. clomiphene citrate) or gonadotrophins—FSH, human menopausal gonadotrophin (HMG)—is frequently successful in inducing ovulation and conception. Androgen suppression with oestrogens or gonadotrophin-releasing hormone (GnRH) analogues prior to ovulation induction is sometimes necessary. Bilateral ovarian wedge resection is at present only rarely performed, since its effectiveness is at best temporary and it may lead to pelvic adhesions and infertility. Laparoscopic ovarian electro-cautery or laser treatment have been proposed for cases of polycystic ovarian disease resistant to medical treatment (McLaughlin, 1984; Vanderweider et al, 1989). Insufficient information is available in the literature to assess the effectiveness, duration of beneficial effect and possible sequelae (i.e. adhesions) of these procedures.

Management of idiopathic glucocorticoid-suppressible hyperandrogenism (IGSH)

For many years we have utilized low-dose glucocorticoid therapy for management of patients with IGSH. When we use prednisone, the initial dose is 7.5 mg daily (2.5 mg in the morning and 5.0 mg in the evening), while with dexamethasone the initial dose is 0.25–0.5 mg nightly. Reduction of dose and cessation of treatment is based on laboratory and clinical response. In patients in whom hyperandrogenism recurs after cessation of therapy, another course of treatment is administered.

Reduction of serum androgen levels results in improvement in the cutaneous manifestation of hyperandrogenism. However, the effects on sebaceous gland activity are more dramatic than the effects on hirsutism. As androgen levels decline, sebaceous gland stimulation is reduced, resulting in a decrease in sebum production, a decrease in oiliness of the scalp and hair, and a decrease in pore size. This may result in amelioration or disappearance of acne (Nader et al, 1984). On the other hand, hirsutism will not disappear. The rate of hair growth slows as androgen levels decline. The reduction in the rate of hair growth and the prevention of new hair growth may result in a considerable improvement.

In hyperandrogenic patients with ovarian dysfunction, reduction of circulating androgen levels is associated with progressive improvement in ovulatory activity (Rodriguez-Rigau et al, 1979a). This improvement is a slow process. For example, in patients with amenorrhoea the first sign of improvement is occurrence of anovulatory cycles. This is followed by ovulatory cycles characterized by long follicular phases and short luteal phases. Eventually normal ovulatory cycles may be established. In patients presenting with less severe forms of ovulatory dysfunction the improvement follows a similar pattern. The extent of improvement of the ovulatory function has been shown to be directly correlated to the degree of suppression of circulating testosterone levels (Rodriguez-Rigau et al, 1979a).

The incidence of hyperandrogenism in female infertility due to ovulatory dysfunction is high (Steinberger et al, 1979). These patients present with varying degrees of ovulatory dysfunction ranging from minor alterations in the length of the phases of the menstrual cycle to amenorrhoea. Treatment with glucocorticoids leads to progressive improvement in ovulatory activity (Steinberger et al, 1981a). The degree of suppression of serum testosterone levels is directly correlated to the incidence of pregnancy and inversely correlated to the time necessary for the pregnancy to occur (Steinberger et al, 1979). In hyperandrogenic women with ovulatory dysfunction, glucocorticoid treatment is associated with lower miscarriage rates than treatment with clomiphene citrate or gonadotrophins (Steinberger et al, 1981a). Clomiphene citrate is effective in treatment of infertile women with ovulatory dysfunction, including women with hyperandrogenism. However, the effectiveness of clomiphene citrate is improved when the circulating androgen levels are also suppressed with glucocorticoids (Radwanska and Sloan, 1979; Lobo et al, 1982; Daly et al, 1984). Even in hyperandrogenic women unresponsive to clomiphene citrate, pretreatment with glucocorticoids to suppress androgen levels results in establishment of an ovulatory response to clomiphene citrate (Lobo et al, 1982).

Side-effects of low-dose glucocorticoid treatment

The adverse effects of prolonged administration of supraphysiological doses of glucocorticoids are numerous and have been well described over the years (Dujovne and Azarhoff, 1973; Rimsza, 1978; Tyrell and Baxter, 1987). The side-effects can be divided into those due to suppression of the hypothalamic–pituitary–adrenal axis and those due to the effects of excess glucocorticoids on other organs such as eye, bone, immune system or on protein, carbohydrate and lipid metabolism.

The side-effects, if any, of physiological replacement doses of glucocorticoids used for treatment of hyperandrogenism are less well defined. Theoretically, at these doses one would not expect any adverse side-effects. When patients report adverse symptoms during treatment, it is often difficult to determine whether the symptoms are related to the glucocorticoid or are a consequence of the underlying disease state for which the medication has been prescribed.

In 1964, Danowski et al reviewed the clinical course of over 150 patients treated with 'replacement/displacement' doses of cortisol or other glucocorticoids for 1–72 months and found no incidents suggestive of adrenal insufficiency, although many patients underwent surgical procedures without supplemental glucocorticoid coverage. Some of these patients failed to respond normally to an intravenous metyrapone challenge test during treatment, but they responded normally 5 weeks after treatment was stopped. Even these patients had no difficulties responding to the stress of surgical procedures while on treatment, when no supplemental glucocorticoids were administered. Fujieda et al (1980) showed that patients on replacement doses of prednisone were able to increase serum cortisol levels in response to insulin-induced hypoglycaemia, but the response was less than that seen prior to treatment. Smith et al (1982) found a normal cortisol response to ACTH during prednisone treatment which was not different from that before treatment. The clinical relevance of slightly diminished pituitary responsiveness to provocative testing in patients treated with physiological doses of glucocorticoids is unclear, since the patients appear to have no clinical difficulty responding to physical stress. We recently investigated 199 patients treated with glucocorticoids for hyperandrogenism. Of these patients, 31 had 35 surgical procedures while on therapy and none had glucocorticoid supplementation during surgery. No patient developed clinical evidence of adrenal insufficiency. These procedures included 14 laparoscopies, ten cases of dilatation and curettage, seven laparotomies (including hysterectomies), and four miscellaneous procedures.

There is a paucity of reports dealing with side-effects during treatment with physiological doses of glucocorticoids. Most reports deal with pharmacological doses or do not mention dose at all. Those reports dealing with physiological doses note the absence of any side-effects. Jeffries (1967) reported no side-effects in 371 patients treated with up to 20 mg of hydrocortisone daily. We reviewed the side-effects reported by a group of hyperandrogenic women treated with glucocorticoids for 1–83 months (mean 20.1 months). Prednisone therapy was employed in 147 women and 79 took dexamethasone (Table 1). The overall incidence of reported side-effects was 21.2%. The most frequently reported side-effects were fluid retention (5.8%) and weight gain (3.1%). None of the other side-effects were reported by more

Table 1. Side-effects reported by hyperandrogenic women during glucocorticoid treatment.

	Prednisone ($n = 147$)	Dexamethasone ($n = 79$)	Total ($n = 226$)
Side-effects*	26 (17.7%)	22 (27.8%)	48 (21.2%)
Fluid retention†	4 (2.7%)	9 (11.4%)	13 (5.8%)
Weight gain‡	0 (0.0%)	7 (8.9%)	7 (3.1%)
Anxiety, depression	3 (2.0%)	2 (2.5%)	5 (2.2%)
Headache	1 (0.6%)	4 (5.1%)	5 (2.2%)
Mastodynia	4 (2.7%)	0 (0.0%)	4 (1.8%)
Gastrointestinal symptoms	2 (1.4%)	2 (2.5%)	4 (1.8%)
Hot flushes	3 (2.0%)	0 (0.0%)	3 (1.3%)
Vaginitis	2 (1.4%)	1 (1.3%)	3 (1.3%)
Decreased libido	3 (2.0%)	0 (0.0%)	3 (1.3%)
Nocturia	1 (0.6%)	1 (1.3%)	2 (0.9%)
Striae	0 (0.0%)	1 (1.3%)	1 (0.4%)
Miscellaneous	6 (4.1%)	3 (3.8%)	9 (4.0%)

* Some patients reported more than one side-effect.
† $P < 0.05$.
‡ $P < 0.005$.

than 2.2% of patients. Treatment with dexamethasone was associated with a significantly higher incidence of complaints of fluid retention and weight gain than was treatment with prednisone.

Since low-dose glucocorticoid treatment is used in hyperandrogenic women desiring pregnancy, frequently patients are receiving glucocorticoids at the time of conception. Reinisch et al (1978) suggested that weight at birth was reduced in offspring of women who had taken 10 mg of prednisone daily throughout pregnancy. However, Smith et al (1979b) showed that there was no effect on birth weight or duration of pregnancy when prednisone treatment was discontinued at the time of the diagnosis of pregnancy. To our knowledge, there are no published data that suggest that glucocorticoids used in this manner have any adverse effects on offspring. As a matter of fact, the incidence of miscarriages in patients treated with prednisone is lower than the miscarriage rate following treatment with ovulation induction agents (Steinberger et al, 1981a).

Long-term follow-up of glucocorticoid treatment

A group of 428 patients with IGSH was studied. Serum testosterone levels after acute dexamethasone suppression test and after initiation of chronic glucocorticoid therapy are presented in Figure 2. Figure 3 presents serum DHEA sulphate data in the same group of patients. Chronic therapy elicited similar degrees of suppression of both androgen levels as the dexamethasone suppression test. Androgen levels within the normal range were maintained (testosterone below 40 ng/dl, DHEA sulphate below 150 µg/dl). It should be noted that in this group of patients treatment was discontinued after various time intervals depending on clinical and laboratory responses. The data in Figures 2 and 3 include the values obtained in many cases after discontinuation of therapy. In patients with recurrence of hyperandrogenism, treatment was re-initiated. Thus, the data presented show that androgen

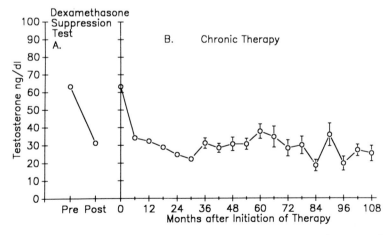

Figure 2. Serum testosterone levels after acute dexamethasone suppression test and after initiation of chronic glucocorticoid therapy in 428 hyperandrogenic females.

levels can be maintained within the normal range in IGSH by proper therapeutic management.

After discontinuation of therapy, androgen levels remained suppressed for long periods of time in some patients. In others, hyperandrogenaemia recurred. In order to investigate the incidence and pattern of recurrence of hyperandrogenism subsequent to cessation of chronic glucocorticoid therapy, we studied in detail a subgroup of 59 patients in whom a minimum of 3 months of follow-up off therapy was available. These patients were treated for an average of 18.2 months and were followed for an average of

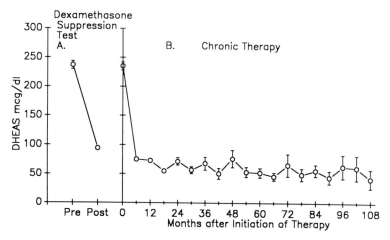

Figure 3. Serum dehydroepiandrosterone sulphate (DHEAS) levels after acute dexamethasone suppression test and after initiation of chronic glucocorticoid therapy in 428 hyperandrogenic females.

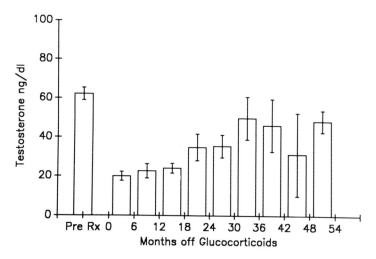

Figure 4. Serum testosterone levels before chronic glucocorticoid treatment and after discontinuation of treatment in 59 hyperandrogenic females.

18.6 months after cessation of the initial course of therapy. Figures 4 and 5 illustrate serum testosterone and DHEA sulphate levels in these patients. This group includes some patients in whom hyperandrogenaemia recurred. In two thirds of patients (Group 1, Table 2) testosterone levels remained suppressed for the duration of follow-up after cessation of therapy (average

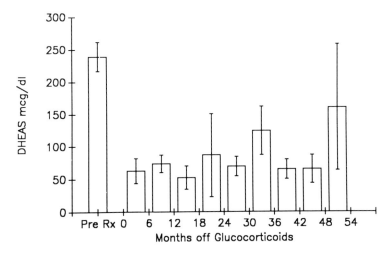

Figure 5. Serum dehydroepiandrosterone sulphate (DHEAS) levels before chronic gluco-corticoid treatment after discontinuation of treatment in 59 hyperandrogenic females.

Table 2. Long-term follow-up of 59 hyperandrogenic women after discontinuation of chronic glucocorticoid therapy.

	Group 1 (n = 39, 66.1%)	Group 2 (n = 9, 15.3%)	Group 3 (n = 11, 18.6%)	Total (n = 59)
Age	29.9 ± 0.8*	28.0 ± 1.6	26.3 ± 2.1	28.8 ± 0.7
Treatment months	20.9 ± 2.9	8.8 ± 2.5	15.5 ± 4.8	18.2 ± 2.2
Post-treatment months	15.7 ± 1.9	24.0 ± 3.3	29.2 ± 6.7	18.6 ± 2.0
Pretreatment testosterone (ng/dl)	60.1 ± 2.7	76.7 ± 15.5	55.6 ± 5.3	61.8 ± 3.1
Treatment testosterone (ng/dl)	25.1 ± 0.2	31.1 ± 9.9	32.6 ± 5.3	26.6 ± 2.3
Post-treatment testosterone (ng/dl)	17.8 ± 1.4	48.1 ± 9.2	51.9 ± 4.5	27.8 ± 2.7
Pretreatment DHEAS (μg/dl)	212.9 ± 22.1	271.1 ± 25.6	242.0 ± 36.7	227.9 ± 19.7
Treatment DHEAS (μg/dl)	30.7 ± 5.5	25.1 ± 4.2	32.0 ± 8.5	30.2 ± 4.2
Post-treatment DHEAS (μg/dl)	52.6 ± 7.9	110.2 ± 20.9	128.3 ± 25.2	74.0 ± 8.9

* Mean ± SE.
Group 1: Normal serum testosterone maintained after discontinuation of therapy.
Group 2: Partial recurrence of hyperandrogenaemia after discontinuation of therapy.
Group 3: Complete recurrence of hyperandrogenaemia after discontinuation of therapy.
DHEAS, dehydroepiandrosterone sulphate.

15.7 months, range 3–83 months). In 18.6% of patients (Group 3) hyperandrogenaemia recurred to pretreatment levels shortly after cessation of therapy. In 15.3% (Group 2), a partial recurrence of hyperandrogenaemia was observed 1–22 months after cessation of therapy. It is of interest that DHEA sulphate levels remained suppressed after cessation of therapy in all groups regardless of recurrence of elevated testosterone levels. These data indicate a remarkably high incidence of long-term remission of the disorder. In patients with partial or complete recurrence of hyperandrogenaemia, re-initiation of therapy leads rapidly to re-establishment of normal androgen levels.

SUMMARY

Hyperandrogenism is a common disorder in the reproductive age female. It is associated with cutaneous manifestations and ovulatory dysfunction. The degree of hyperandrogenaemia is directly related to the severity of ovulatory dysfunction. The ovulatory dysfunction frequently leads to infertility. The most common form of hyperandrogenism is idiopathic glucocorticoid-suppressible hyperandrogenism (IGSH). The management of this disorder involves appropriate use of physiological doses of glucocorticoids. This treatment leads not only to normalization of serum androgen levels but also to amelioration of cutaneous symptoms and improvement in ovulatory function. In infertile women with ovulatory dysfunction secondary to IGSH, occurrence of pregnancy after treatment with glucocorticoids is directly related to the degree of the suppression of serum androgen levels. In other words, this treatment does not 'induce ovulation', but its effectiveness in improving ovulatory function is a result of a correction of the hyperandrogenic state. At physiological doses glucocorticoid therapy does not appear to be associated with significant side-effects. With appropriate management, androgen levels can be maintained within the normal range indefinitely. Furthermore, in a majority of patients, androgen levels remain within the normal range for a long time (years) after discontinuation of chronic glucocorticoid therapy.

REFERENCES

Bardin CW, Hembree WC & Lipsett MB (1968) Suppression of testosterone and androstenedione production rates with dexamethasone in women with idiopathic hirsutism and polycystic ovaries. Journal of Clinical Endocrinology and Metabolism 28: 1300–1306.

Bartter FC, Albright F, Forbers AP, Leaf A, Dempsey E & Carroll E (1951) The effects of adrenocorticotropic hormone and cortisone in the adrenogenital syndrome associated with congenital adrenal hyperplasia: an attempt to correct its disordered hormonal pattern. Journal of Clinical Investigation 30: 237–251.

Biffignandi P, Manieri C, Massobrio M, Mazzocchi S, Messina M & Molinatti GM (1981) Androgen receptors: a quantitative investigation in female unexplained hirsutism. Panminerva Medica 23: 1–4.

Biffignandi P, Massucchetti C & Molinatti GM (1984) Female hirsutism: pathophysiological considerations and therapeutic implications. Endocrine Reviews 5: 498–513.

Daly DC, Walters CA, Soto-Albers CE, Tolian N & Riddick DH (1984) A randomized study of dexamethasone in ovulation induction with clomiphene citrate. *Fertility and Sterility* **41:** 844–848.

Danowski TS, Bonessi JV, Sabeh G, Sutton RD, Webster MW & Sarver ME (1964) Probabilities of pituitary–adrenal responsiveness after steroids therapy. *Annals of Internal Medicine* **61:** 11–26.

Dujovne CA & Azarhoff DL (1973) Clinical complications of corticosteroid therapy: a selected review. *Medical Clinics of North America* **57:** 133–142.

Ferriman P & Gallwey JD (1961) Clinical assessment of body hair growth in women. *Journal of Clinical Endocrinology and Metabolism* **21:** 1440–1447.

Fujieda K, Reyes FI, Blankstein J & Faiman C (1980) Pituitary–adrenal function in women treated with low doses of prednisone. *American Journal of Obstetrics and Gynecology* **137:** 962–965.

Greenblatt RB (1953) Cortisone in the treatment of the hirsute woman. *American Journal of Obstetrics and Gynecology* **66:** 700–710.

Greenblatt RB, Barfield WE & Lampros CP (1956) Cortisone in the treatment of infertility. *Fertility and Sterility* **7:** 203–212.

Hay JB & Hodgins MB (1978) Distribution of androgen metabolizing enzymes in isolated tissues of human forehead and axillary skin. *Journal of Endocrinology* **79:** 29–39.

Helfer EL, Miller JL & Rose LI (1988) Side effects of spironolactone therapy in the hirsute woman. *Journal of Clinical Endocrinology and Metabolism* **66:** 208–211.

Horton R & Neisler J (1968) Plasma androgens in patients with the polycystic ovary syndrome. *Journal of Clinical Endocrinology and Metabolism* **28:** 479–484.

Jeffries WM (1967) Low dosage glucocorticoid therapy. *Archives of Internal Medicine* **119:** 265–278.

Jones GES, Howard JE & Langford H (1953) The use of cortisone in follicular phase disturbance. *Fertility and Sterility* **4:** 49–62.

Karpas AE, Rodriguez-Rigau LJ, Smith KD & Steinberger E (1984) Effect of acute and chronic androgen suppression by glucocorticoids on gonadotropin levels in hirsute women. *Journal of Clinical Endocrinology and Metabolism* **59:** 780–784.

Kligman AM (1974) An overview of acne. *Journal of Investigative Dermatology* **62:** 268–287.

Koksal A, Pabucca R & Akyurek C (1987) Spironolactone in the treatment of hirsutism. *Archives of Gynecology* **240:** 95–100.

Lardinois C & Mazzaferri E (1985) Cimetidine blocks testosterone synthesis. *Archives of Internal Medicine* **145:** 920–922.

Lobo RA (1984) The role of the adrenal in polycystic ovary syndrome. *Seminars in Reproductive Endocrinology* **2:** 251–262.

Lobo RA, Paul W, March CM, Granger L & Kletzky OA (1982) Clomiphene and dexamethasone in women unresponsive to clomiphene alone. *Obstetrics and Gynecology* **60:** 497–501.

Lorenzo EM (1970) Familial study of hirsutism. *Journal of Clinical Endocrinology and Metabolism* **31:** 556–564.

Martikainen H, Heikkinen J, Ruokonen A & Kauppila A (1988) Hormonal and clinical effects of ketoconazole in hirsute women. *Journal of Clinical Endocrinology and Metabolism* **66:** 987–991.

Marynick SP, Chakmakjian ZH, McCaffree DL & Herndon JH (1983) Androgen excess in cystic acne. *New England Journal of Medicine* **308:** 981–986.

McLaughlin DS (1984) Evaluation of adhesion reformation by early second-look laparoscopy following microlaser ovarian wedge resection. *Fertility and Sterility* **42:** 531–537.

Mowszowicz I, Riahi M, Wright F, Bouchard PH, Kutten F & Mauvais-Jarvis P (1983) Androgen receptor in human skin cytosol. *Journal of Clinical Endocrinology and Metabolism* **52:** 338–344.

Nader S, Rodriguez-Rigau LJ, Smith KD & Steinberger E (1984) Acne and hyperandrogenism: impact of lowering androgen levels with glucocorticoid treatment. *Journal of the American Academy of Dermatology* **11:** 256–259.

Parker LN (ed.) (1989) Obesity. In *Adrenal Androgens in Clinical Medicine*, pp 246–262. San Diego: Academic Press.

Paulson JD, Keller DW, Weist WG & Warren JC (1977) Free testosterone concentration in serum. Elevation is the hallmark of hirsutism. *American Journal of Obstetrics and Gynecology* **128:** 851–857.

Perloff WH & Channick BJ (1959) Effect of prednisone on abnormal menstrual function. *American Journal of Obstetrics and Gynecology* **77**: 138–143.

Perloff WH, Smith KD & Steinberger E (1965) Effect of prednisone on female infertility. *International Journal of Fertility* **10**: 31–40.

Radwanska E & Sloan C (1979) Serum testosterone levels in infertile women. *International Journal of Fertility* **24**: 176–181.

Reingold SB & Rosenfield RL (1987) The relationship of mild hirsutism or acne in women to androgens. *Archives of Dermatology* **123**: 209–212.

Reinisch JM, Simon NG, Karow WG & Gandelman R (1978) Prenatal exposure to prednisone in humans and animals retards intrauterine growth. *Science* **202**: 436–438.

Rimsza ME (1978) Complications of corticosteroid therapy. *American Journal of Diseases of Children* **132**: 806–810.

Rodriguez-Rigau LJ, Smith KD, Tcholakian RK & Steinberger E (1979a) Effect of prednisone on plasma testosterone levels and on duration of phases of the menstrual cycle in hyperandrogenic women. *Fertility and Sterility* **32**: 408–413.

Rodriguez-Rigau LJ, Steinberger E, Atkins BJ & Lucci JA (1979b) Effect of testosterone on human corpus luteum steroidogenesis in vitro. *Fertility and Sterility* **31**: 448–450.

Rodriguez-Rigau LJ, Smith KD & Steinberger E (1986) Management of polycystic ovarian dysfunction. In Steinberger E, Frajese G & Steinberger A (eds) *Reproductive Medicine*, pp 277–281. New York: Raven Press.

Rodriguez-Rigau LJ, Petak SM, Leite Z, Smith KD & Steinberger E (1989) Therapy of hyperandrogenism. In Frajese G, Steinberger E & Rodriguez-Rigau LJ (eds) *Reproductive Medicine: Medical Therapy*, pp 69–77. Amsterdam: Excerpta Medica.

Rosenfield RL (1975) Studies of the relation of plasma androgen levels to androgen activity in women. *Journal of Steroid Biochemistry* **6**: 695–702.

Rosenfield RL & Moll GW (1983) The role of proteins in the distribution of plasma androgens and estradiol. In Molinatti GM, Martini L & James UHT (eds) *Androgenization in Women*, pp 25–46. New York: Raven Press.

Smith KD, Steinberger E & Perloff WH (1965) Polycystic ovarian disease: a report of 301 patients. *American Journal of Obstetrics and Gynecology* **93**: 994–1001.

Smith KD, Rodriguez-Rigau LJ, Tcholakian RK & Steinberger E (1979a) The relation between plasma testosterone levels and the lengths of phases of the menstrual cycle. *Fertility and Sterility* **32**: 403–407.

Smith KD, Steinberger E & Rodriguez-Rigau LJ (1979b) Prednisone therapy and birth weight. *Science* **206**: 96–97.

Smith KD, Rodriguez-Rigau LJ & Steinberger E (1982) Response of the adrenal to ACTH in hyperandrogenic women treated chronically with low doses of prednisone. *Fertility and Sterility* **38**: 202–206.

Steinberger E, Smith KD, Tcholakian RK & Rodriguez-Rigau LJ (1979) Testosterone levels in female partners of infertile couples. *American Journal of Obstetrics and Gynecology* **133**: 133–138.

Steinberger E, Smith KD & Rodriguez-Rigau LJ (1981a) Hyperandrogenism and female infertility. In Crosignani PG & Rubin B (eds) *Endocrinology of Human Infertility: New Aspects*, pp 327–342. London: Academic Press.

Steinberger E, Rodriguez-Rigau LJ, Smith KD & Held B (1981b) The menstrual cycle and plasma testosterone levels in women with acne. *Journal of the American Academy of Dermatology* **4**: 54–58.

Steinberger E, Smith KD & Rodriguez-Rigau LJ (1984) Testosterone, dehydroepiandrosterone and dehydroepiandrosterone sulfate in hyperandrogenic women. *Journal of Clinical Endocrinology and Metabolism* **59**: 471–477.

Tyrell B & Baxter JD (1987) Glucocorticoid therapy. In Felig P, Baxter JD, Broadus AE & Frohman LA (eds) *Endocrinology and Metabolism*, 2nd edn, pp 788–817. New York: McGraw-Hill.

Vanderweider RM, Alberda AT, DeJong FH & Brandenburg H (1989) Endocrine effects of laparoscopic ovarian electrocautery in patients with PCO resistant to clomiphene citrate. *European Journal of Obstetrics, Gynaecology and Reproductive Biology* **32**: 157–162.

Wilkins L, Lewis RA, Klein R & Rosemberg E (1950) The suppression of androgen secretion by cortisone in a case of congenital adrenal hyperplasia. *Bulletin of the Johns Hopkins Hospital* **86**: 249–252.

Wright F, Mowszowicz I & Mauvais-Jarvis P (1978) Urinary 5α-androstane, 3α,17β-diol radioimmunoassay: a new clinical evaluation. *Journal of Clinical Endocrinology and Metabolism* **47:** 850–860.
Yen SSC (1980) The polycystic ovary syndrome. *Clinical Endocrinology* **12:** 177–207.

4

Induction of ovulation: historical aspects

BRUNO LUNENFELD
VACLAV INSLER

Since the beginning of recorded history the human race has placed emphasis on fertility. In the Judeo-Christian tradition the importance of procreation is inherent in man's very creation: 'So God created man in His own image, in the image of God created He him; male and female created He them. And God blessed them, and God said unto them: Be fruitful and multiply and replenish the earth and subdue it' (Genesis **1:** 27–28). Nothing more vividly demonstrates the importance of fertility to the individual than the reaction by and to those who do not have children. The grief of a woman who has failed to bear a live-born child is no less in modern society than it was for our forefathers.

Infertility is seldom, if ever, a physically debilitating disease. It may, however, severely affect the couple's psychological harmony, sexual life, and social function. Even in those societies which made family planning and birth control their official policy and social vogue, the individual couple desiring a child but unable to conceive one feels demeaned, deprived and bitter. In some cultures childlessness may cast a heavy shadow on the physiological and social adequacy of the female and diminish the social standing of the male partner. Whatever the demographic policy of the government, and regardless of the aims proclaimed and/or pursued by the society, the individual family perceives its freedom to procreate as a most basic human right. By most cultures, children are regarded as an extension of self, as bearers and perpetuators of the family name and tradition, as well as an expansion of one's hopes, aims and strivings. The inability to procreate is thus always perceived as a denial of basic rights, an injustice and a disappointment, sometimes bordering on grief.

Most childless couples must cope with difficult psychological, family and social problems. The examination and treatment of infertility may pose additional psychological difficulties, interfere with the sexual life of the couple, and impose a financial burden on the family or on society.

DIMENSION OF THE PROBLEM

The estimates of prevalence of infertility are based on either demographic data or on health service statistics. These sources produce diverse and

Baillière's Clinical Obstetrics and Gynaecology—
Vol. 4, No. 3, September 1990
ISBN 0–7020–1478–8

inaccurate assessments. Belsey (1976), using data collected by the World Health Organization (WHO), projected the prevalence of infertility in the world population. Arithmetic recalculation of those data indicated that according to demographic estimates the prevalence of infertility among the female population in the fertile age groups would be approximately 45% (including women who are fertile but perceive themselves as infertile and those of unproven fertility). As reported by health services the incidence of infertility was calculated to be approximately 15%.

The percentage of childless marriages, voluntary or involuntary, varies considerably according to society and time period. In most Western societies the figure is about 10%, although much higher percentages are found in some countries. The range in the index of primary infertility of married women varies greatly demographically. In Thailand (World Fertility Survey, 1977) and Korea (Korean Institute for Family Planning, 1971) only 1–1.5% of married women 35–39 years of age have never been pregnant. The same category of women in urban areas of Columbia have an index of infertility as high as 13–23%. The higher levels of both childlessness or nulliparity in urban areas (Veevers, 1972) suggest that either voluntary infertility is higher in urban areas or that certain 'acquired' causes of infertility, such as pelvic inflammatory disease, are more common in these areas. In developing countries a wide range of infertility prevalence exists in different regions and/or tribes within a country, and great variation is also found between neighbouring nations. The prevalence of childlessness among married women who have completed their reproductive years varies from as low as 1.1% to as high as 42.5% for different districts in the Sudan

Table 1. Women aged 19–34 years in 1990 and estimated number of infertile women.

Country	Women	Infertile women
West Europe	39 500 000	3 160 000
East Europe	45 200 000	3 620 000
USA	27 700 000	2 220 000
Canada	2 900 000	230 000
Japan	12 800 000	1 020 000
Australia	1 900 000	150 000
Total	130 000 000	10 400 000

Table 2. Women entering 'fertile age pool' every year, 1990–1995.

Country	New women	New infertile women
West Europe	2 630 000	210 000
East Europe	3 010 000	240 000
USA	1 850 000	150 000
Canada	190 000	15 000
Japan	850 000	68 000
Australia	130 000	10 000
Total	8 660 000	693 000

(Sudan Population and Census Office, 1958). Similarly wide ranges of childlessness are noted in other areas of Africa (Belsey, 1976). In England and Wales the percentage of married women with no children after 12 years of marriage fell from 13% in 1953 to 8% in 1960. In the USA the proportion of married women who remained childless rose from 8% among those women married in the latter half of the 19th century and approached 20% in the period between the two world wars. In the post-war years the proportion of women that remained childless decreased sharply, but it has risen since. In Israel, 12.2% of women who married in 1966 remained childless after ten years of marriage.

From figures published by the United Nations Population Division we have estimated that the population size of women between the ages of 19 and 34 years in the developed world in 1990 will be about 130 million. If we assume that at least 8% will be infertile, then the pool of the infertile population will be above 10 million (Table 1), with about 700 000 new patients entering this pool every year between the years 1990 and 1995 (Table 2).

The estimation of incidence of different infertility causes varies extremely between the reported series. Table 3 summarizes the diagnostic categories established in 6549 infertile couples managed by different authors in five

Table 3. Incidence of different infertility causes.

Author, year and country	Number of couples (years observed)	Tubal	Ovulation disturbances	Cervix/ uterus	Other	Unexplained	Male
Nakamura et al, 1975, Brazil	1000 (19)	34.9	10.9	18.4	8.5	NS	27.9
Cox, 1975, Australia	900 (9)	11.0	42.9	NS	8.9	17.6	26.2
Newton et al, 1974, UK	872 (2)	18.0	27.0	NS	8.0	NS	NS
Cocev, 1972, Bulgaria	744 (4)	76.7	12.4	3.2	4.2	3.5	40.9
Ratnam et al, 1976, Singapore	709 (4)	11.7	22.5	5.8	14.7	22.1	23.1
Dor et al, 1977, Israel	665 (15)	16.2	33.4	5.1	1.2	16.1	27.9
Insler et al, 1981, Israel	583 (4)	21.4	49.1	NS	0.7	12.0	30.2
Raymont et al, 1969, Canada	500 (10)	32.2	16.9	25.6	26.2	NS	26.2
Gunaratne, 1979, Sri Lanka	393 (1)	15.3	16.2	16.6	NS	NS	41.6
Anderson, 1968, Denmark	183 (3)	36.1	29.5	48.0	NS	6.0	46.6

NS, not stated.

continents. The follow-up period was between 1 and 20 years, exceeding 4 years in the majority of series. The incidence of tubal factor ranged from 11.0 to 76.7%. Ovulation disturbances were detected in 10.9% of women by Nakamura et al (1975) in Brazil, in 42.9% by Cox (1975) in Australia, and in 49.1% by Insler et al (1981) in Israel. The incidence of cervical or uterine causes of infertility ranged between 3.2 and 48.0%. The cause of infertility was reported as unknown (i.e. unexplained or idiopathic) in 3.5–22.1% of couples. Male infertility ranged from 26.2 to 46.6%. The incidence of multifactorial (combined) infertility is about 10% (Dor et al, 1977; Insler et al, 1981). Analysis of the above data implies that the incidence of different fertility disturbances in each infertility clinic depends on the following elements:

1. the type of population served, considering general health, endemic diseases, socio-economic and cultural factors;
2. the availability and utilization of different diagnostic tests and procedures; and
3. the technical know-how and scientific interest of the medical staff.

It is obvious that the primary task of the infertility clinic is to diagnose the main cause (or causes) of infertility in each couple in order to be able to institute appropriate therapy within a reasonable time.

THE LANDMARKS FOR UNDERSTANDING THE PATHOPHYSIOLOGY OF FUNCTIONAL INFERTILITY

The cornerstone to the conquest of infertility was laid in the beginning of this century. However, it took nearly 80 years of work by many scientists from all over the globe to slowly unravel the puzzle of nature's most guarded secret, the control of the reproductive processes. Physiologists, biochemists, surgeons and physicians engaged in fundamental and applied research funded by international and national organizations, hand in hand with the pharmaceutical and diagnostic industries, have slowly been able to reduce the often-quoted figures of 8–12% infertility to a point where barely 2% of previously infertile women will not be able to experience motherhood.

Probably the most far-reaching discovery in reproductive biology was made by Crowe et al (1909) who showed that the male and female reproductive systems are under the functional control of the anterior hypophysis. They demonstrated that partial hypophysectomy in the adult dog provoked atrophy of the reproductive organs and prevented sexual development in juvenile animals. However, only 20 years later Zondek and Ascheim (1927) in Europe and Smith and Engel (1927) in the USA discovered the gonadotrophic hormones: follicle-stimulating hormone (FSH), luteinizing hormone (LH) and human chorionic gonadotrophin (hCG) and obtained firm evidence that the male and female reproductive systems were under the functional control of gonadotrophins secreted by the pituitary gland. It took 30 more years to realize that the pituitary–ovarian axis was controlled by the hypothalamus, and a further 20 years to identify the gonadotrophin-releasing hormone (GnRH) and recognize its pulsatile release by the arcuate nucleus.

Within the last decade the non-steroidal gonadal factors such as inhibins, activins and insulin-like growth factors have been discovered, and their importance for the regulation (or modulation) of ovarian responses to gonadotrophin stimulation has been recognized.

THE MILESTONES IN CLASSIFICATION OF ANOVULATORY STATES AND DEVELOPMENT OF EFFECTIVE THERAPY

Gonadotrophins

In the early 1950s the first attempts were made to use gonadotrophins obtained from pregnant mares' serum (PMS) and animal pituitaries for ovulation induction in anovulatory women. Gonadotrophins of animal origin are no longer used for this purpose since humans rapidly produce antibodies to non-primate gonadotrophins which neutralize their clinical effects. In 1954, Borth et al demonstrated that kaolin extracts from pooled menopausal urine contained FSH and LH activity in comparable amounts. These extracts prevented Leydig cell atrophy and maintained complete spermatogenesis in hypophysectomized male rats, and were capable of inducing follicular growth and promotion of multiple corpora lutea in hypo-physectomized female rats (Borth et al, 1957). On the basis of these obser-vations we had already predicted in 1954 (Borth et al, 1954) that such extracts could open up interesting therapeutic possibilities. The recognition of the therapeutic potential of human gonadotrophins stimulated the search for sources suitable for extraction of these hormones in amounts adequate for clinical use. Most investigators were purifying gonadotrophins from menopausal urine (hMG); however, the Stockholm group led by Carl Gemzell (Gemzell et al, 1958) took the shorter route and obtained active gonadotrophins by processing human pituitaries (hPG). Due to the scarcity of postmortem pituitary glands, however, the possibility of their wide-scale use was limited. Thus, attention of pharmaceutical companies (Serono and Organon) was directed towards preparation of purified extracts from menopausal urine (Donini et al, 1964). Borth et al (1961) reported that this preparation was a potent ovarian stimulant in the human, capable of promoting multiple follicular development. A survey of over 22 000 gonadotrophin treatments published during the last several years indicates that this therapy has become universally accepted for induction of ovulation in anovulatory infertile women (Insler, 1988; Lunenfeld and Lunenfeld, 1988).

Experimental and clinical data obtained over the years also showed that FSH is capable of increasing the recruitment rate of new crops of small follicles, of maintaining the normal development of multiple follicles to the preovulatory stage and, consequently, of enlarging the yield of fertilizable eggs. These findings prompted the use of gonadotrophins as the preferred treatment modality in most in vitro fertilization (IVF) programmes.

With the use of gonadotrophins for induction of superovulation in normally ovulating women conceptual changes in the monitoring schemes had to be introduced. When attempting to induce ovulation in anovulatory women the challenge is to imitate as much as possible the normal cycle and to aim at the development of a single dominant follicle. This approach has been directed at achieving ovulation and pregnancy in many patients while preventing multiple follicular growth, multiple pregnancies and hyperstimulation in most of them. In contrast, the conceptual idea of IVF, gamete intrafallopian transfer (GIFT) or tubal embryo transfer (TET) programmes is to use a super-physiological dosage in order to obtain a large number of fertilizable eggs. For this purpose many different protocols have emerged, each with its own merits and disadvantages and all using ultrasonographic scanning to estimate both the number and size of the growing follicles and oestradiol assays to assess their functional integrity.

Clomiphene citrate and related drugs

In 1937, Robson and Schonberg reported in Nature that triphenylethylene and triphenylchloroethylene are oestrogen agonists of low potency but of long duration of action. These observations received little attention until 1953, when Shelton et al demonstrated that the biological potency of the oestrogen agonists could be augmented by alkoxy substitution. Six years later, Allen et al (1959) obtained a patent for clomiphene citrate, a triphenylethylene derivative substituted with a chloride anion and an aminoalkoxyl. Although 4951 papers have been published about this compound, its site(s) and mechanism of action have not been fully elucidated.

The first clinical trials of ovulation induction were carried out in 1961 by Kistner and Smith using MER-25, a close structural analogue of clomiphene. It was in October 1961 that Robert Greenblatt et al reported the first results of clinical testing with clomiphene which was then known as MRL-41. This was the first publication on the clinical action of this drug. Greenblatt reported that 'although the mechanism of action of this compound is not clear at the present time, it is heartening to find a drug which holds much promise of inducing ovulatory type menses with considerable regularity in anovulatory women'. Greenblatt et al (1961) were the first to report the successful induction of ovulation and pregnancies following clomiphene therapy. Subsequently, other pharmacological agents for ovulation induction were developed, but clomiphene citrate has probably helped more infertile women to conceive than any other therapy.

The mode of action of clomiphene in the induction of ovulation may be tentatively described as follows. 'Blinded' by clomiphene molecules occupying the oestrogen receptor sites, the hypothalamus and pituitary are unable to correctly perceive the real level of oestrogens in the blood. A false message of insufficient oestrogen concentration is registered and acted upon, resulting in exaggerated secretion of FSH and LH. When clomiphene citrate is given during the early follicular phase to ovulating women, an increase in LH and a milder enhancement of FSH can be seen (Vandenberg and Yen, 1973). It seems that clomiphene increases the amplitude of the pulsatile discharge of gonadotrophins from the pituitary. The exaggerated FSH levels in responsive patients probably stimulate the growth of a greater crop of follicles. These follicles, in the presence of increased LH levels, produce more oestrogens than are synthesized in normal cycles. Oestrogens enhance the pituitary response to GnRH and increase ovarian sensitivity to gonadotrophins. Highly sensitized preovulatory follicles exposed to exaggerated gonadotrophic stimulation are thus compelled to ovulate. The occupation of hypothalamic oestrogen receptors by clomiphene is a time-limited process of rather short duration. A fair chance exists that by the time ovarian follicles that are stimulated by the clomiphene-induced gonadotrophin elevation reach the preovulatory stage, the hypothalamus is already free of clomiphene influence and ready to perceive the correct steroid signal. From this moment on, the events are regulated and controlled by the endogenous feedback mechanism within the hypothalamic–pituitary–ovarian axis. In ovulation-inducing therapy, clomiphene acts essentially as a primary gonadotrophin releaser, creating the first push necessary for recruiting a follicular cohort and initiating their growth.

Prolactin-inhibiting agents

It has been apparent for a long time that inappropriate prolactin secretion may be of clinical importance in humans. However, significant progress in this area was made possible only after specific assays of human prolactin were made available for clinical use. Friesen et al (1972) showed that primate pituitaries synthesize and secrete prolactin and that this hormone may be immunologically distinguished and separated from growth hormone. The primate prolactin is immunologically related to prolactin from other species.

Prolactin has been characterized (Lewis et al, 1971) and purified (Hwang et al, 1972), and radio-immunoassays for the measurement of prolactin levels in serum have been developed (Hwang et al, 1972). This has helped in the elucidation of the control mechanism of the hormone.

It has been demonstrated that excessive secretion of prolactin can cause amenorrhoea with or without galactorrhoea, and that it may also lead to anovulation or disturbed corpus luteum function. Mild hyperprolactinaemia has also been found in 18–27% of patients with polycystic ovarian disease. Lactotroph cell stimulation by continuous and excessive oestrogen secretion is a logical cause for this phenomenon.

It may now be presumed that in hyperprolactinaemic women pulsatility of GnRH secretion is disturbed, leading to disarrayed gonadotrophin secretion and consequently to the functional ovarian disturbances described above. Depending on the relative concentrations of prolactin, the LH surge may be completely neutralized, resulting in anovulation, or it may be partially inhibited, resulting in corpus luteum insufficiency. It has been shown that the positive feedback effect of oestrogen on LH secretion is suppressed in women with hyperprolactinaemia (Nyboe Andersen et al, 1982) and that pulsatile secretion of LH was either abolished or reduced in amplitude during periods of maximal prolactin secretion. Abolishment or impairment of pulsatile release of LH was also reported by Bohnet et al (1976). Moult et al (1982) showed that institution of bromocryptine therapy in women with hyperprolactinaemic amenorrhoea restored the normal rate of LH pulsatility. Leyendecker et al (1980) reported that ovulation could be successfully induced in hyperprolactinaemic women by pulsatile administration of LH releasing hormone (LHRH) despite persistent elevation of prolactin concentrations. This report supports the conjecture that the mechanism of the impairment of fertility in hyperprolactinaemic states involves deranged pulsatility of gonadotrophin secretion.

Elevated prolactin levels may also cause ovarian refractoriness to gonadotrophins. Thorner et al (1975) have observed resistance to the effect of exogenous gonadotrophins in hyperprolactinaemic women, which disappeared after prolactin levels were lowered. Others have shown the same phenomenon of ovarian refractoriness to exogenous gonadotrophins in the physiologically hyperprolactinaemic state of the puerperium. In addition, McNatty et al (1977) have shown experimentally that prolactin may exert a specific effect on ovarian steroidogenesis in vitro, and that there appears to be an inverse relationship between prevailing prolactin levels and the steroidogenic potential of the follicular cells.

Kauppilla et al (1982), using both ultrasonographic and endocrinological investigations, demonstrated that metoclopramide-induced hyperprolactinaemia interferes with follicular maturation. They found irregularities in follicular size, selection of the dominant follicle, and follicular and corpus luteum steroidogenesis in women treated with this drug. In contrast, other authors have suggested that prolactin has no direct effect upon the ovary, since stimulation of the ovaries of hyperprolactinaemic amenorrhoeic patients with gonadotrophins has induced ovulation and pregnancy. Lunenfeld et al (1970) were able to show that patients with amenorrhoea and galactorrhoea could be efficiently treated with human gonadotrophins (hMG); moreover, the required doses were lower than in amenorrhoeic women without galactorrhoea.

Gonadotrophin releasing hormone (GnRH) and its analogues

Native GnRH

Information arising in the central nervous system (CNS) or travelling through the bloodstream from other parts of the body culminates at the hypothalamus. The overall summation of these stimulatory and inhibiting signals results in the secretion of specific peptides from highly specialized hypothalamic neurones. These secretions, the releasing hormones, then stream along the neurone axons and are released at the nerve terminals located in the median eminence. There they are collected by the venous portal system and travel along the pituitary stalk to the anterior pituitary gland where they exert their action.

In 1971 the groups of Schally and of Guillemin reported the isolation, amino acid content, and later the sequence of luteinizing hormone releasing factor (LRF) (Burgus et al, 1971; Guillemin, 1978; Schally et al, 1978).

GnRH is secreted from the hypothalamus in a pulsatile fashion (i.e. short periods of high secretion separated by longer periods of low or undetectable levels). Recently the plasma levels of immunoreactive endogenous LHRH in women were measured by Elkind-Hirsch et al (1982) and found to be cyclic with a frequency approximating one pulse per hour. The frequency and amplitude of the GnRH pulse are crucial for release of LH and FSH. Knobil's group (Pohl et al, 1983) demonstrated that intermittent administration of exogenous GnRH to monkeys with arcuate nucleus lesions re-established the pulsatile secretion and peripheral plasma level of gonadotrophins. Continuous administration of the releasing hormone at different infusion rates failed to restore gonadotrophin secretion. Furthermore, in ovariectomized hypothalamic-lesioned monkeys changing the GnRH pulse frequency or amplitude had a direct influence on the secretion and relative amount of each of the gonadotrophins. Thus, raising the frequency from the 'physiological' one-pulse-per-hour rate to three or five pulses per hour reduced the secretion of both LH and FSH. Lowering the frequency to one pulse every 3 h caused a variable decline in LH levels but not in FSH levels, which, in fact, rose. Lowering the exogenous GnRH pulse amplitude while keeping the pulse frequency at the 'physiological' rate resulted in a decline of both gonadotrophins to undetectable levels. Raising the pulse amplitude under these conditions lowered the FSH levels but not the LH levels. It seems from this experimental model that the fashion in which the pituitary is challenged by GnRH determines its secretory reaction.

The use of GnRH can be considered for patients lacking endogenous gonadotrophins who have a pituitary gland capable of responding to this medication. Thus, GnRH has a place in the treatment of hypothalamic amenorrhoea.

A search of the early literature regarding the clinical use of non-pulsatile GnRH therapy revealed that in 218 trials only 67 ovulations and 14 conceptions occurred. Thus, the initial high hopes for GnRH therapy were not fulfilled, and the general interest in this treatment approach declined. Lack of the expected clinical responses to non-pulsatile administration of GnRH, even in high doses, is not surprising in view of the concept of down-regulation. Early experiments with GnRH agonist showed that initial stimulation of gonadotrophin release was followed by return to baseline levels or below. Receptor binding studies showed that the latter effect was due to a decrease in the number of receptors on the cell and not to an alteration of the affinity of receptors for GnRH.

Following Knobil's (1980) demonstration that imitation of the physiological pulsatile pattern of GnRH could restore ovarian function in hypothalamus-lesioned monkeys, interest in the therapeutic use of GnRH was again stimulated. Leyendecker et al (1980) showed that it was possible to induce ovulation followed by pregnancy in an amenorrhoeic patient with hypothalamic failure by pulsatile intravenous administration of GnRH through a computerized infusion pump. During the last few years a number of reports on the pulsatile administration of GnRH have appeared.

Reviewing 36 papers published between 1980 and 1984 (Blankstein et al, 1986), 916 treatment cycles in 388 patients could be assessed. The conception rate was 56%, multiple gestation rate 7.3%, abortion rate 14.5% and hyperstimulation rate 1.1%. Although it appears that careful monitoring will reduce the appearance of hyperstimulation, more cases have to be evaluated before definite conclusions can be drawn. From reviews of the available literature it seems that doses between 3.4 and 20.0 μg, with pulse intervals between 62.5 and 120.0 min, are capable of eliciting a pituitary response sufficient for follicular stimulation resulting in ovulation.

GnRH analogues: agonists and antagonists

The main reason for the tremendous amount of interest in GnRH and its analogues during the past decade is the fact that, depending on their mode of application, they can either stimulate pituitary gonadotrophin secretion or be potent inhibitors. When administered in a precise pulsatile pattern GnRH can restore the normal cyclic gonadotrophin secretion. When administered chronically, GnRH or its agonists proved to be potent inhibitors of gonadotrophin secretion, providing a gonadotrophin-specific, temporary (fully reversible) medical hypophysectomy (Cetel et al, 1983; Karten and Rivier, 1986; Shadmi et al, 1987; Insler et al, 1988).

The possibility of achieving a temporary medical hypophysectomy has been used as a rationale for consequently attaining a 'medical gonadectomy', i.e. to temporarily shut off the gonadal steroid production. This could be of value in the treatment of diseases dependent on gonadal steroids. To date, indeed, this approach has proved its efficacy in the treatment of metastatic prostatic cancer (Soloway, 1988), precocious puberty (Aubert et al, 1988; Laron et al, 1988) and endometriosis (Brosens and Cornillie, 1988; Dmowski et al, 1988). It has been shown to reduce the volume of uterine fibroids (leiomyomas) and has been suggested as a medical therapy for this condition in high-risk surgical cases of perimenopausal women (Healy, 1986) or in some young patients who still desire pregnancy. It is being investigated for hormone-dependent breast cancer (Klijn, 1984; Robertson and Blamey, 1988) and for ovarian cancer (Jaeger, 1988).

In the management of infertile patients in whom conventional treatment regimes had failed, GnRH agonists have been successfully utilized to suppress the pituitary ovarian axis prior to and concomitantly with stimulation of follicular growth and induction of ovulation by exogenous gonadotrophins. This therapeutic regime has also been efficiently used for the stimulation of multiple follicular development in in vitro fertilization programmes to prevent cancellations due to an untimely LH surge. GnRH agonists have been dispersed in biocompatible biodegradable polymeric matrices of DL-lactide-coglycolide in the form of microcapsules or microspheres. Alternatively they are incorporated in a matrix of a lactide-glycolide copolymer in the form of biodegradable implants. The introduction of potent and long-acting agonists and delayed-release formulations has permitted application on a once-per-month basis for long-term treatment of gonadal steroid-dependent diseases described above (Max et al, 1988). This has improved their usefulness and acceptance.

While the potent GnRH agonists have been widely applied during the last few years, the production of suitable antagonists working by receptor occupancy has been disappointing. Progress in the synthesis of antagonists was slower since several amino acids have to be substituted on the GnRH molecule. Antagonists also require precise topological features for high binding affinity to the receptor. Use of GnRH antagonists with their immediate inhibitory actions may be useful for contraception and in treatment of hormone-dependent disorders as described above, avoiding the initial stimulatory phase of the agonist.

The present disadvantages of antagonists are that their effective dose is approximately 1000 times that of agonists. Furthermore, the introduction of D-arginine or other basic side-chains into position 6 has been shown to trigger histamine release from rat mast cells and to induce an anaphylactoid-like reaction. Recently, attempts have been made to synthesize GnRH antagonists lacking the histamine-releasing activity. This was achieved by either switching the residues between positions 5 and 6 or by reducing the overall hydrophobicity and shielding the side-chain basic groups. The new third-generation analogues induce a long duration of gonadotrophin inhibition by single-dose administration and are virtually free of the histamine release side-effect. The duration of inhibition of gonadotrophin secretion has been shown to be dose-dependent, permitting treatment regimens to be tailored to specific clinical indications. Their action is conveniently reversible by intravenous administration of native GnRH. Ultimate restoration of FSH/LH secretion to pretreatment levels occurs. These characteristics promise an immediate inhibition of pituitary gonadotrophin secretion without the initial flare-up effect of GnRH agonists.

With all the tremendous potential of GnRH analogues in the treatment of a wide variety of sex steroid-dependent disorders, prolonged decrease of oestrogen may lead to deleterious metabolic disturbances. Changes in lipid metabolism and decrease in bone mineral content have been observed with prolonged use. The development of adjunctive treatment regimes may be necessary to prevent these effects. If long-acting formulations become available and long-term safety is assured, GnRH agonists (and possibly also antagonists) could also provide an effective alternative in male and female contraception.

Well-controlled long-term postmarketing surveillance will be necessary to demonstrate that long-term GnRH analogue therapy is safe. If so proven, these agents can provide a revolutionary approach to sex hormone-dependent diseases and a manifold impact on present therapy.

Intraovarian function of growth factors

Even with the best protocols for inducing ovulation in anovulatory patients and superovulation in in vitro procedures, a number of patients will need excessive amounts of gonadotrophins and some of them, despite this, will be poor responders. During the last few years the importance of intraovarian regulation and the potentiating effect of growth hormone (GH) and various growth factors on granulosa cell response to FSH has been demonstrated (Advis et al, 1981). The action of GH on the granulosa cells may be direct

(Jia et al, 1986) or may occur via an increase in ovarian concentration or production of growth factors (Davoren and Hsueh, 1986). It has been demonstrated that somatomedin-C potentiates gonadotrophin-stimulated progesterone and oestrogen biosynthesis (Adashi et al, 1985, a, b) and luteinizing hormone (LH) receptor binding by cultured rat granulosa cells. Furthermore, two recent observations claimed that GH administration increased the sensitivity of the ovary to gonadotrophin stimulation (Homburg et al, 1988; Blumenfeld and Lunenfeld, 1989).

These findings prompted us to assess whether the level of GH reserve is correlated to the ovarian response to human menopausal gonadotrophin (hMG) and may serve as an indicator for the effective dose of hMG in ovulation induction protocols. Methods of inducing GH release have included arginine stimulation and insulin-induced hypoglycaemia (Fass et al, 1979). The use of clonidine as a provocative agent for GH stimulation is based on a large number of studies demonstrating an α-adrenergic action in men (Lancranjan and Marbach, 1977; Slover et al, 1984). Due to its simplicity and relative lack of side-effects, the clonidine test has been used.

A prospective study (Menashe et al, 1989, 1990) demonstrated that all patients who responded to clonidine with elevation of GH responded normally to hMG therapy with a mean total dose of 870 ± 98 IU FSH/LH (11.6 ± 1.3 ampoules). Patients who did not respond to clonidine with elevation of GH either needed excessive amounts of gonadotrophins— 2737 ± 413 IU FSH/LH (36.5 ± 5.5 ampoules)—to obtain an acceptable response or, despite higher doses of hMG, responded inadequately as expressed by either low oestradiol level or lack of sufficient follicular development or both. The combined GH/gonadotrophin therapy in clonidine-

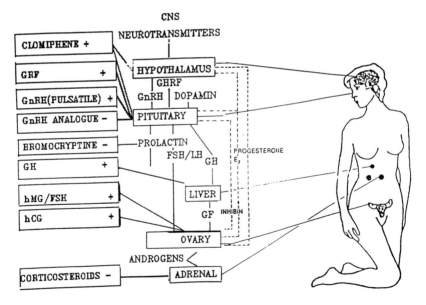

Figure 1. Drugs used in the treatment of anovulation.

negative patients improved the response despite the significant reduction in hMG dose requirement. In some women, repeated assays of endogenous FSH showed excessive values, resembling perimenopausal levels.

CONCLUSIONS

We have attempted to review briefly the regulation of follicular development, particularly with regard to new findings demonstrating the potentiating effect of growth hormone and/or various growth factors on ovarian sensitivity to FSH. This new knowledge, as well as availability of potent GnRH analogues, will evidently refine our clinical approach to treatment of functional infertility.

Continuous advances in the understanding of mechanisms regulating reproductive processes and the better recognition of underlying causes of infertility will lead to the optimal choice of first-, second- and third-line routine therapies (Figure 1) which will apply to the majority of patients. Furthermore, it will become possible to design tailor-made ovulation-inducing protocols for specific patients who do not respond properly to the routine treatment.

SUMMARY

The cornerstone of the conquest of infertility was laid in the beginning of this century. It took, however, nearly 80 years of work of many scientists from all over the globe to slowly unravel the puzzle of nature's most guarded secret, the control of the reproductive processes.

The estimated population size of women between the ages 19 and 34 years in the developed world in 1990 will be about 130 million. If we assume that at least 8% will be infertile, then the pool of the infertile population will be above 10 million, with about 700 000 new patients entering this pool every year between the years 1990 and 1995.

In the past only about 40% of infertile patients benefited from ovulation induction regimens. With the advent of assisted reproduction this population increased to about 80%. With the use of gonadotrophins for induction of superovulation in normally ovulating women conceptual changes in treatment regimens and monitoring schemes had to be introduced.

It is obvious that the primary task of infertility clinics is to diagnose the main cause (or causes) of infertility in each couple in order to be able to institute appropriate therapy within a reasonable time.

We have attempted to review briefly the regulation of follicular development, particularly with regard to new findings demonstrating the potentiating effect of growth hormone and/or various growth factors on ovarian sensitivity to FSH. This new knowledge, as well as availability of potent GnRH analogues, will evidently refine our clinical approach to treatment of functional infertility.

Continuous advances in the understanding of mechanisms regulating reproductive processes and the better recognition of underlying causes of infertility will lead to the optimal choice of first-, second- and third-line routine therapies which will apply to the majority of patients. Furthermore, it will become possible to design tailor-made ovulation-inducing protocols for specific patients who do not respond properly to the routine treatment.

REFERENCES

Adashi EY, Resnick CE, Svoboda ME & Van Wyk JJ (1985a) Somatomedin C synergizes with FSH in the acquisition of projection biosynthetic capacity by cultured rat granulosa cells. *Endocrinology* **116**: 2135.

Adashi EY, Resnick CE, Svoboda ME & Van Wyk JJ (1985b) Somatomedin C enhances induction of LH receptors by FSH in cultured rat granulosa cells. *Endocrinology* **116**: 2369.

Advis JP, Smith White S & Ojeda SR (1981) Activation of growth hormone short loop negative feedback delays puberty in the female rat. *Endocrinology* **108**: 1343.

Allen RE, Palopoli FP, Schumann EL et al (1959) *US Patent* **2**: 561, 914.

Anderson AJB (1968) Infertilitaet. *Ugeskrift for Laeger* **130**: 663.

Aubert ML, Kreuter R & Syzoneko PC (1988) Mechanism of action of GnRH and GnRH analogues in sexual maturation and function. *Gynecological Endocrinology* **2 (supplement 1)**: 35.

Belsey MA (1976) The epidemiology of infertility: a review with particular reference to sub-Saharan Africa. *Bulletin of the World Health Organization* **54**: 321.

Blankstein J, Mashaih S & Lunenfeld B (1986) *Ovulation Induction and In Vitro Fertilization*, pp 131–150. Chicago: Year Book Medical Publishers.

Blumenfeld Z & Lunenfeld B (1989) The potential effect of growth hormone on follicle stimulation with human menopausal gonadotropin in a panhypopituitary patient. *Fertility and Sterility* **52**: 328.

Bohnet HG, Dahlen HG, Wultke W et al (1976) Hyperprolactinemic anovulatory syndrome. *Journal of Clinical Endocrinology* **42**: 132.

Borth R, Lunenfeld B & de Watteville H (1954) Activite gonadotrope d'un extrait d'urines de femmes en menopause. *Experientia* **10**: 266.

Borth R, Lunenfeld B, Riotton G et al (1957) Activite gonadotrope d'un extrait d'urines de femmes en menopause. *Experientia* **13**: 115.

Borth R, Lunenfeld B & Menzi (1961) Pharmacologic and clinical effects of a gonadotropin preparation from human postmenopausal urine. In Albert A (ed.) *Human Pituitary Gonadotropins*, pp 266–271. Springfield, Illinois: Charles C. Thomas.

Brosens I & Cornillie F (1988) Is there a rationale for GnRH analogues therapy in endometriosis? *Gynecological Endocrinology* **2 (supplement 1)**: 28.

Burgus R, Butcher M, Ling N et al (1971) Structure moleculaire du facteur hypothalamique (LRF) d'origine ovine controlant la secretion de l'hormone gonadotrope hypophysaire de luteinisation (LH). *Compte Rendue Academie de Science [D]* **273**: 1611.

Cetel NS, Rivier J, Valwe W & Yen SSC (1983) The dynamics of gonadotropin inhibition in women induced by an antagonistic analog of gonadotropin-releasing hormone. *Journal of Clinical Endocrinology and Metabolism* **57**: 62.

Cocev D (1972) Results of studies and treatment of sterility in families in Blagoengrade district during a period of five years. *Akusherstwo i Ginekologia (Sofia)* **11**: 133.

Collins JA, Wrixon W & Janes LB (1983) Treatment-independent pregnancy among infertile couples. *New England Journal of Medicine* **309**: 20.

Cox L (1975) Infertility: a comprehensive programme. *British Journal of Obstetrics and Gynecology* **82**: 2.

Crowe SJ, Cushing H & Homans J (1909) Cited in Lunenfeld B & Donini P (1966) Historic aspects of gonadotrophins. In Greenblatt B (ed.) *Ovulation*, pp 9–34. Toronto: Lippincott.

Davoren JB & Hsueh AJW (1986) Growth hormone increased ovarian levels of immunoreactive somatomedin C/insulin-like growth factor I in vivo. *Endocrinology* **118**: 888.

Dmowski WP, Radwanska E, Binor Z, Tumon I & Pepping P (1988) GnRH analogues in the management of endometriosis. *Gynecological Endocrinology* **2 (supplement 1)**: 29.

Donini P, Puzzuoli D & Montezemolo R (1964) Purification of gonadotropin from human menopausal urine. *Acta Endocrinologica* **45**: 329.

Dor J, Homburg R & Rabau E (1977) An evaluation of etiologic factors and therapy in 665 infertile couples. *Fertility and Sterility* **28**: 718.

Elkind-Hirsch K, Schiff I, Ravnikar V et al (1982) Determinations of endogenous immunoreactive luteinizing hormone releasing hormone in human plasma. *Journal of Clinical Endocrinology and Metabolism* **54**: 602.

Fass B, Lippe BM & Kaplan SA (1979) Relative usefulness of three growth hormone stimulation screening tests. *American Journal of Diseases of Children* **133**: 931.

Franchimont P, Almer S, Mannaerts B, Boen P & Kicivic PM (1989) New GnRH antagonist ORG 30850: the first clinical experience. *Gynecological Endocrinology* **3 (supplement 1)**: 13.

Friedman S (1977) Artificial donor insemination with frozen semen. *Fertility and Sterility* **28**: 1230.

Friesen H, Belanger C, Guyda H & Hwang P (1972) The synthesis and secretion of placental lactogen and pituitary prolactin. In Wolstenholme GEW & Knight J (eds) *Lactogenic Hormones*, pp 83–103. Edinburgh, London: Churchill Livingstone.

Gemzell CA, Diczfalusy E & Tillinger G (1958) Clinical effect of human pituitary follicle-stimulating hormone (FSH). *Journal of Clinical Endocrinology* **29**: 1333.

Greenblatt RB, Barfield WE, Jungck EC et al (1961) Induction of ovulation with MRL/41, preliminary report. *Journal of the American Medical Association* **178**: 101.

Guillemin R (1978) Peptides in the brain: the new endocrinology of the neuron. *Science* **202**: 390.

Gunaratne M (1979) The epidemiology of infertility: a selected clinic study. *Ceylon Medical Journal* **24**: 36.

Healy DL, Lawons SR, Abbott M, Baird DT & Fraser HM (1986) Toward removing uterine fibroids without surgery: subcutaneous infusion of a luteinizing hormone-releasing hormone agonist commencing in the luteal phase. *Journal of Clinical Endocrinology and Metabolism* **63**: 619.

Homburg R, Eshel A, Abdallah HI & Jacobs HS (1988) Growth hormone facilitates ovulation induction by gonadotropines. *Clinical Endocrinology* **29**: 113.

Hwang P, Guyda H & Friesen HG (1972) Purification of human prolactin. *Journal of Biochemistry* **247**: 1955.

Insler V (1988) Gonadotropin therapy: new trends and insights. *International Journal of Fertility* **33**: 85–97.

Insler V, Potashnik G & Glassner M (1981) Some epidemiological aspects of fertility evaluation. In Insler V, Bettendorf G & Geissler KH (eds) *Advances in Diagnosis and Treatment of Infertility*, p 165. New York: Elsevier, North-Holland.

Insler V, Potashnik G, Lunenfeld E et al (1988) Ovulation induction with hMG following down regulation of the hypothalamic pituitary axis by LHRH analogs. *Gynecological Endocrinology* **2 (supplement 1)**: 67.

Jaeger WH (1988) GnRH analogues in treatment of ovarian carcinoma. *Gynecological Endocrinology* **2 (supplement 1)**: 41.

Jia XCH, Kalmijin J & Hsueh AJW (1986) Growth hormone enhances FSH induced differentiation of cultured rat granulosa cells. *Endocrinology* **118**: 1401.

Karten MJ & Rivier JE (1986) Gonadotropin-releasing hormone analog design. Structure–function studies toward the development of agonists and antagonists: rationale and perspective *Endocrinological Review* **7**: 44.

Kauppila A, Leinonen P, Vihko R et al (1982) Metoclopramide-induced hyperprolactinemia impairs ovarian follicle maturation and corpus luteum function in women. *Journal of Clinical Endocrinology and Metabolism* **54**: 955.

Kistner RW & Smith OW (1961) Observations on the use of nonsteroidal estrogen antagonist MER-25: effects in endometrial hyperplasia and Stein–Leventhal syndrome. *Fertility and Sterility* **12**: 121.

Klijn JGM (1984) Long-term LHRH agonist treatment in metastatic breast cancer as a single treatment and in combination with other additive endocrine treatments. *Medical Oncology and Tumor Pharmacotherapy* **1**: 1234.

488 B. LUNENFELD AND V. INSLER

Knobil E (1980) Neuroendocrine control of the menstrual cycle. *Recent Progress in Hormone Research* **36**: 53.
Korean Institute for Family Planning (1971) *Fertility–Abortion Survey*, Seoul.
Lancranjan I & Marbach P (1977) New evidence for growth hormone modulation by the alpha-adrenergic system in man. *Metabolism* **26**: 1225.
Laron Z, Kauli R & Schally AV (1988) Long term experience with a superactive GnRH analog (D-Trp-6-LH-RH) in the treatment of precocious puberty—review of 46 patients. *Gynecological Endocrinology* **2 (supplement 1)**: 39.
Leal JA, Williams RF, Danforth DR et al (1988) Prolonged duration of gonadotropin inhibition by a third generation GnRH antagonist. *Journal of Clinical Endocrinology and Metabolism* **87**: 1325.
Lewis UJ, Singh RNP, Sinha YN et al (1971) Electrophoretic evidence for human prolactin. *Journal of Clinical Endocrinology* **32**: 153.
Leyendecker G, Struve T & Plotz EJ (1980) Induction of ovulation with chronic intermittent (pulsatile) administration of LHRH in women with hypothalamic and hyperprolactinemic amenorrhea. *Archives in Gynecology* **229**: 177.
Lunenfeld E & Lunenfeld B (1988) Modern approaches to the diagnosis and management of anovulation. *International Journal of Fertility* **33**: 308.
Lunenfeld B, Insler V & Rabau E (1970) Die Pinzipien der Gonadotropintherpie. *Acta Endocrinologica* **148 (supplement)**: 52–101.
Matsuo H, Baba Y, Nair RMG et al (1971) Structure of the porcine LH and FSH releasing factor: I. The proposed amino acid sequence. *Biochemical and Biophysical Research Communications* **43**: 1334.
Max D, Seely J, Swanson L & Brauneller R (1988) Clinical studies of leuprolide depot formulation in metastatic prostatic cancer. *Gynecological Endocrinology* **2 (supplement 1)**: 80.
McNatty KP, McNeilly AS & Sawers RS (1977) Prolactin and progesterone secretion by human granulosa cells in vitro. In Crosignani PG & Robyn C (eds) *Prolactin and Human Reproduction*, volume 11. London: Academic Press, Serono Symposia Proceedings.
Menashe Y, Pariente C, Lunenfeld B et al (1989) Does endogenous growth hormone reserve correlate to ovarian response to human menopausal hormone gonadotropins? *Israel Journal of Medical Sciences* **25**: 296.
Menashe Y, Lunenfeld B, Pariente C, Frenkel Y & Mashiach S (1990) Can growth hormone increase, after clonidine administration, predict the dose of human menopausal hormone needed for induction of ovulation? *Fertility and Sterility* **53**: 432–435.
Moult PJA, Rees LH & Besser GM (1982) Pulsatile gonadotrophin secretion in hyperprolactinemic amenorrhea and the response to bromocriptine therapy. *Clinical Endocrinology* **16**: 153.
Nakamura MS et al (1975) Etiologia da esterilidade conjugal no Departamento de Ginecologia da Facultade de Medicina da Universidade de Sao Paulo. *Reproduction* **2**: 39.
Newton J, Craig S & Joyce D (1974) The changing patterns of a comprehensive infertility clinic. *Journal of Biosocial Science* **6**: 477–482.
Nyboe Andersen A, Schioler V, Hertz J et al (1982) Effect of metoclopramide induced hyperprolactinemia on the gonadotrophic response to estradiol and LRH. *Acta Endocrinologica* **100**: 1.
Pohl CR, Richardson DW, Hutchinson JS et al (1983) Hypophysiotropic signal frequency and the functioning of the pituitary–ovarian system in the rhesus monkey. *Endocrinology* **112**: 2076.
Ratnam SS et al (1976) Experience of a comprehensive infertility clinic in the department of obstetrics and gynaecology, University of Singapore. *Singapore Medical Journal* **17**: 157.
Raymont A et al (1969) Review of 500 cases of infertility. *International Journal of Fertility* **14**: 141.
Robertson JFR & Blamey RW (1988) GnRH analogues in breast cancer. *Gynecological Endocrinology* **2 (supplement 1)** 50.
Robson JM & Schonberg A (1937) Oestrons reactions, including mating, produced by triphenyl ethylene. *Nature* **140**: 196.
Schally AV, Coy DH & Meyers CA (1978) Hypothalamic regulatory hormones. *Annual Review of Biochemistry* **47**: 89–128.
Shadmi AL, Lunenfeld B, Bahari C et al (1987) Abolishment of the positive feedback

mechanism: a criterion for temporary medical hypophysectomy by LH-RH agonist. *Gynecological Endocrinology* **1:** 1.

Shelton RS, van Campen MG Jr, Meisner DF et al (1953) Synthetic estrogens: halotriphenylethylene derivatives. *Journal of the American Chemical Society* **75:** 5491.

Slover RH, Klingensmith GJ, Gotlin RW & Radcliffe J (1984) A comparison of Clonidine and standard provocative agents of growth hormone. *American Journal of Diseases of Children* **138:** 314.

Smith PE & Engle ET (1927) Experimental evidence regarding role of anterior pituitary in development and regulation of genital system. *American Journal of Anatomy* **40:** 159.

Soloway M (1988) A phase III, multicenter comparison of depot zoladex and orchiectomy in patients with previously untreated stage D-2 prostate cancer. *Gynecological Endocrinology* **2 (supplement 1):** 50.

Sudan Population and Census Office (1958) *The first population census of Sudan, 1955.* Ministry of Social Affairs, Khartoum.

Thorner MO, Besser GM, Jones A et al (1975) Bromocryptine treatment of female infertility: report of 13 pregnancies. *British Medical Journal* **4:** 694.

Vandenberg G & Yen SSC (1973) Effect of anti-estrogenic action of clomiphene during the menstrual cycle: evidence for a change in the feedback sensitivity. *Journal of Clinical Endocrinology and Metabolism* **37:** 356.

Veevers JE (1972) Declining childlessness and age at marriage: a test of a hypothesis. *Social Biology* **19:** 285.

WHO Scientific Group (1975) *The epidemiology of infertility.* Technical Report Series No. 582.

World Fertility Survey (1977) *The survey of fertility in Thailand: Country Report.* Report No. 1, Institute of Population Studies, Chulalongkorn University and Population Survey Division, National Statistical Office.

Zondek B & Ascheim S (1927) Das Hormon des Hypophysenvorderlappens; Testobject zum Nachweis des Hormons. *Klinische Wochenschrift* **6:** 248.

5

Clomiphene citrate

ANNA F. GLASIER

Clomiphene citrate is a triarylethylene compound (Figure 1) similar in structure to the potent synthetic oestrogen diethylstilboestrol. Introduced for the treatment of anovulation in the 1950s, clinically available preparations are a racemic mixture of two isomers: the zu (*cis*) isomer, which is thought to act as a weak oestrogen, and the en (*trans*) isomer which has potent anti-oestrogenic properties. Current preparations contain about 40% zuclomiphene and 60% enclomiphene.

MECHANISM OF ACTION

Clomiphene citrate acts as an anti-oestrogen by interacting with the oestradiol receptor. Like other anti-hormones, it has been suggested that it acts

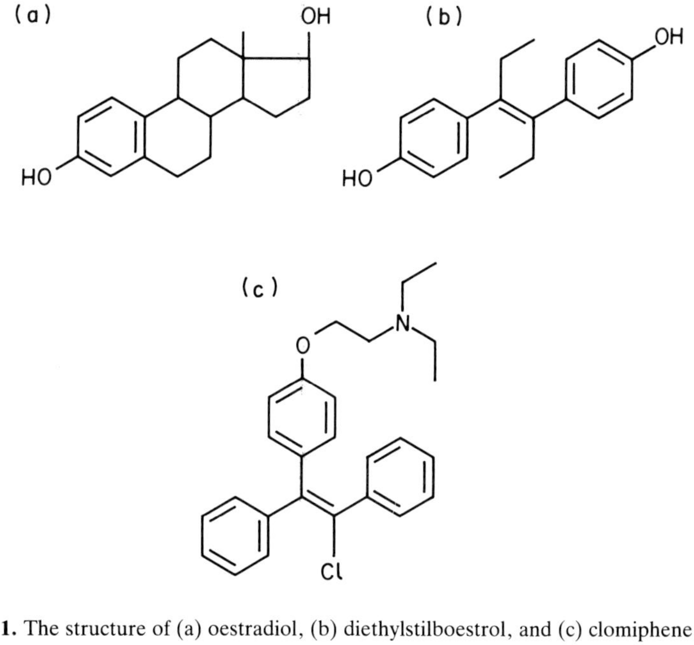

Figure 1. The structure of (a) oestradiol, (b) diethylstilboestrol, and (c) clomiphene citrate.

Baillière's Clinical Obstetrics and Gynaecology—
Vol. 4, No. 3, September 1990
ISBN 0–7020–1478–8

initially—at least in the rat (Clarke et al, 1974)—as a weak agonist when it binds to the cytoplasmic oestradiol receptor. Once bound, however, clomiphene inhibits or delays replenishment of the receptor, causing oestrogen insensitivity in the target cell (Taubert and Kuhl, 1986) and thus acting as an anti-oestrogen. Whether its action is principally agonistic or antagonistic appears to depend on the dose of clomiphene used (Clark and Markaverich, 1982) and on the endogenous oestrogenic status of the recipient; in post-menopausal women clomiphene citrate can act as an oestrogen, suppressing the release of pituitary/gonadotrophins (Hashimoto et al, 1976).

Effects on the hypothalamus and pituitary

The main mode of action of clomiphene citrate with respect to its ability to induce ovulation is to increase gonadotrophin-releasing hormone (GnRH)

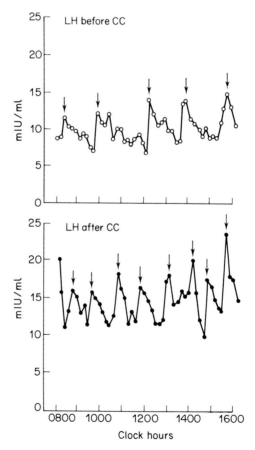

Figure 2. Serum concentrations of luteinizing hormone (LH) in a single subject during 8 h of blood sampling at 10 min intervals before and after clomiphene citrate (CC) treatment. From Kerin et al (1985) with permission.

pulse frequency by acting directly on the hypothalamus (Kerin et al, 1985; Judd et al, 1987). This results in an increase in luteinizing hormone (LH) and, to a lesser extent, in follicle-stimulating hormone (FSH). In an elegant study giving 50 mg clomiphene in the early follicular phase of the cycle, Kerin et al (1985) demonstrated a clear increase in the frequency rather than in the amplitude of pulses of gonadotrophin secretion (Figure 2). Increased gonadotrophins stimulate multiple follicular development with a consequent rise in serum oestrogen concentrations. In a comparison between spontaneous cycles following clomiphene administration in a group of normally ovulating women, Glasier et al (1989) demonstrated a mean of 2.4 ± 0.3 preovulatory follicles on the day of the onset of the LH surge in clomiphene-treated cycles compared with a mean of 1.2 ± 0.3 follicles in spontaneous cycles. Serum oestradiol concentrations on the day of the LH peak were more than doubled in clomiphene-treated cycles. There is some evidence (Hsueh et al, 1978) that clomiphene also acts directly on the pituitary, increasing the sensitivity of the gonadotrophs to GnRH. Littman and Hodgen (1985) have also demonstrated in the Rhesus monkey an effect on positive feedback with a delay in the midcycle LH surge despite oestradiol (E_2) levels which rose higher and more rapidly than in untreated monkeys. In women, too, the day of the LH peak occurs later following treatment with either clomiphene citrate or with the en isomer alone when compared with normal cycles (Glasier et al, 1989). Interestingly, in the same study treatment with the zu isomer alone appeared to advance the timing of the surge when compared with single spontaneous cycles.

Ovarian effects

There is some evidence that clomiphene citrate may have a direct effect on the ovary in some animals. Kessel and Hsueh (1987) demonstrated an enhancement of FSH-stimulated aromatase activity in primary cultures of rat granulosa cells. In the human in vivo it is virtually impossible to separate the effects resulting from increased LH and FSH from a possible direct effect. Yuen et al (1988) have recently demonstrated an inhibitory effect of clomiphene citrate on the accumulation of progesterone and 20α-hydroxy-4-pregnen-3-one in cultured granulosa cells obtained from women undergoing in vitro fertilization (IVF). While this may not reflect an instrumental role of ovarian effects of clomiphene citrate in the mechanism of action, the investigators suggest that this effect on ovarian steroidogenesis may contribute to the luteal phase deficiency experienced by some women treated with clomiphene citrate.

PHARMACOKINETICS

The main route of excretion of clomiphene citrate is via the faeces, with a small amount being excreted in the urine and some sequestered into an enterohepatic circulation. The half-life of clomiphene citrate is about 5 days, but some activity can be measured in the circulation up to 30 days after standard treatment (Lunenfeld et al, 1986). It would appear that the en isomer is absorbed faster and eliminated more completely than the zu isomer. In a study of the pharmacokinetics of a single dose of 50 mg clomiphene citrate administered to healthy volunteers, Mikkelson et al (1986) showed that after 24 h the mean plasma concentration of the zu isomer was around 4.0 ng/ml (maximum concentration at 6 h around 7.5 ng/ml) while less than 0.5 ng/ml of the en isomer was measurable in the circulation (maximum concentration around 4.2 ml at 4 h). Moreover, repeated administration of a single 50 mg dose at monthly intervals showed a significant accumulation of zu isomer (Figure 3).

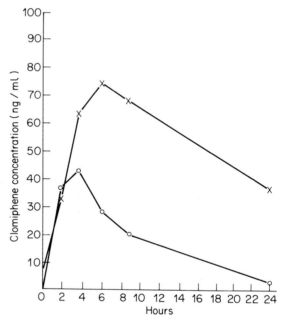

Figure 3. Mean plasma concentrations of zuclomiphene (×——×) and enclomiphene (○——○) after oral administration of one 50 mg tablet of clomiphene citrate (n = 23). From Mikkelson et al (1986) with permission of the publisher, the American Fertility Society.

INDICATIONS

It is clear that since the main mechanism of action of clomiphene citrate is to increase gonadotrophin section, it can only be effective in inducing ovulation in the presence of an intact hypothalamo–pituitary–ovarian axis, particularly with respect to the positive feedback effects of oestradiol. Ovulation can rarely, if ever, be achieved in women who are hypo-oestrogenic. Thus clomiphene citrate is indicated in women with failure of ovulation who either bleed spontaneously, whether regularly or irregularly, or who bleed in response to a progestagen challenge. Clomiphene is therefore useful in women with normogonadotropic amenorrhoea or with amenorrhoea or oligomenorrhoea associated with an elevated LH:FSH ratio as in polycystic ovarian syndrome. Women with hypogonadotrophic hypogonadism do not generally respond to clomiphene citrate and those with hyperprolactinaemia are better treated with bromocriptine.

In practice, the use of clomiphene citrate is not limited to women with anovulatory infertility. It is fairly widely used empirically to treat women with unexplained infertility. While a case can perhaps be made for increasing the ovulation rate in such women in an attempt to achieve a pregnancy, the disadvantages of clomiphene citrate—the effects on cervical mucus and the endometrium—probably outweigh the benefits.

Clomiphene citrate has also been used to treat women with proven or suspected luteal phase defects. Results of treatment are variable. Luteal phase deficiency is poorly understood and may be multifactorial in origin, probably occurs inconsistently even in infertile women, and is extremely time-consuming to diagnose. The rationale for using clomiphene citrate lies in the fact that an endogenous or experimentally induced deficiency of FSH in the early follicular phase is known to result in low or inadequate concentrations of progesterone in the luteal phase; thus a drug which increases serum FSH is thought to be beneficial. In a group of 41 women treated for well-characterized luteal phase deficiency, Downs and Gibson (1983) reported a conception rate of 39%, approaching normal. Those women with severe luteal phase deficiency were said to have the best response. However, since clomiphene citrate administration is associated with inadequate luteal phase levels of progesterone (Jones et al, 1970) many clinicians prefer to use other methods of treatment such as exogenous luteal phase progesterone administration (Soules et al, 1977).

Clomiphene citrate has also been widely used, alone or in combination with gonadotrophins, for the induction of superovulation for IVF and gamete intrafallopian transfer (GIFT). In many superovulation programmes it has now been superseded by a combination of GnRH analogues and gonadotrophins; recent reports of a possible toxic effect on oocytes and embryos (see below) have led to the avoidance of clomiphene citrate by many clinicians.

MODE OF ADMINISTRATION

A wide variety of treatment regimes has been proposed, varying particularly with regard to timing, none proving to be superior to another. It is generally argued that the lowest dose to achieve ovulation should be administered. Most clinicians start at a dose of 50 mg given daily, orally, for 5 days in the early follicular phase. In Edinburgh we start on day 3 of the cycle. Occasionally in women who are underweight and who complain of abdominal pain and distension around midcycle we have reduced the dose and achieved ovulation with 25 mg/day. If there is no response to 50 mg the dose is increased to 100 mg and then 150 mg. In many centres if 150 mg fails to induce ovulation an alternative treatment is instituted rather than increasing the dose further, although doses up to 250 mg have been used (O'Herlihy et al, 1981). The ovarian response to clomiphene should be monitored either by measuring basal body temperature or by biochemical means such as luteal phase progesterone or pregnanediol (urinary) estimations. Women are advised to have intercourse from day 9 or 10 of the cycle until a rise in basal body temperature (BBT) is observed or for at least 1 week. Ultrasound examination of the ovaries for follicular development may be undertaken in some centres, particularly when clomiphene is used in combination with another agent.

CLOMIPHENE IN COMBINATION

Some women taking clomiphene show evidence of follicular development— rising serum oestradiol concentrations and follicle growth on ultrasound— but do not ovulate as a result of failure of positive feedback induction of the midcycle LH surge. In these cases human chorionic gonadotrophin (hCG) can be given to induce ovulation at a dose of 5000 IU. The timing of hCG is obviously important. Ovulation is induced within 34–40 h of injection when it is given in the presence of a mature follicle. Given prematurely or too late it will be ineffective. O'Herlihy et al (1981) achieved a 66% conception rate in a group of women given hCG in combination with clomiphene citrate when hCG administration was timed by ultrasound scan. An LH surge can also be induced with a single dose of 1 mg oestradiol benzoate (Canales et al, 1978), but the use of hCG is more physiological. In women with an elevated serum testosterone with or without clinical signs of hyperandrogenism, clomiphene can be given in combination with an anti-androgen. Dexamethasone 0.5 mg daily given throughout the cycle may be used, or a higher dose for a shorter period (2 mg/day, days 5–14) is sometimes given. Fayez (1976) reported ovulation in 84.5% and conception in 46% of women resistant to clomiphene alone when dexamethasone was added to the regime.

Clomiphene has been used in combination with human menopausal gonadotrophin (hMG) as a means of reducing the dose of gonadotrophins and therefore theoretically the risk of hyperstimulation and multiple pregnancy. Usually clomiphene is given as a pretreatment (doses up to 200 mg have been used) followed by daily injections of hMG. Reports of success rates have varied, but Ron-El et al (1989) recently published a series of 47 pregnancies achieved with a hyperstimulation rate of only 2.6% and multiple pregnancy rate of 7.7% per cycle, significantly lower than for hMG alone.

Pulsatile GnRH and bromocriptine have both been used in combination with clomiphene citrate, with no very good physiological rationale for doing so. Their use is reviewed by Taubert and Kuhl (1986). Oestradiol in combination with clomiphene citrate has been given in an attempt to improve the quality of cervical mucus either for 3 months before treatment or during the same cycle, but it can cause extreme ovarian hyperstimulation and is rarely used.

SIDE-EFFECTS

Minor side-effects due to the pharmacological effects of clomiphene citrate on various tissues do occur, but it is rare that they interfere with treatment. About 10% of women complain of hot flushes during clomiphene citrate administration. Interestingly, the concomitant administration of oestrogen (Greenblatt, 1968) does not alleviate the flushes. Among almost 4000 women reviewed by Kistner (1968) less than 2% of women complained of other minor side-effects such as nausea, vomiting, breast tenderness, dizziness, mild skin reactions and reversible hair loss. Clomiphene citrate does have a mydriatic action, and 1.6% noted mild visual disturbances such as blurred vision or decreased visual acuity which resolved once the drug was withdrawn.

Two other major side-effects of clomiphene administration are the side-effects of ovarian stimulation and ovulation induction. Clomiphene citrate induces multiple follicular development, and ovarian hyperstimulation can occur. It is much less common than following ovulation induction with gonadotrophin therapy. Gysler et al (1982) reported palpable ovarian enlargement in 5.1% of patients, and Rust et al (1974) reported ovarian cysts in 6.7% of women studied. The duration of therapy is probably more important (Lunenfeld and Insler, 1978) than the dose of clomiphene used. Cysts usually resolve spontaneously in a few weeks, and cases of full-blown hyperstimulation with nausea, vomiting, ascites and hydrothorax are rare.

As a consequence of multiple follicular development, multiple pregnancy does occur after ovulation induction with clomiphene citrate. A multiple pregnancy rate of 6–7% has been reported (World Health Organization, 1973), although higher incidences have also been reported—Hull et al (1979) reported 17.8%—and clomiphene in combination with hCG is said to be associated with an increased multiple pregnancy rate. While the majority are twin pregnancies, triplets, quads and quins have been reported.

RESULTS OF TREATMENT

When given to normoprolactinaemic women who bleed either spontaneously or in response to progestagen withdrawal, an ovulation rate of around 70% can be achieved. Of the women who do ovulate, 50% will do so on a dose of 50 mg, and few will require more than 150 mg. Women who have oligomenorrhoea in general respond better than those with amenorrhoea; whether infertility is primary or secondary seems to make little difference. Reported pregnancy rates vary greatly: 25–35% (World Health Organization, 1973), 11.1–45.5% (from a number of studies reviewed by Lunenfeld and Insler, 1978), and 100% (Barrett and Hakim, 1974). It is almost universally agreed, however, that there is a significant discrepancy between the ovulation rate and the pregnancy rate achieved by clomiphene citrate. The reasons for this discrepancy are multiple. The selection of patients, the regimen used and the monitoring of treatment vary widely between centres, and it is also quite clear that many women being treated with clomiphene have other problems associated with infertility such as endometriosis, mild tubal disease or adhesions. Moreover, in a multicentre study of infertile couples carried out by the World Health Organization (Farley, 1986) more than 30% of couples had factors involving both partners.

Clomiphene citrate has pharmacological effects on all oestrogen-dependent tissues, and an effect on tubal transport (Whitelaw et al, 1970) has been postulated to explain the low pregnancy rates. It is quite clear that clomiphene has an adverse effect on cervical mucus with suppression of both the quantity and quality of mucus and an increase in cervical mucus hostility (Insler et al, 1973). In our own studies we have demonstrated a significant reduction in spinnbarkeit (Glasier et al, 1989) and modified Katz–Overstreet tests of sperm–mucus interaction, the former being more affected by the zu rather than the en isomer.

The inadequacy of the luteal phase occurring after successful induction of ovulation in some women may also contribute to the disappointing pregnancy rate. Morever, even if ovulation is achieved there may be some factors which interfere with implantation. Garcia et al (1977) reported endometrium which was 'out of date' for the time in the cycle in 50% of women treated with clomiphene. More recently Markiewicz et al (1988) have described significant increases in endometrial prostaglandin production in human tissue exposed to clomiphene citrate in vitro. In vivo administration of clomiphene resulted in minor differences in mitotic rate and basal vacuolation of glandular epithelium in endometrial biopsies taken by Thatcher et al (1988), although this group was unable to identify a specific deleterious effect of clomiphene.

With the recent availability of human oocytes and early embryos for experimentation more information is now available on the effects of clomiphene citrate on gametes. Yoshimura et al (1988) demonstrated no effect of clomiphene citrate administered to perfused rabbit ovaries on either ovulation or fertilization rates, but a significant reduction in the number of offspring resulting from embryo transfer. Administration of oestrogen to the perfusate reversed this effect, suggesting that the anti-oestrogenic effects of clomiphene may affect post-fertilization development. Clomiphene has also been shown to have deleterious effects on mouse oocytes in which a decrease in the fertilization rate has been described (Laufer et al, 1983). In the human, Oelsner et al (1987) have measured high concentrations of clomiphene isomers, particularly the zu isomer, in follicular fluid obtained at the time of oocyte recovery in women undergoing IVF with clomiphene citrate for superovulation. The group report a direct relationship between the rate of degeneration of blastocysts and the concentrations of clomiphene. Wramsby et al (1987) report a 50% incidence of abnormal chromosome karyotype in 23 human oocytes obtained at laparoscopy from women treated with clomiphene citrate. While reports to date are largely preliminary, these and similar studies suggest that clomiphene has widespread effects which may help to explain the low pregnancy rate.

These possible effects on oocytes and embryos may also help to explain the increased abortion rate associated with clomiphene. While reported rates vary, there is general agreement that rates of 20–25% occur. While all the adverse effects of clomiphene listed above may contribute to early pregnancy loss, it is true to say that the abortion rate is high in all groups of infertility patients. A 25% rate is quoted for women undergoing IVF, for example.

SAFETY OF CLOMIPHENE CITRATE

In addition to the concerns raised by information regarding the effects of clomiphene on oocytes and embryos, there are theoretical possibilities that the drug may have adverse effects in early pregnancy. The zu isomer of clomiphene is structurally similar to diethylstilboestrol (DES). Roughly 60% of offspring exposed to DES in vitro have uterine, cervical or vaginal abnormalities, including vaginal adenosis and clear cell carcinoma. For this reason clomiphene citrate should be avoided in early pregnancy. It is also of interest to speculate whether the anti-oestrogenic effects of clomiphene may have any adverse effect on oestrogen-dependent tissues developing during embryogenesis.

Despite these concerns, normal births have been reported in women taking clomiphene up to day 35 of gestation, and a survey of 2369 women conceiving on clomiphene carried out by Merrell National Laboratories reported no significant increase in congenital malformation rates (Merrell National Laboratories Product Information Bulletin). McKenna and Pepperell (1988) reviewed three studies combined to provide 1263 babies delivered after clomiphene citrate and found no difference in the incidence of anomalies compared with controls. Recently there has been some concern over an increase in the incidence of neural tube defects in the offspring of women who undergo ovulation induction. Czeizel (1989) reported three cases of neural tube defect in 3 of 852 pregnancies (0.4%) compared with 12 in 18 904 controls (0.1%). Cuckle and Wald (1989), however, suggested that present evidence is too slight to judge whether the association is real. In a recent review of the safety of drugs used in ovulation, Lunenfeld et al (1986) concluded that clomiphene citrate is 'relatively safe to both patients and offspring if administered to properly selected patients in correct dosage and following effective mode of treatment'. This group does, however, add that the final conclusions with regard to long-term side-effects must wait until sufficiently large surveys of post-pubertal offspring are completed.

REFERENCES

Barrett CA & Hakim CA (1974) Low dosage clomiphene therapy in the treatment of infertility due to defective ovulation. *African Medical Journal* **48:** 1456–1460.
Canales ES, Cabezas A, Vazquez-Matute L & Zarate A (1978) Induction of ovulation with clomiphene and oestradiol benzoate in anovulatory women refractory to clomiphene alone. *Fertility and Sterility* **29:** 496–499.
Clark JH & Markaverich BM (1982) The agonistic–antagonistic properties of clomiphene: a review. *Pharmacology and Therapeutics* **15:** 467–478.
Clark HJ, Peck EJ & Anderson JN (1974) Oestrogen receptors and antagonism of steroid hormone action. *Nature* **251:** 446–448.

Cuckle H & Wald N (1989) Ovulation induction and neural tube defects. *Lancet* **ii**: 1281.

Czeizel A (1989) Ovulation induction and neural tube defects. *Lancet* **ii**: 167.

Downs DE & Gibson M (1983) Clomiphene citrate therapy for luteal phase defect. *Fertility and Sterility* **39**: 34–38.

Farley TMM (1986) The WHO standardised investigation of the infertile couple In Ratnam SC, Teoh E-S & Anandakumar C (eds) *Infertility Male and Female. Proceedings of the 12th World Congress on Fertility and Sterility*, Singapore, October 1986. Advances in Fertility and Sterility, Series 4, pp 7–19.

Fayez JA (1976) Selection of patients for clomiphene citrate therapy. *Obstetrics and Gynecology* **47**: 671–676.

Garcia J, Seegar-Jones G & Wentz AC (1977) The use of clomiphene citrate. *Fertility and Sterility* **28**: 707–717.

Glasier AF, Irvine DS, Wickings EJ, Hillier SG & Baird DT (1989) A comparison of the effects on follicular development between clomiphene citrate, its two separate isomers and spontaneous cycles. *Human Reproduction* **4**: 252–256.

Greenblatt RB (1968) Experimental studies using clomiphene citrate. In Behrman SJ & Kistner RW (eds) *Progress in Infertility*, pp 455–466. Boston: Little Brown.

Gysler M, March CM, Mishell DR & Bailey EJ (1982) A decade's experience with an individualized clomiphene treatment regimen including its effect on the post coital test. *Fertility and Sterility* **37**: 161–167.

Hashimoto T, Miyai K, Izumi K & Kumahara Y (1976) Effect of clomiphene citrate on basal and LHRH-induced gonadotropin secretion in post menopausal women. *Journal of Clinical Endocrinology and Metabolism* **42**: 593–594.

Hsueh AJW, Erickson GF & Yenss C (1978) Sensitisation of pituitary cells to luteinizing hormone releasing hormone by clomiphene citrate in vitro. *Nature* **273**: 57–59.

Hull MGR, Savage PE & Jacobs HS (1979) Investigation and treatment of amenorrhoea resulting in normal fertility. *British Medical Journal* **i**: 1257–1261.

Insler V, Zakut H & Serr DM (1973) Cycle pattern and pregnancy rate following combined clomiphene–estrogen therapy. *Obstetrics and Gynecology* **41**: 602–607.

Jones GS, Maffezzoli RD, Strott CA, Ross GT & Kaplan G (1970) Pathophysiology of reproductive failure after clomiphene-induced ovulation. *American Journal of Obstetrics and Gynecology* **108**: 847–867.

Judd SJ, Alderman J, Bowden J & Michailov L (1987) Evidence against the involvement of opiate neurons in mediating the effect of clomiphene citrate on gonadotrophin-releasing hormone neurons. *Fertility and Sterility* **47**: 574–578.

Kerin JF, Liu JH, Phillipou G & Yen SSC (1985) Evidence for a hypothalamic site of action of clomiphene citrate in women. *Journal of Clinical Endocrinology and Metabolism* **61**: 265–268.

Kessel B & Hsueh AJW (1987) Clomiphene citrate augments follicle-stimulating hormone-induced luteinizing hormone receptor content in rat granulosa cells. *Fertility and Sterility* **47**: 334–340.

Kistner RW (1965) Induction of ovulation with clomiphene citrate (clomid). *Obstetrical and Gynecological Survey* **20**: 873–900.

Kistner RW (1968) Induction of ovulation with clomiphene citrate. In Behrman SJ & Kistner RW (eds) *Progress in Infertility*, pp 407–453. Boston: Little, Brown.

Laufer N, Pratt BM, Decherney AH, Naftolin F, Merino M & Markert CL (1983) The in vivo and in vitro effects of clomiphene citrate on ovulation, fertilization and development of cultured mouse oocytes. *American Journal of Obstetrics and Gynecology* **147**: 633–639.

Littman BA & Hodgen GD (1985) A comprehensive dose–response study of clomiphene citrate for enhancement of the primate ovarian/menstrual cycle. *Fertility and Sterility* **43**: 463–469.

Lunenfeld B & Insler V (eds) (1978). *Diagnosis and Treatment of Functional Infertility*, pp 33–55. Berlin: Grosse Verlag.

Lunenfeld B, Blankstein J, Koter-Emeth S, Kokia E & Geier A (1986) Drugs used in ovulation induction. Safety of patient and offspring. *Human Reproduction* **1**: 435–439.

Markiewicz L, Laufer N & Gurpide E (1988). In vitro effects of clomiphene citrate on human endometrium. *Fertility and Sterility* **50**: 772–776.

McKenna KM & Pepperell RJ (1988) Anti-oestrogens: their clinical physiology and use in reproductive medicine. *Baillière's Clinical Obstetrics and Gynaecology* **2(3)**: 545–566.

Mikkelson TJ, Kroboth PD, Cameron WJ, Dittert LW, Chungi V & Manberg PJ (1986) Single-dose pharmacokinetics of clomiphene citrate in normal volunteers. *Fertility and Sterility* **46:** 392–396.

Oelsner G, Barnea ER, Admon D, Mikkelson TJ & De Cherney AH (1987) Letter to the editor, *New England Journal of Medicine* **316:** 318.

O'Herlihy C, Pepperell RJ, Brown JB, Smith MA, Sandri L & McBain JC (1981) Incremental clomiphene therapy: a new method for treating persistent anovulation. *Obstetrics and Gynecology* **58:** 533–542.

Ron-El R, Soffer Y, Langer R, Herman A, Weintraub Z & Caspi E (1989) Low multiple pregnancy rate in combined clomiphene citrate–human menopausal gonadotrophin treatment for ovulation induction or enhancement. *Human Reproduction* **4:** 495–500.

Rust LA, Israel R & Mishell DR (1974) An individualized graduated therapeutic regimen for clomiphene citrate. *American Journal of Obstetrics and Gynecology* **120:** 785–790.

Soules MR, Wiebe RH, Aksel S & Hammond CB (1977) The diagnosis and therapy of luteal phase deficiency. *Fertility and Sterility* **28:** 1033–1037.

Taubert HHD & Kuhl H (1986) Steroids and steroid-like compounds. In Insler V & Lunenfeld B (eds) *Infertility: Male and Female*, pp 413–449. Edinburgh, London, Melbourne, New York: Churchill Livingstone.

Thatcher SS, Donachie KM, Glasier A, Hillier SG & Baird DT (1988) The effects of clomiphene citrate on the histology of human endometrium in regularly cycling women undergoing in vitro fertilization. *Fertility and Sterility* **49:** 296–301.

Whitelaw MJ, Kalman CF & Grams LR (1970) The significance of the high ovulation rate versus the low pregnancy rate with clomid. *American Journal of Obstetrics and Gynecology* **107:** 865–877.

World Health Organisation (1973) *Agents stimulating gonadal function in the human.* Technical Report Series No. 153, p 15, Geneva.

Wramsby H, Fredga K & Liedholm P (1987) Chromosome analysis of human oocytes recovered from preovulatory follicles in stimulated cycles. *New England Journal of Medicine* **316:** 120–124.

Yoshimura Y, Hosoi Y, Atlas SJ, Dharmarajan AM, Adachi T & Wallach EE (1988) Effect of the exposure of intrafollicular oocytes to clomiphene citrate on pregnancy outcome in the rabbit. *Fertility and Sterility* **50:** 153–158.

Yuen BH, Mari N, Duleba AJ & Moon YS (1988) Direct effects of clomiphene citrate on the steroidogenic capability of human granulosa cells. *Fertility and Sterility* **49:** 626–631.

6

Human gonadotrophins

LARS NILSSON
LARS HAMBERGER

GONADOTROPHIN PREPARATIONS

The first gonadotrophin preparations utilized for ovarian stimulation in the human were of pituitary origin (Gemzell et al, 1958; Gemzell, 1962). Both follicle-stimulating hormone (FSH) and luteinizing hormone (LH) are known today to be compact glycosylated globular proteins with molecular weights of 28 000–29 000. The molecules are composed of two subunits which are internally cross-linked and stabilized by disulphide bonds. The gonadotrophic activity was estimated initially using in vivo bio-assays and later using in vitro bio-assays. After the introduction of immunological and radio-immunological assays (RIAs) these methods became utilized more and more, particularly in clinical practice, because of their simplicity. However, it soon became evident that biologically inactive subunits of the gonadotrophins were also being measured in the RIAs. The half-life as well as the biological activity of the gonadotrophins were further shown to be dependent on, e.g., the pH, the content of sialic acid and the electrical charge of the molecules (for references see Cook et al, 1988).

No gonadotrophins from pituitary extracts are commercially available for clinical use. Among the gonadotrophins from urinary extracts of post-menopausal women, other molecular structures have been identified (Graesslin et al, 1973). The three human menopausal gonadotrophins commercially available today (Pergonal®, Serono; Humegon®, Organon, and Inductor®, Searle) are charactized by using somewhat different assay systems, and this makes an objective comparison troublesome. The ratio between FSH and LH has been set at 1:1 in all preparations, and the activity of each at 75 IU per ampoule. Independent investigators utilizing bio-assays and/or RIAs have revealed considerable variations between the preparations, as well as a batch-to-batch variation, both in gonadotrophic activity measured as IU and in the ratio between FSH and LH (Harlin et al, 1986).

During the last decade it has been considered favourable to utilize more FSH relative to LH, at least for early follicular stimulation, even though it was previously claimed that the ratio between FSH and LH was un-important. For such reasons the market has been provided with so called 'pure FSH' preparations with an FSH:LH ratio of approximately 75:1

(Metrodin®, Serono; Fertiline®, Searle). This degree of purity, however, is seldom needed or even wanted, and has led to the development of stimulation mixtures with FSH:LH ratios of 3:1 or 2:1. Some investigators even shift the FSH:LH ratio during the stimulation starting with 'pure FSH' and ending with a 1:1 ratio of FSH:LH.

PRINCIPAL MODES OF ADMINISTRATION

In the stimulation schedules used for patients with hypothalamic–hypophyseal insufficiency, the amount of gonadotrophins administered daily is generally increased stepwise, at least during the first cycle. In normal cycling women the gonadotrophins are either administered at a constant dose level, or occasionally increased, but more often decreased, towards the end of the stimulation. Efforts have been made to change the gonadotrophin administration model from one intramuscular injection every 24 h to the injection of lower amounts twice daily, or even to use pulsatile pumps for subcutaneous or intravenous administration since it is well known that both FSH and LH are physiologically secreted in episodic bursts. A certain increase in the treatment success rate has been seen with these more laborious administration regimens in the terms of clinical pregnancies (Nakamura et al, 1986, 1989). Moreover, it has been convincingly shown that the total dose of administered gonadotrophin needed for full follicular development is reduced if pulsatile pumps are utilized rather than daily injections (Ho Yuen and Pride, 1984). A certain difference between pulsatile administration of pure FSH compared to human menopausal gonadotrophin (hMG) has also been reported from these studies, especially in patients known to be 'poor responders' (see below).

CLINICAL APPLICATIONS

Gonadotrophin treatment of anovulatory infertility dates back to the late 1950s and is today an established principle in infertility practice. The main indications for treatment remain anovulatory infertility of World Health Organization (WHO) group I (low gonadotrophin–low oestrogen, no withdrawal bleeding after progestogen medication) and WHO group II (normal gonadotrophin or slightly elevated LH levels, more or less normal oestrogen level, cyclic bleeding or bleeding after progestogen medication). Within group II the polycystic ovary (PCO) syndrome is the most common diagnosis. Large case materials present cumulative success rates, in group I of approximately 90% viable pregnancies and in group II of approximately 50% (e.g. Dor et al, 1980).

Since anovulatory infertility due to hyperprolactinaemia today can be more efficiently treated with bromocriptine, this group of patients is seldom treated with human gonadotrophins. Furthermore, patients belonging to WHO group II may preferably be treated with clomiphene citrate (CC), provided that they react to this drug. On the other hand, gonadotrophin therapy has been successfully used in the treatment of other causes of infertility, e.g. luteal phase deficiency and cervical mucus hostility. Above all, different stimulation protocols, partly or completely based on gonadotrophin administration, are being used in connection with assisted reproduction, e.g. in vitro fertilization (IVF), gamete intrafallopian transfer (GIFT), direct intraperitoneal insemination (DIPI), intrauterine insemination (AIH and AID) etc., whenever dating of the ovulation and/or follicular hyperstimulation are desirable.

The principles for treatment of either anovulatory or ovulatory women are basically the same, although the management of the induced cycles differs, as will be discussed below.

NORMAL FOLLICLE DEVELOPMENT

From early prenatal life up to the time of menopause the follicles of the woman's ovaries are under constant development. Primary follicles present in the ovarian cortex are continuously recruited for growth and development from a pool of non-growing follicles. Once a follicle has started to grow it will either degenerate or develop further to reach the 0.5–4 mm stage (large preantral and early antral follicles) within about 60 days (Gougeon, 1982).

Very little is known about the mechanisms governing the early follicle development, until the main follicular cell types (granulosa and thecal cells) gradually become sensitive to the gonadotrophins FSH and LH. Various regulatory peptides—e.g. insulin-like growth factor (IGF), epidermal growth factor (EGF), inhibin, activin and follicular regulatory protein (FRP)—have been implicated, as well as prostaglandin E, insulin and growth hormone. However, it is still not clear whether these substances exert their influences before or in parallel with the gonadotrophins (e.g. DiZerega et al, 1982; Westergaard et al, 1984; Westergaard, 1988). The position of the follicle within the ovary as well as ovarian circulation and innervation have also been suggested to be of selective importance.

Theoretically, several critical levels of development exist (Figure 1), and large cohorts of growing follicles are believed to go through repeated waves of recruitment and selection. Consequently, only a small fraction of the follicles reach the 'surface' (Figure 1) and become 0.5–4 mm follicles. At this stage they become sensitive to gonadotrophin stimulation and thus ready for the final recruitment into a natural menstrual cycle (e.g. McNatty, 1981; DiZerega and Hodgen, 1981). In the presence of a certain threshold level of FSH and LH, or similar activity as e.g. in the PCO syndrome, during pregnancy and during childhood, follicular development may proceed somewhat further, up to the 6–8 mm stage. In the absence of *cyclic* FSH and LH activity these follicles cannot develop further but remain relatively immature, producing mainly androgenic steroids. Sometimes such immature follicles may undergo cystic degeneration and become larger, while remaining atretic with a low steroid production.

In the natural cycle, on the other hand, the FSH and LH levels are very low in the luteal phase and do not allow follicles to proceed beyond the 4 mm

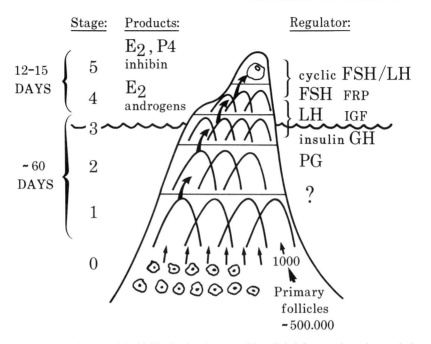

Figure 1. The iceberg model of follicular development. Very little is known about the regulation of development below the 'water surface'. Stages 4–5 correspond to the normal menstrual cycle. At puberty, approximately 500 000 primary follicles are present in the ovarian cortex. During each menstrual cycle, about 1000 of these are lost; only one will ovulate. Manipulation of stages 4–5 may bring 10–30 follicles close to the ovulatory stage. E₂, oestradiol; P4, progesterone; FSH, follicle-stimulating hormone; LH, luteinizing hormone; FRP, follicular regulatory protein; IGF, insulin-like growth factor; GH, growth hormone; PG, prostaglandin.

stage. Towards the end of the luteal phase the serum concentrations of FSH and LH begin to rise and serve to recruit a cohort of follicles in the sensitive 0.5–4 mm stage, FSH acting to stimulate granulosa cell proliferation and the formation of follicular fluid. LH stimulates the thecal cells of the follicle to produce androgens, whereas FSH is also considered to stimulate the aromatization of androgens to oestrogens within the granulosa cells. In the leading follicle(s) the increasing production of oestradiol (E_2) promotes further binding of FSH which, in turn, accelerates the granulosa cells' production of E_2 and inhibin and other peptides. The rising concentrations of E_2 and inhibin in serum cause a decrease in the production and release of FSH by the pituitary by means of a negative feedback mechanism. Thus, a local self-amplifying mechanism within the leading follicle(s) becomes counterbalanced by a central inhibitory mechanism. Only follicles capable of binding the available FSH molecules in sufficient quantities will continue to grow. Some evidence exists to show that the inhibin concentration at the end of the previous luteal phase determines the number of leading follicles in the growing cohort (Baird, personal communication; Roseff et al, 1989).

In the natural menstrual cycle only one follicle usually passes through this

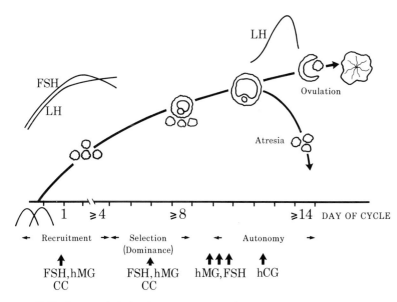

Figure 2. Follicular growth during the menstrual cycle (after DiZerega and Hodgen, 1981). This corresponds to stages 4–5 in Figure 1. Follicle-stimulating hormone (FSH), human menopausal gonadotrophin (hMG) and clomiphene citrate (CC) can be used to influence the phases of recruitment and selection of the dominant follicle. At most, some 10–30 follicles may reach preovulatory size. The ensuing luteal phase is usually of a constant time period (12–16 days).

final selection to reach preovulatory maturity (Figure 2) (DiZerega and Hodgen, 1981; McNatty, 1981). At a certain maturational stage of the dominant follicle its granulosa cells start to express LH receptors on their surface. The rising E_2 concentrations in serum reach the critical level and duration to elicit a positive feedback effect on the pituitary, releasing bursts of LH into the circulation. This peak of LH triggers the complete ovulatory response: completion of oocyte meiosis, luteinization of the follicular cells and rupture of the follicle wall to release the fertilizable oocyte.

All but the leading follicle of the cohort undergo atresia at this time, theoretically because these follicles cannot aromatize their androgen burden into E_2. The development of a 0.5–4 mm follicle into a preovulatory one takes another 10–15 days from the start of the FSH rise to ovulation. A longer follicular phase may result, when no recruitable follicles are immediately available, e.g. after long periods of gonadotrophin deficiency as in WHO anovulation group I.

Whenever a normal ovulation takes place and a normal corpus luteum is formed from the ruptured follicle, the luteal phase is remarkably constant: 12–16 days. The mechanisms underlying luteal regression in the human are still incompletely understood. For normal function of the corpus luteum, at least some LH—or human chorionic gonadotrophin (hCG)—activity is required, and the prolactin levels should be neither too high nor too low (McNatty et al, 1974; Henderson and McNatty, 1975). The demise of the corpus luteum after approximately 14 days is accompanied by decreasing concentrations of progesterone (P4) and E_2, and possibly also inhibin (Roseff et al, 1989), allowing the pituitary to escape from negative feedback and to again secrete increasing amounts of FSH and LH for the next cycle of follicle recruitment.

INDUCTION OF FOLLICULAR DEVELOPMENT

Hitherto, manipulation of follicular development has only been possible with stages 'above the surface', somewhere between stages 2 and 4 (Figure 1), coinciding with the development of gonadotrophin receptors on follicular cells. Even in a state of gonadotrophin deficiency, as in anovulation of WHO group I, follicular development continues up to but not above the 'surface'. Gonadotrophin therapy can substitute for this deficiency and allow development to stages 3–5 (Figures 1 and 2). When low doses are given, more or less physiological numbers of preovulatory follicles develop.

In anovulation of WHO group II, unco-ordinated but normal or slightly elevated gonadotrophin (LH) concentrations prevail, allowing for follicular development up to and into stage 4 (Figure 1) but not further. The presence of several follicles between 4 and 8 mm, some of these in a growing state, means that gonadotrophin therapy can elicit a response very quickly, with the possibility of many follicles starting to grow into stage 5 being high. This is in contrast to the situation in anovulation of WHO group I, in which few follicles are in a recruitable stage, and where a considerable latency may exist before a clinical response can be elicited.

In the regularly ovulating woman, gonadotrophin therapy is usually used to induce multifollicular development. All stimulation protocols designed for this purpose are aimed at augmenting the normal gonadotrophin signals. Exogenous FSH, usually in the form of hMG, or endogenous FSH augmented by the use of CC or gonadotrophin-releasing hormone (GnRH) should be administered concomitant with the spontaneous FSH rise at the end of the previous luteal phase or at the beginning of the current follicular phase. By keeping the FSH level high during the early and mid-follicular phases (Figure 2), the normal selection of one follicle is usually replaced by several follicles being rescued from atresia and reaching the preovulatory stage (level no 5, Figure 1). Usually, the FSH therapy is continued even into the phase of follicular autonomy (Figure 2) to prevent atresia of some follicles, even if many of the largest follicles continue to grow independent of the decreasing FSH levels.

Irrespective of the reason for gonadotrophin therapy the long-standing stimulation creates problems related to the asynchrony of different follicle cohorts (Figure 3). As the FSH stimulation proceeds, new cohorts of follicles appear at the recruitable 'surface' about every second to fourth day, and the prolonged increase in FSH serves not only to block the selection of a dominant follicle but also to recruit new cohorts of follicles. Provided that the last phases (4 and 5) of follicular development take place at a more or less constant pace, which seems to be the case, these follicles (with their enclosed

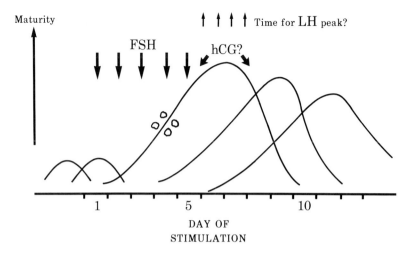

Figure 3. Asynchrony of follicle cohorts. Human menopausal gonadotrophin (hMG) or clomiphene citrate (CC) may, through the action of follicle-stimulating hormone (FSH), not only recruit a single cohort but may act continuously to recruit new cohorts. However, the correct moment of injecting human chorionic gonadotrophin (hCG) may be difficult to decide. A spontaneous LH peak may occur before hCG is injected. At ovulation or oocyte pick-up, a mixture of immature, mature and postmature oocytes may be present.

oocytes) will reach optimal maturity at different points of time. When hCG is given to induce final maturation of the oocytes, or even when a spontaneous LH surge is induced by the rising E_2 concentrations, only the most mature follicles ovulate, while the others go into atresia. Still other follicles may be less responsive to LH/hCG and even continue their growth into the luteal phase, and thereby causing abnormalities in steroid secretion (see below) during this phase, resulting in asynchronous maturation of the endometrium.

MONITORING THE RESPONSE

Non-invasive methods of judging the maturity of the oocytes in the cycle do not exist, irrespective of whether the cycle is spontaneous or induced. In spontaneous cycles the control mechanisms usually guarantee a mature oocyte when the endogenous LH peak induces the ovulation. In cycles manipulated or induced by CC and/or gonadotrophins, LH peaks may occur prematurely or be delayed and may not be synchronized with oocyte maturation. In anovulation of WHO group I, LH peaks may not occur at all. For this reason, as well as for the purpose of scheduling ovulation to a convenient time, the LH is often substituted by an injection of hCG (Figure 3). In order to give this injection at the correct time (Williams and Hodgen, 1980), monitoring is mandatory. Ultrasound scanning of the ovaries demonstrates the growth and enlargement of several follicles, and these follicles may be of different sizes, may belong to different cohorts and contain

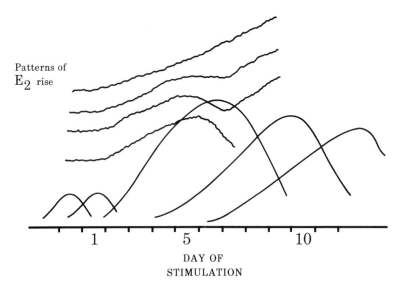

Patterns of
E_2 rise

DAY OF
STIMULATION

Figure 4. Asynchrony of follicular development as mirrored in the pattern of serum oestradiol (E_2). Note that different cohorts of follicles may contribute to the net sum of E_2. The resulting pattern may be different despite the degeneration of follicles of the first cohort.

oocytes of different maturities. The serum or urinary concentrations of E_2 determined daily or even more frequently give a good indication of the strength of the response to stimulation. However, after a few days the E_2 value represents the net sum of E_2 production from different follicle cohorts (Figure 4) as well as from peripheral aromatization of androgens. A fixed value of E_2, therefore, is not by itself a good indicator of follicular maturity.

Although the correlation between follicle size and oocyte maturity in multifollicular cycles is far from absolute, follicles of 18–25 mm in diameter usually contain fertilizable oocytes, whereas follicles below 15 or above 26 mm seldom do. Cystic follicles are usually, but not always, large, contain few granulosa cells, provide very little E_2 and seldom contain healthy oocytes.

Even if the absolute level of E_2 does not indicate oocyte maturity, there is a correlation between the maximum E_2 level and the number of large, healthy follicles. A progressive rise in E_2 for at least 5–6 days, starting at a minimum of 150% of the baseline level, usually indicates maturity of the oocytes of the first follicle cohort (cf. McBain and Trounson, 1984). More than 6 days of rising E_2 is likely to induce an LH peak, and the monitoring of serum LH concentrations at least twice daily is recommendable after 4–5 days of increasing E_2 in order to avoid a 'surprise' ovulation. Earlier determinations of LH and/or P4 may help to identify premature LH secretion and a premature luteinization. Combinations of repeated ultrasound scanning of follicles and endometrium and daily E_2 and/or LH determinations, plus standard clinical examinations, are usually necessary to perform a good gonadotrophin stimulation. Furthermore, an endometrial thickness of at least 9–10 mm and a mature cervical response are valuable extra indicators of preovulatory maturity.

ASYNCHRONY

One of the major problems in stimulated cycles is the asynchronous development of follicles (Figure 3). Recently, an interesting approach to this problem was described by Shorham et al (1989). These authors suggested that a single leading follicle with a diameter more than 6 mm larger than that of the other follicles should be aspirated early during the ovarian stimulation (as a mean on day 8.1) to allow a greater number of synchronous follicles to develop. When this regime was used, three of seven patients in a smaller series became pregnant after IVF treatment.

GONADOTROPHIN STIMULATION IN ANOVULATORY INFERTILITY

The indication for treatment is anovulatory infertility and the object is to achieve ovulation of a few (one to three) mature oocytes. In *WHO group I anovulation*, gonadotrophin therapy may be regarded as a substitution therapy. FSH, usually in the form of hMG (FSH/LH ratio approximately 1:1) is injected on a daily basis, the dosage being increased by 1 ampoule of hMG (75 IU) per day every 3–5 days until a steady slow rise in the E_2 concentrations in serum or urine can be measured. This clinically mute latency phase corresponds roughly to the recruitment phase (Figure 2). When the threshold dose of hMG has been found, it is generally kept constant or slightly reduced up to assumed follicular maturity. When an E_2 concentration of 1–3 nmol/litre is reached in serum after 5–8 days of steadily increasing, an ultrasound examination of the ovaries shows 1–3 follicles with a diameter of 15–20 mm, and if the cervical response is sufficient, hCG (5000–10 000 IU) is injected to induce ovulation. Serum or urinary levels of LH may be measured to detect an LH peak, although in this group of patients LH surges do not usually occur. Since these patients have a deficiency in gonadotrophin secretion, they should preferably be given luteal support in the form of hCG (Messinis et al, 1988), 1250 to 5000 IU every 3–4 days for at least 9–12 days following ovulation. If the patient does not become pregnant in her first treatment cycle, gonadotrophic stimulation can be reinstituted for at least six consecutive cycles. In the subsequent cycles, the dose of hMG known to give a threshold response may be used directly to save time, even if the patient may react slightly differently the next time. Excellent cumulative conception rates may be expected in this group of patients (e.g. Dor et al, 1980).

In *WHO group II anovulation*, the hMG therapy should be given with caution to avoid clinical hyperstimulation. In the first treatment cycle, a very low dose of hMG, 'pure' FSH or a mixture of these (FSH/LH ratio 1:1 to 75:1) should be given for the first 5 days, gradually increasing the daily dosage by 37.5–75 IU every 5 days, until the threshold dose is found. The latency phase may be very short (see above) and several follicles develop almost inevitably. Using only ultrasound it may be difficult in the beginning to see which follicle(s) in the 4–8 mm range are starting to grow. A slow and steady rise in serum E_2 for 5–8 days is a good prognostic sign. Human CG is administered on the same indications as for WHO group I patients, although somewhat higher E_2 levels may have to be accepted, as well as more follicles above 10 mm. Monitoring the LH is recommendable, since spontaneous LH surges are not infrequent and they may occur before optimal follicular maturity is reached. Although ovulation can usually be induced, clinical overstimulation is more frequent and the conception rate per cycle is much lower than in WHO group I patients. Luteal support with hCG is not logical in WHO group II patients and carries a risk of worsening an overstimulation while not seeming to improve the birth rates (Messinis et al, 1988). It seems wise to start the stimulation in WHO group II patients after a progestogen withdrawal bleeding or after a course of contraceptive pills in order to obtain a defined starting point preferably with a moderate starting level of E_2 (below 0.20 nmol/litre).

In the last few years, many fertility specialists have advocated the use of GnRH agonists (see below) in these patients to down-regulate pituitary gonadotrophin secretion before hMG therapy is instituted. This will bring the follicles down to or below the 'surface' (Figure 1) and correct the dominance of LH secretion often found in this group of patients. Some authorities consider an increased LH secretion harmful to oocyte maturation and embryo development (see Howles et al, 1986). Even after down-regulation with GnRH agonists, many patients retain their tendency for overstimulation (Breckwoldt et al, 1988), and the same caution in increasing the dose of hMG should be applied after treatment with a GnRH agonist. Some authors have reported very good conception rates in the WHO group II patients, especially PCO patients, after treatment with 'pure' FSH (e.g. Birkhäuser et al, 1988). Perhaps down-regulation with GnRH agonists followed by more or less 'pure' FSH treatment would improve the results in these patients. In the presence of a GnRH agonist, the amount of hMG needed for full stimulation is higher since desialated gonadotrophic molecules are often not effectively blocked and may occupy the gonadotrophic receptors without a biological effect. When the treatment with a GnRH agonist is maintained up to or close to the time of hCG injection, spontaneous LH surges can be completely avoided. Therefore, luteal support is probably necessary.

GONADOTROPHIN THERAPY IN OVULATORY WOMEN

The indication for treatment in this group of patients is usually the wish to obtain many ovulatory oocytes and/or to fix the time of ovulation, and not to cure anovulation. Since these patients have a more or less regular cyclic pattern of gonadotrophin secretion, hormonal augmentation must be given in a synchronized fashion. FSH/hMG and/or CC are given so as to amplify

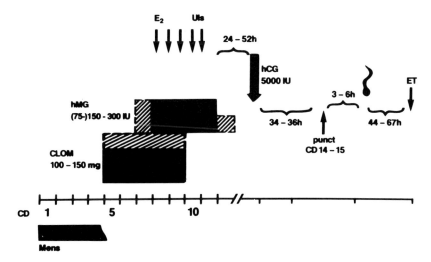

Figure 5. The stimulated cycle for in vitro fertilization (IVF): clomiphene (CLOM) and human menopausal gonadotrophin (hMG). E_2, oestradiol; Uls, ultrasound examination; ET, embryo transfer; CD, cycle day; hCG, human chorionic gonadotrophin.

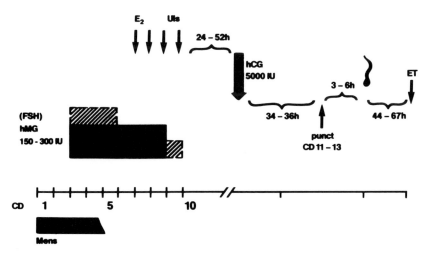

Figure 6. The stimulated cycle for in vitro fertilization (IVF): human menopausal gonadotrophin (hMG). FSH, follicle-stimulating hormone; E_2, oestradiol, Uls, ultrasound examination; hCG, human chorionic gonadotrophin; CD, cycle day; ET, embryo transfer.

and prolong the endogenous FSH secretion. Figures 5 and 6 show two standard stimulation protocols designed to induce multiple follicular development, usually for the purpose of IVF.

CC may be given from cycle day 2–5 for 5 days, depending on the woman's spontaneous cycle length, the hMG and/or 'pure' FSH injected to overlap more or less with the CC medication, depending on the strength of stimulation wanted. A daily CC dose exceeding 100 mg is seldom used nowadays. When a more forceful stimulation is necessary, the hMG dose and/or the overlap with CC is increased.

Gonadotrophins alone (hMG and/or 'pure' FSH) may be given in the same fashion without CC. In fact, higher doses are often given the first 2–4 days to recruit more follicles, and the dose is adjusted according to the response. Although CC has been suspected to induce unfavourable endometrial effects also in the secretory phase, and to increase the secretion of LH more than that of FSH in the follicular phase, most IVF centres report better results with stimulation protocols containing CC and hMG than with hMG alone protocols. In both of these protocols hCG is usually administered when follicles over 18 mm are found using ultrasound and when the E_2 level has risen to adequate values for an adequate length of time. Determination of the LH level is recommendable, so that the procedures involved in assisted reproduction, i.e. follicle aspiration in IVF, may be performed at the optimal time, 28–32 h after the LH peak or 32–36 h after the injection of hCG.

One of the major problems in cycling women exposed to hormonal hyperstimulation is the appearance of endogenous gonadotrophic bursts. In principle, these bursts can cause premature rupture of the follicle(s) or luteinization. So far, interest has been focused predominantly on LH, although the endogenous release of FSH may also induce unwanted biological effects. Growing follicles primarily have only FSH receptors on their granulosa cells and respond with an increased E_2 formation. Thus, an endogenous burst of FSH close to follicular aspiration or rupture can cause an increased oestrogen production in the smaller follicles. In turn, this may lead to a low progesterone/oestradiol ratio in the systemic circulation which interferes with the shift of the endometrium from a proliferative to a secretory phase. In addition, the tonus of the uterine musculature remains elevated and may cause uterine contractions in connection with embryo transfer in IVF patients.

This unfavourable steroid ratio may prevail for several days during which time a cohort of smaller follicles continues to grow. Since their capacity to rupture is small in the existing hormonal environment, they either become atretic or remain for prolonged periods as follicular cysts.

GONADOTROPHIN AND GnRH ANALOGUES

GnRH agonists may be used in either of two ways. Especially English IVF teams (see Macnamee et al, 1989) use an agonist for 'flare up' stimulation, substituting 5 days of CC medication with 3 days of the analogue and overlapping with hMG. This provides a stimulated cycle which usually has a favourable FSH/LH ratio, and such treatment is claimed to block LH surges for a long time, giving time for an hCG injection when the appropriate follicle diameters and E_2 levels are reached. According to Macnamee et al (1989), the E_2 levels in serum are somewhat lower with this type of stimulation. GnRH agonists (or antagonists) may instead be administered to block pituitary FSH/LH secretion. The agonists must then be given for some weeks to allow the stimulated response to pass. Subsequently, the patient can be treated as an anovulatory patient group I (WHO), since only low endogenous gonadotrophin secretion is likely to occur. When the GnRH agonist treatment is prolonged, no LH surge can occur and hCG may be injected to induce final oocyte maturation and ovulation. In the case of IVF treatment, the hMG (or FSH) preparation is injected in doses sufficient to create multifollicular development, and follicle aspiration is performed within 36 h after hCG injection to avoid ovulation.

OVARIAN HYPERSTIMULATION

The hyperstimulation syndrome is believed to result from the over-production of oestrogen. When gonadotrophins are used to induce follicle development there is always a risk of pronounced hyperstimulation, which is much less when only CC is used. In IVF and GIFT treatment the puncture of follicles may reduce the risk of hyperstimulation even if it cannot completely block its occurrence (Friedman et al, 1984). Moreover, ovulatory women seem to run a lower risk than anovulatory women. GnRH treatment before stimulation appears to increase this risk of hyperstimulation. Patients with PCO-like ovaries run an even higher risk.

To avoid severe hyperstimulation, gonadotrophin treatment should be provided at the lowest possible daily dose and should not be continued longer than necessary. When the first cohort of follicles is believed to have reached optimal maturity further stimulation will only cause new cohorts to grow, with an increased net production of E_2, and unruptured, less mature follicles will continue to produce high amounts of E_2 into the luteal phase. The unfavourable E_2:P4 ratio will probably derange the endometrial maturation and is likely to cause premature demise of the corpora lutea, in addition to inducing hyperstimulation. Whenever the E_2 curve rises too quickly during the stimulation phase and/or whenever ultrasound exami-nation shows many growing follicles of 10–12 mm in diameter, the gonado-trophin medication should be reduced or stopped. If the process still con-tinues, hCG should not be injected. Although hyperstimulation may occur after a spontaneous LH peak, this risk is much less than after the long-acting hCG preparations. Luteal support with hCG should be avoided. Instead, medication with high doses of progesterone may counteract the negative effects of E_2.

If a full-blown hyperstimulation syndrome develops, pregnancy should be suspected and confirmed or ruled out. If the patient is not pregnant, a quick-acting GnRH antagonist may be given to reduce the pituitary drive. Otherwise symptomatic treatment should be given to correct water and salt balance and coagulation perturbations. Indomethacin may be of value to reduce the increased vascular permeability. In rare cases of life-threatening hyperstimulation during an early pregnancy, therapeutic abortion must be considered.

Fortunately, severe clinical hyperstimulation is rare (approximately 1%) with proper management of the gonadotrophin treatment (Insler et al, 1987; Schenker and Navot, 1987).

INDIVIDUAL TREATMENT

Shortly after the introduction of hyperstimulated cycles in IVF it was realized that the intra-individual response variation to a given stimulation was strikingly small while the inter-individual response variation was large. The Norfolk group classified the patient response in three categories: low, intermediate and high responders.

The intermediate responders showed the best results in terms of clinical pregnancies, and the high responders could rather easily be turned into intermediates by lowering the gonadotrophin dose or modifying the length of the stimulation.

The low responders have often been called poor responders but should perhaps rather be regarded as atypical responders. In this latter group, an individualized stimulation schedule seems necessary, while the other groups probably can be treated in fixed stimulation schedules with relative success, no doubt, making life easier for the doctor and cheaper for the patient (Muasher, 1988).

The question then arises, can the poor responders be identified even prior to hyperstimulation treatment to avoid a gonadotrophin-stimulated test cycle where the stimulation has to be discontinued. Two groups of patients can probably be suspected of being atypical responders, i.e. those with PCO syndromes and those over 40 years old. Women with irregular cycles may also belong to this group.

Determinations of the serum E_2 and prolactin levels prior to, as well as the ratio between FSH and LH during or prior to, the start of gonadotrophic stimulation seem important. Numerous treatment combinations have been suggested during the last decade involving anti-oestrogens, oestrogens, GnRH agonists. antagonists or growth hormone.

In the future, gonadotrophic treatment will probably be recommended solely to WHO group I patients where excellent results can be elicited. In WHO group II patients, as well as in irregularly cycling women stimulated in association to assisted reproduction procedures, the gonadotrophic treatment will most probably be combined with other drugs to meet with the problems created by interference of the endogenous gonadotrophins.

SUMMARY

Treatment with exogenous gonadotrophic hormones to overcome certain cases of female infertility has been used for more than 30 years. Children born after such treatment have not shown any increased incidence of abnormalities (genetic or otherwise) and their reproductive ability seems normal. Furthermore, no increase in malignant disease (breast, ovarian, endometrial) have been reported following such repetitive gonadotrophic stimulations. Thus it seems the treatment can be regarded as safe. Two categories of patients are treated today. Firstly, hypothalamic–hypophyseal insufficiencies (WHO group I), where treatment is compulsory for attaining fertility, and secondly (including anovulation WHO group II), more or less regularly cycling women, where gonadotrophic treatment is used to augment fertility. Especially in the latter group, caution must be taken not to induce adverse effects. To meet these demands, exogenous gonadotrophic stimulation needs to be combined with other drugs and regimens that take into consideration the problems created by the concomitant presence of endogenous gonadotrophins.

Acknowledgements

The included figures have been published earlier by the authors in sales promotion activities by Pharmacia Ltd and Organon Ltd, Sweden. These Companies have kindly permitted copyrights.

REFERENCES

Birkäuser MH, Huber PR, Neuenschwander E & Napflin S (1988) Induktion der Follikelreifung mit 'reinen' FSH beim Polyzystischen Ovar-Syndrom. *Geburtshilfe und Frauenheilkunde* **48:** 220–227.

Breckwoldt M, Geisthövel F, Neulen J & Schillinger H (1988) Management of multiple conceptions after gonadotrophin releasing hormone analog/human menopausal gonadotropin/human chorionic gonadotropin therapy. *Fertility and Sterility* **49:** 713–715.

Cook AS, Webster BW, Terranova PF & Brooks AK (1988) Variation in the biological and biochemical characteristics of human menopausal gonadotropin. *Fertility and Sterility* **49:** 704–712.

DiZerega GS & Hodgen GD (1981) Folliculogenesis in the primate ovarian cycle. *Endocrine Reviews* **2:** 27–49.

DiZerega GS, Goebelsmann U & Nakamura R (1982) Identification of protein(s) secreted by preovulatory ovary which suppress follicular response to gonadotropins. *Journal of Clinical Endocrinology and Metabolism* **54:** 1091–1096.

Dor J, Itzkowic DJ, Mashiach S, Lunenfeldt B & Serr DM (1980) Cumulative conception rates following gonadotrophin therapy. *American Journal of Obstetrics and Gynaecology* **136:** 102–105.

Friedman Ch, Schmidt I, Chang GE & Kim MH (1984) Severe ovarian hyperstimulation following follicular aspiration. *American Journal of Obstetrics and Gynaecology* **15:** 436.

Gemzell CA (1962) Induction of ovulation with human pituitary gonadotropins. *Fertility and Sterility* **13:** 153–168.

Gemzell CA, Diczfalusy E & Tillinger KG (1958) Clinical effect of human pituitary follicle stimulating hormone. *Journal of Clinical Endocrinology and Metabolism* **18:** 1333.

Gougeon A (1982) Rate of follicular growth in the human ovary. In Rolland R, van Hall EV, Hillier SG et al (eds) *Follicular Maturation and Ovulation.* International Congress Series, Volume 560, pp 155–163. Amsterdam: Excerpta Medica.

Graesslin D, Spies A, Weise HC & Bettendorf G (1973) Properties of human pituitary and urinary LH. *Acta Endocrinologica* **173:** 53.

Harlin J, Khan SA & Diczfalusy E (1986) Molecular composition of luteinizing hormone and follicle-stimulating hormone in commercial gonadotropin preparations. *Fertility and Sterility* **46:** 1055–1061.

Henderson KM & McNatty KP (1975) A biochemical hypothesis to explain the mechanism of luteal regression. *Prostaglandins* **9:** 779–797.

Howles CM, Macnamee MC, Edwards RG, Goswamy R & Steptoe PC (1986) Effect of high tonic levels of luteinizing hormone on outcome of in vitro fertilization. *Lancet* **ii:** 521.

518 L. NILSSON AND L. HAMBERGER

Ho Yuen B & Pride SM (1984) Successful induction of ovulation and conception with pulsatile intravenous administration of human menopausal gonadotropins in anovulatory infertile women resistant to clomiphene and pulsatile gonadotropin-releasing hormone therapy. *American Journal of Obstetrics and Gynecology* **148:** 508–512.

Insler V, Lunenfeld G, Potashnik G & Meizner I (1987) The hyperstimulated cycle: analysis of ultrasonic and functional parameters. In Eng-Soon T, Shan Ratnam S & Peng Cheang Wong (eds) *Advances in Fertility and Sterility, Ovulation and Early Pregnancy,* pp 39–47. London: Parthenon.

Macnamee MC, Howles CM, Edwards RG, Taylor PJ & Elder KT (1989) Short-term luteinizing hormone-releasing hormone agonist treatment: prospective trial of a novel ovarian stimulation regimen for in vitro fertilization. *Fertility and Sterility* **52:** 264–269.

McBain JC & Trounson AO (1984) Patient management–treatment cycle. In Wood C & Trounson AO (eds) *Clinical In Vitro Fertilization,* pp 49–66. New York: Springer.

McNatty KP (1981) *The selection of an ovarian follicle for ovulation: some speculations on the underlying mechanisms of action.* Universitaire Pers Leiden.

McNatty KP, Sawers RS & McNeilly AS (1974) A possible role for prolactin in control of steroid secretion by the human Graafian follicle. *Nature* **250:** 653–655.

Messinis I, Bergh T & Wide L (1988) The importance of human chorionic gonadotropin support of the corpus luteum during human gonadotropin therapy in women with anovulatory infertility. *Fertility and Sterility* **50:** 31–35.

Muasher SJ (1988) Stimulation protocols for patients with 'atypical response' *Annals of the New York Academy of Sciences* **541:** 82–95.

Nakamura Y, Yoshimura Y, Tanabe K & Iizuka R (1986) Induction of ovulation with pulsatile subcutaneous administration of human menopausal gonadotropin in anovulatory infertile women. *Fertility and Sterility* **46:** 46–54.

Nakamura Y, Yoshimura Y, Yamada H et al (1989) Clinical experience in the induction of ovulation and pregnancy with pulsatile subcutaneous administration of human menopausal gonadotropin: a low incidence of multiple pregnancy. *Fertility and Sterility* **51:** 423–429.

Polson DW, Watsworth J, Adams J & Franks S (1988) Polycystic ovaries—a common finding in normal women. *Lancet* **i:** 870–872.

Roseff SJ, Bangah ML, Kettel LM et al (1989) Dynamic changes in circulating inhibin levels during the luteal–follicular transition of the human menstrual cycle. *Journal of Clinical Endocrinology and Metabolism* **69:** 1033–1036.

Schenker JG & Navot D (1987) Complications of induction of ovulation. In Eng-Soon T, Shan Ratnam S & Peng Cheang Wong (eds) *Advances in Fertility and Sterility, Ovulation and Early Pregnancy,* pp 53–61. London: Parthenon.

Shorham Z, Barash A, Lunenfeld B et al (1989) Prevention of unwanted LH surge by aspiration of the leading follicle in an IVF-ET program. In Tsafriri A & Dekel N (eds) *Follicular Development and the Ovulatory Response.* Serono Symposia No. 23, pp 301–306.

Westergaard LG (1988) Intrafollicular factors regulating human ovarian follicular development and oocyte meiosis. Thesis. *Danish Medical Bulletin.*

Westergaard L, Byskov AG, Andersen CY, Grinsted J & McNatty KP (1984) Is resumption of meiosis in the human preovulatory oocyte triggered by a meiosis-inducing substance (MIS) in the follicular fluid. *Fertility and Sterility* **41:** 377–384.

Williams RF & Hodgen GD (1980) Disparate effects of human chorionic gonadotropin during the late follicular phase in monkeys: normal ovulation, follicular atresia, ovarian acyclicity, and hypersection of follicle-stimulating hormone. *Fertility and Sterility* **33:** 64–68.

7

Special preparations: pure FSH and desialo-hCG

GERHARD BETTENDORF

In the 1920s it was conclusively shown that ovarian function is dependent on stimulation by pituitary gonadotrophins (Aschheim and Zondek, 1928). Two factors were described: prolan A, the follicle-stimulating principle, and prolan B, the luteinizing factor. The question arose whether these observations in rodents were applicable to the human being. Results with preparations from human pregnancy urine, were disappointing. Zondek suggested that better results could be achieved by using gonadotrophins prepared from human pituitaries or from urines of castrated or climacteric women or from pregnant mare serum. He stated that clinical results depend on the quality of the preparation and the adequacy of the dosage. Gonadotrophins from animal urine, and even more, pregnant mare serum gonadotrophin gave inconsistent results. This could be attributed to the formation of antibodies to the heterologous gonadotrophins following repeated or prolonged administration. In clinical studies it was found that human chorionic gonadotrophin (hCG) administration induced luteinization. When it was administered following spontaneous follicular maturation, ovulation could be induced and the life-span of corpora lutea prolonged.

HUMAN GONADOTROPHINS

Research based on this knowledge of species-specific gonadotrophin preparation was intensified. The first publication that deals with the preparation of gonadotrophins from the urine of menopausal women was published in 1949 by Donini (Donini, 1970). The clinical effects of this preparation were reported by Borth et al (1961). Gemzell was the first to use human pituitary extracts containing both follicle-stimulating hormone (FSH) and luteinizing hormone (LH), (Gemzell et al, 1958). We used a very simple extraction procedure to prepare a preparation from human postmortem pituitaries with varying FSH/LH ratios (Bettendorf et al, 1962). The first clinical studies by several groups resulted in the successful induction of ovulation and pregnancy with all preparations in combination with hCG (Lunenfeld et al, 1960; Buxton and Herrmann 1961; Apostolakis et al,

1962). Of special interest was the observation that a human gonadotrophin preparation could induce ovulation even in hypophysectomized patients, resulting in a pregnancy (Bettendorf et al, 1964).

Between 1960 and 1970 numerous treatment schedules were tested. It must be mentioned that at this time no reliable methods for the evaluation of the increasing ovarian reaction during a stimulation were available. In addition, very little was known about the functional events in the normal ovarian cycle. It is amazing that under these circumstances the observations in clinical studies of this time became the basis of gonadotrophin therapy, for the indications as well as for the schedule and monitoring of treatment.

Human menopausal gonadotrophin (hMG) preparations became commercially available in the late sixties: Pergonal (Serono) and Humegon (Organon). The potencies per ampoule stated by the manufacturers are based on the results of in vivo bio-assays: each ampoule contains 75 IU FSH and 75 IU LH. Donini in Serono laboratories (Rome) prepared highly purified FSH from hMG using anti-hCG antibodies to selectively bind the LH (Donini et al, 1966a, b).

FSH AND LH ACTIVITY

The FSH:LH ratio is a problem dating back to the early days of gonado-

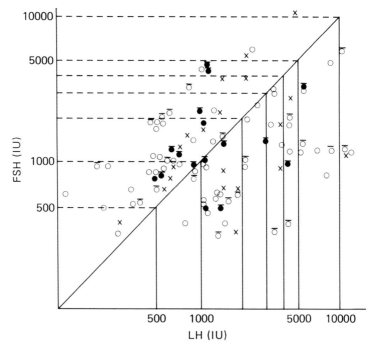

Figure 1. Range of total follicle-stimulating hormone (FSH) and luteinizing hormone (LH) doses and corresponding ovarian reaction. From Bettendorf et al (1968). (O), Ovulation; (●), pregnancy; (×), no ovulation; (−), hyperstimulation.

trophin therapy. Investigations of the role of FSH:LH ratios of hMG preparations used clinically were carried out by several people (Bettendorf et al, 1968; Jones et al, 1985; Berger et al, 1972; Bertrand et al, 1972; Rosemberg et al, 1972; Taymor 1973). The clinical effectiveness of the various gonadotrophin preparations used at that time was found to be a function of the amount of FSH activity administered. The preparations exhibited remarkable differences in FSH:LH ratios. However, a difference of more than tenfold in this ratio did not interfere with the clinical effectiveness provided that a large enough dose of FSH was given (Diczfalusy et al, 1964). Extracts of human pituitary gonadotrophins resulted in preparations with FSH:LH ratios between 0.05 and 10. With each of these preparations, ovarian stimulation could be induced (Figure 1) (Bettendorf et al, 1968).

Gonadotrophin preparations with an FSH:LH ratio of around 1 seemed to be the most suitable with respect to induction of ovulation and to incidence of hyperstimulation.

During the spontaneous ovulatory cycle, there are significant variations in the ratio of FSH to LH. In the first part of the follicular phase of the menstrual cycle, the FSH:LH ratio in serum and in urine was found to be about 2:1. In the second part of the follicular phase but before the ovulatory peak, the FSH:LH ratio is about 0.3:1. In the luteal phase, the ratio is around 1:1 and becomes greater than 1 with increasing premenstrual FSH levels. The change in FSH:LH ratio is important for normal follicular maturation and ovulation.

THE 'POLYCYSTIC OVARY SYNDROME'

In a group of patients with ovulatory dysfunction and infertility, disturbed FSH:LH ratios can be found. Mostly, the LH levels are elevated. This symptom is found in patients with a great variety of other symptoms and the patients are classified as having polycystic ovary (PCO) syndrome. Clomiphene is the drug of choice for induction of ovulation, and in the majority of patients it is successful. Only a small group respond to administration of glucocorticoids. The results of treatment with gonadotrophin-releasing hormone (GnRH) are contradictory. The treatment originally described by Stein and Leventhal (1935), wedge resection of the ovaries, should be abandoned because of the additional risks of the operation, its tendency to cause pelvic adhesions, and the poor results in terms of ovulations and pregnancies. Whether laser surgery or ovarian electrodiathermy will be effective methods remains to be seen.

Those PCO patients who do not respond to one of the drugs mentioned before become candidates for gonadotrophin treatment. However, in these women, especially, additional exogenous FSH and LH induce unpredictable alterations. Therefore, treatment of this group of patients with hMG is difficult, the results are poor, and the risk of hyperstimulation is high.

The administration of additional exogenous gonadotrophins may influence the delicate endogenous balance. Obviously this occurs predominantly in patients with spontaneous ovulatory function. The most regular response to the administration of hMG is seen in hypogonadotrophic patients, who therefore have the greatest chance of becoming pregnant with this therapy.

After purified FSH became available, a new strategy for treatment of the group of patients with an elevated LH : FS ratio could be studied. Since these women characteristically have a high endogenous LH level, they should need a substitution with FSH to correct the balance between FSH and LH. The experimental basis for clinical use of FSH to correct the biochemical imbalance in PCO is the observation that granulosa cells from patients with PCO are able to respond to FSH with conversion of androgens to oestrogens. Since these patients have high serum LH levels, giving additional LH, as was found for hMG, should be unnecessary and contribute additionally to the development of serious sequelae.

FSH THERAPY

There are two main problems in a critical examination of the efficacy of FSH therapy. The first is the selection of patients; the effect of this treatment has been studied mostly in patients who were classified in the group of PCO syndrome.

Although the diagnosis of PCO is used daily by clinicians and researchers, it is not possible to designate a concrete set of rules that can be used to identify a homogeneous group of patients with PCO. PCO is a syndrome 'with limits less well defined than those of the Sahara or Sudan' (Barbieri et al, 1988). Since the effect of purified FSH was studied mainly in those patients, one has to consider that each investigator had his own diagnostic criteria. The only symptoms which most but not all of the investigators consider relevant are elevated LH and testosterone levels. The heterogeneity of the findings after FSH administration is not, therefore, surprising, as the single classification 'PCO' is obviously based on different symptoms and never uniform (Givens, 1984; Jacobs, 1987; Seibel et al, 1985).

The second problem is monitoring of the therapy. From the long-standing experience with stimulation by hMG we know quite well that individually adjusted treatment is the only one which should be used when ovarian stimulation is indicated for infertility patients. To achieve the best clinical results and the fewest detrimental side-effects, fixed treatment schemes should be abandoned.

Results of FSH therapy

It is obvious that the clinical results of FSH therapy must be compared with those of hMG treatment. In hypogonadotrophic patients, an ovulation rate of 90% and a pregnancy rate of 60–80% can be achieved by hMG (Bettendorf et al, 1981; Zimmermann et al, 1982; Blankstein et al, 1986). The only study dealing with the effects of FSH in hypogonadotrophic patients was reported by Couzinet et al (1988). Six women had panhypopituitarism secondary to surgical removal of central nervous system tumour process and four women had congenital isolated gonadotrophin deficiency. Each woman was given both FSH and hMG. The regimen employed in the first period was randomly chosen: either FSH or hMG at a fixed dose of 225 IU FSH/day for 10 days. The women volunteered for the study to learn their ovulatory potentials; they had no immediate desire to conceive. In the hMG cycles, hCG was not administered to two cases because of ovarian hyper-stimulation, but ovulation occurred in all other cases after hCG. Following FSH, hCG was administered to nine women and ovulation occurred in six. According to the endocrine effects of the two therapeutic principles as discussed by the investigators, pharmacological doses of FSH with minute LH contamination are able to stimulate ovarian follicular maturation, underlining the key role of FSH in folliculogenesis. So far there has been no study in which FSH was used or tested in hypogonadotrophic infertile patients. The ovulation rate of 60% achieved by FSH in the study mentioned of hypogonadotrophic volunteers is lower than that after hMG. Unfortunately, a fixed dose regimen was used and the number of women studied is small.

In collected data for hMG treatment, the ovulation rate is around 80% and the pregnancy rate around 40%. These studies include patients with a variety of ovulatory dysfunctions, classified as amenorrhoea, oligomenorrhoea, anovulation, luteal phase defect, and also PCO. For selected groups of patients with so-called PCO treated with hMG, the higher risk of hyperstimulation and multiple pregnancies was mentioned. It is more difficult to monitor this subgroup, and the rate of dropout is greater. It is a general observation that the results in investigative studies are always better than those that can be achieved in routine clinical use.

The patients selected for treatment with FSH in all studies were diagnosed as having PCO, but it must be remembered that this classification is not uniform (Table 1). The treatment schedules were: individually adjusted, fixed dosage, pulsatile FSH or FSH following GnRH-A pretreatment. The GnRH-A and FSH combined treatments and those in which no hCG was administered must be discussed separately. In the other treatments, the ovulation rate ranged from 45 to 90%, the pregnancy rate in most of the studies 20 to 30%. Lower pregnancy rates were found in the studies in which FSH administration was pulsatile or in fixed dosage. We know that this schedule is less effective in hMG therapy too. The incidence of ovarian hyperstimulation (OHS) is not given by all the authors. It can happen in up to 40% of the cycles. The number of pregnancies is too small for calculation of the multiple pregnancies. The number given is 26–28% of all pregnancies.

The largest study of FSH stimulation was reported by Birkhäuser (personal communication, 1989). FSH treatment was given to 40 patients, who were carefully classified: long-standing infertility, secondary amenorrhoea or oligomenorrhoea with anovulation, clomiphene-resistant, elevated testosterone, elevated LH : FSH (>2) and no other female or male infertility factors. In contrast to other studies, most of the patients were treated more than once. The mean number of treatments was 2.2. Twenty-three pregnancies were achieved, that is 57% per patient and 25.8% per cycle. The

Table 1. Results of follicle-stimulating hormone (FSH) therapy.

Reference	Diagnosis	Treatment	Number of patients	Number of cycles	Ovulations n/cycle (%)	Pregnancies n/cycle (%)	OHS n (%)	Multiple n (%)
Braendle et al, 1985	Clomiphene failure hyperandrogenism LH:FSH >2	Individual high-dose FSH + hMG	18 9 5	25 23 10	22 (88) 12 (52) 9 (90)	6 (24) 0 0	1 (4) 0 0	0 – –
Flamigni et al, 1985	PCO	Individual	21	25	22 (88)	8 (32)	10 (40)	–
Garcea et al, 1985	PCO	Individual	18	43	39 (90)	9 (21)	9 (21)	–
Hoffmann et al, 1985	Anovulation clomiphene failure	Fixed dosage	15	16		4 (25)	0	–
Seibel et al, 1985	PCO, amenorrhoea elevated LH	Fixed dosage	10	11	5 (45)	1 (9)	0	0
Murdock et al, 1985	Amenorrhoea PCO, clomiphene failure	Pulsatile	5	8	4 (50)	1 (12)	2 (25)	?
Claman et al, 1985	PCO LH:FSH >2.5	Individual with hCG	4	8	8 (100)	3 (38)	0	?
Lanzone et al, 1987	PCO LH:FSH >2.5	GnRH-A–FSH fixed dosage	5 16	5 31	5 (100) ?	3 (60) 7 (22)	? 8 (25)	1 1

Author	Indication	Protocol						
Ayalon et al, 1988	PCO LH:FSH >1.5 testosterone >1 ng	GnRH-A FSH individual	17	17	15 (88)	7 (41)	14 (82)	2 (28)
Birkhäuser et al, 1988	PCO, clomiphene failure LH:FSH >2	Individual	30	68	54 (79)	17 (25)	13 (19)	5 (29)
Butt, 1988	PCO	Individual	9	22	19 (86)	4 (18)	0	?
Couzinet et al, 1988	Hypogonadotrophic panhypopituitarism	Fixed	10	10	6 (60)	–	–	–
Franks et al, 1988	PCO	Pulsatile	10	33	23 (69)	6 (18)	?	?
Birkhäuser, personal communication	PCO LH:FSH >2 elevated testosterone	Individual	40	89	74 (83)	23 (26)	9 (10)	6 (26)
		GnRH-A-FSH	10	17	14 (82)	7 (41)	2 (11)	2 (28)
Buvat et al, 1989	PCO elevated LH + testosterone	Individual conventional	17	21	?	2 (9,5)	?	0
		slow protocol	23	44	?	7 (15,9)	?	0
Quartero et al, 1989	PCO, clomiphene failure LH:FSH >3	Fixed	12	16	?	2 (12)	5 (31)	?
		Pulsatile		15	?	?	?	?

OHS, ovarian hyperstimulation; LH, luteinizing hormone; hMG, human menopausal gonadotrophin; PCO, polycystic ovary syndrome; GnRH-A, gonadotrophin-releasing hormone-analogue.

Table 2. Results of follicle-stimulating hormone (FSH) in in vitro fertilization (IVF) and gamete intrafallopian transfer (GIFT)

References	Treatment	Number of patients	Number of cycles	Number of pregnancies/cycle (%)
Jones et al, 1985	IVF, fixed dosage	12	12	5 (41)
Polan et al, 1986	IVF, fixed dosage	15	15	6 (40)
Neveu et al, 1987	IVF, fixed dosage	10	10	1 (10)
	GnRH-A–FSH	10	10	6 (60)
Scoccia et al, 1987	IVF, fixed dosage	16	23	3 (13)
Benadiva et al, 1988	IVF, FSH + hMG	45	39	7 (17, 9)
Bentick et al, 1988	IVF, GnRH-A–FSH	13	13	5 (38)
Brzyski et al, 1988	IVF/GnRH-A–FSH	12	12	1 (8, 3)
Lavy et al, 1988	IVF, FSH individual	20	20	2 (10)
Palermo et al, 1988	IVF, GnRH-A–FSH + hMG	8	8	4 (33)
	GIFT, individual	4	4	
Grillo et al, 1989	IVF, GnRH-A individual	63	63	12 (19)
Remorgida et al, 1989	GIFT, GnRH-A short individual FSH	82	87	25 (30)
	GnRH-A long individual FSH	96	96	31 (32)

GnRH-A, gonadotrophin-releasing hormone A; hMG, human menopausal gonadotrophin.

ovulation rate was 83%. These figures are similar to those for 30 patients treated by the same authors (Birkhäuser et al, 1988). The incidences of OHS in these studies were 19 and 10%. Multiple pregnancies occurred in 29 and 26%.

In three studies FSH administration was pulsatile, and the pregnancy rate reported was 6.6 and 18% per cycle (Murdoch et al, 1985; Franks et al, 1988; Quartero et al, 1989).

In the study by Claman (1986) ten patients were stimulated with FSH but no hCG was administered additionally. In 28 cycles, nine ovulations and three pregnancies occurred.

Of special interest is the combination of GnRH-A followed by FSH. The administration of GnRH-A induces a hypogonadotrophic state. The pregnancy rates in all three studies were significantly higher than those mentioned before: in two studies 41% and in one study 60% per cycle (Table 1). The authors of these three studies give no convincing explanations for the higher success rate. They refer to the detrimental effects of LH during folliculogenesis and the premature LH increase. A better success rate could also be achieved with the combination GnRH-A and hMG (Bettendorf et al, 1986, 1990).

FSH for superovulation

Recently, there has been interest in the use of FSH for inducing super-ovulation in ovulatory women scheduled for in vitro fertilization (IVF) or gamete intrafallopian transfer (GIFT) (Table 2). The results published so far are difficult to compare because of the small number of patients treated and the various treatment protocols. Jones et al (1985) and Polan et al (1986) reported pregnancy rates of 40 and 41%. In all the other studies, the pregnancy rate has been below 20%.

Several investigators used the combination of GnRH-A followed by FSH for IVF. Here again, in most studies the pregnancy rate was high. Only in one study was it 8.3% (Brzyski et al, 1988), and in three reports it was around 30% (Bentick et al, 1988, Palermo et al, 1988, Remorgida et al, 1989) and in one even 60% (Neveu et al, 1987). It is useless to compare the other data of these studies, because there were many differences in the treatment modalities.

Conclusion

To date, it is still very difficult to judge the value of FSH for treatment of infertility patients. The results must be compared with the well-documented data for hMG treatment. The endocrine data obtained during FSH stimulation are very interesting, but there are no hard data that definitely support the efficacy of FSH as being superior to that of hMG. It is always difficult to test a new technique when effective therapeutic tools are already available. Therefore it will be difficult to perform a well-controlled, double-blind study to settle the issue. It is a general observation that the results in investigations are always better than those that can be achieved in routine clinical use. The data for the combination treatment GnRH-A and FSH are of special interest, but those studies also have to be compared with GnRH-A and hMG protocols.

DESIALO-hCG FOR INDUCTION OF OVULATION

The final stimulus for ovulation is a well-timed LH surge. This impulse is controlled by appropriate oestrogen levels produced by the 'full-term' follicle. In exogenous gonadotrophin-stimulated follicular maturation, an intact pituitary function also reacts with an endogenous spontaneous LH surge and ovulation is induced. In clinical studies it was found that the pregnancy rate following hMG treatment without an additional exogenous LH stimulus was low (Apostolakis et al, 1962; Bettendorf and Lehmann, 1977). The same observation was made in patients who were treated with hMG for IVF (Claman et al, 1986). The exact time of the LH increase is difficult to detect, and proper timing of follicle puncture will be difficult.

hCG is LH-like in its biological effect and can be used for induction of ovulation either when there has been spontaneous follicular maturation without a succeeding LH surge or following hMG stimulation of follicular growth. LH and hCG, however, differ in many ways; the half-life of hCG is much longer than that of LH, and the metabolic clearance rate of LH is about ten times that of hCG. Therefore, it is possible that such undesired side-effects of hMG–hCG therapy as overstimulation and multiple pregnancies are a consequence of the long-lasting luteinizing effect of hCG.

hCG, produced by the trophoblast in large amounts, plays a decisive role in the maintenance of early pregnancy by supporting the function of the corpus luteum as a progesterone producer. The corpus luteum contains specific high-affinity receptors for hCG. The extensive homology of the amino acid sequences of human lutropin (hLH) and hCG allows hCG to be used as an alternative to LH. Both hormones bind to the same receptor. hCG is a glycoprotein with a molecular weight of 38000 daltons and a carbohydrate content of about 33%. The hormone-specific β-subunit and the α-subunit, identical with those of the other gonadotrophins and thyroid-stimulating hormone (TSH), are non-covalently bound.

There is a surprising similarity between 94 of the original 115 amino acids of the hCG β-chain and LH-β. A unique property of the polypeptide core of hCG-β is the presence of an additional 30 amino acids. The carbohydrates (in total 55–60 sugar residues per hCG molecule) are covalently bound to the protein core via eight side-chains. The carbohydrate chains are predominantly terminated by N-acetylneuraminic acid (NANA), responsible for the relatively acidic isoelectric point range of hCG, for the longer half-life than hLH, and for protection against enzymatic digestion by liver cells. Finally, NANA is the main source of the microheterogeneity of hCG (Graesslin et al, 1973) (Figure 2).

Different attempts of modification have shown that a number of amino acid and carbohydrate residues or regions of the structure are important in

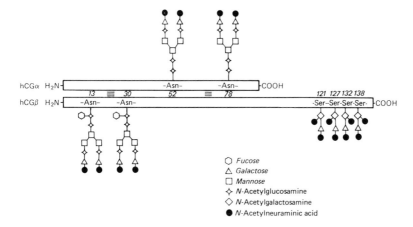

Figure 2. Structure of human chorionic gonadotrophin (hCG).

receptor interaction and subsequent response. One of the most interesting modification was for the terminal residues of the carbohydrate side-chains: NANA. It is known (Hall et al, 1971) that removal of NANA from hCG results in a drastically reduced half-life in blood, leading to apparent inactivation in long-term in vivo assays. In vitro responses, however, including cyclic AMP (cAMP) production and steroidogenesis, are largely retained. There are studies showing differences in the ratio of biological to immunological activity for forms of hCG that contain different amounts of NANA. After complete deglycosylation, however, there is an enhanced ability to bind to the receptor, and the potency for stimulating cAMP and steroid production is drastically reduced (Sairam and Manjunath, 1985).

These data strongly indicate an important functional role for the carbohydrates in hCG. Desialylated hCG was prepared by Donini with neuraminidase. The half-life of native hCG in the human was found to be 215 min and that of partially desialylated hCG 75 min (Crosignani et al, 1982). Two clinical studies were performed with this preparation. Ten patients with secondary normogonadotrophic amenorrhoea (four), secondary hypogonadotrophic amenorhoea (one), anovulatory cycles (four) and luteal insufficiency (one) entered the first study (Bettendorf and Leidenberger, 1975). hMG was administered according to individual response. DesialohCG was injected at a dose of 10 000 IU when appropriate oestrogen levels were reached. Ovulation occurred in all cycles and three patients became pregnant (Figure 3). Ovarian enlargement occurred in the conception cycle and also in others.

In the second study (Crosignani et al, 1980), 24 patients with primary (five) or secondary (nine) hypogonadotrophic, normoprolactinaemic amenorrhoea were treated with hMG. Desialo-hCG was administered when the oestrogen levels were in the range of 400–600 pg/ml. In 39 cycles, 31 ovulations and five pregnancies occurred. Two of the patients had single pregnancies, one a twin pregnancy and two aborted, one of them aborting triplets. No clinical signs of hyperstimulation were seen.

These schedules with desialo-hCG tried to mimic the physiological events occurring around ovulation. Similar clinical studies have been performed with human LH (Bettendorf et al, 1970; Neale and Bettendorf, 1970; Vande Wiele et al, 1970; Rosemberg et al, 1972; Jewelewicz, 1973). Although small numbers of patients were studied, it could be shown that after adequate stimulation with an FSH/LH preparation, hLH administration was followed by ovulation and corpus luteum formation. Some pregnancies occurred.

For both of the new treatments—desialo-hCG and hLH—the clinical efficiency was investigated only in small numbers of patients. It might be worthwhile to carry out well-designed studies in selected groups of patients to evaluate the theoretically indicated advantage over the effects of hCG.

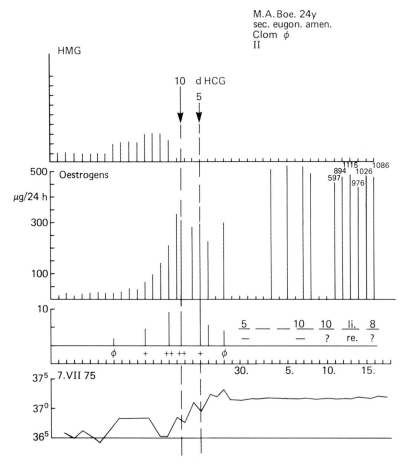

Figure 3. Ovarian stimulation with hMG followed by desialylated human chorionic gonadotrophin (dHCG) in a patient with secondary amenorrhoea, resulting in ovulation and pregnancy.

REFERENCES

Apostolakis M, Bettendorf G & Voigt KD (1962) Klinisch-experimentelle Studien mit menschlichem hypophysärem Gonadotropin. *Acta Endocrinologica* **41**: 14–30.

Aschheim MF & Zondek KM (1928) Das Hormon des Hypophysenvorderlappens. Darstellung, chemische Eigenschaft, biologische Wirkungen. *Klinische Wochenschrift* **7**: 831–835.

Ayalon D, Ben-David M, Wohl R et al (1988) Induction of ovulation with D-Trip^6-LHRH combined with purified FSH in patients with polycystic ovarian disease. *Gynecological Endocrinology* **2**: 319–330.

Barbieri RL, Smith S & Ryan KJ (1988) The role of hyperinsulinemia in the pathogenesis of ovarian hyperandrogenism. *Fertility and Sterility* **50**: 197–212.

Benadiva CA, Ben-Rafel Z, Blasco L, Tureck R, Mastroianni L Jr & Flickinger GL (1988) An increased initial follicle-stimulating hormone/luteinizing hormone ratio does not affect ovarian responses and the outcomes of in vitro fertilization. *Fertility and Sterility* **50**: 771–781.

Bentick B, Shaw RW, Iffland CA, Burford G & Bernard A (1988) A randomized comparative study of purified follicle stimulating hormone and human menopausal gonadotropin after pituitary desensitization with Buserelin for superovulation and in vitro fertilization. *Fertility and Sterility* **50**(1): 79–84.

Berger MJ & Taymor ML (1973) The relative roles of follicle stimulating hormone (FSH) and luteinizing hormone (LH) in ovarian function. In Rosemberg E (ed.) *Gonadotropin Therapy in Female Infertility*, pp 161–167. Amsterdam: Excerpta Medica.

Berger JJ, Taymor ML, Karam K & Nudemberg F (1972) The relative roles of exogenous and endogenous follicle stimulating hormone (FSH) and luteinizing hormone (LH) in human follicular maturation and ovulation induction. *Fertility and Sterility* **23**: 783.

Bertrand PV, Coleman JR, Crooke AC, MacNaughton MC & Mills IH (1972) Human ovarian response to gonadotrophins with different ratios of follicle-stimulating hormone:luteinizing hormone assessed by different parameters. *Journal of Endocrinology* **53**: 231–248.

Bettendorf G & Leidenberger F (1975) Use of desialo-hCG in induction of ovulation. In Crosignani PG and Mischell DR (eds) *Ovulation in the Human*, pp 289–293. London, New York, San Francisco: Academic Press.

Bettendorf G & Lehmann F (1977) Hormonal treatment of female infertility. in Diczfalusy E (ed.) *Regulation of Human Fertility*, p 155. Copenhagen: Scriptor.

Bettendorf G, Apostolakis M & Voigt KD (1962) Darstellung von Gonadotropin aus menschlichen Hypophysen. *Acta Endocrinologica* **41**: 1–13.

Bettendorf G, Breckwoldt M, Knörr K & Stegner HE (1964) Gravidität nach Hypophysektomie und Behandlung mit hypophysärem Humangonadotropin. *Deutsche Medizinische Wochenschrift* **41**: 1952–1957.

Bettendorf G, Breckwoldt M & Neale Ch (1968) FSH and LH dose response relationship in ovulation induction with human gonadotropins. In Rosemberg E (ed.) *Gonadotropins*, pp 453–458. Los Altos, CA: Geron-X Inc.

Bettendorf G, Breckwoldt M & Neale Ch (1970) Erfahrungen mit Human Hypophysären Gonadotropinen (hHG) *Acta Endocrinologica* **Supplement 148**: 102–125.

Bettendorf G, Braendle W, Sprotte Ch, Weise Ch & Zimmermann R (1981) Overall results of gonadotropin therapy. In Insler V & Bettendorf G (eds) *Advances in Diagnosis and Treatment of Infertility*, pp 21–26. New York, Amsterdam, Oxford: Elsevier North-Holland.

Bettendorf G, Braendle W, Sprotte Ch, Poels W, Lichtenberg V & Lindner C (1986) Pharmacologic hypogonadotropism—an advantage for hMG-induced follicular maturation and succeeding fertilization. *Hormone and Metabolic Research* **18**: 656–657.

Bettendorf G, Braendle W, Lindner Ch, Lichtenberg V, Luckhardt M & Schlotfeld T (1990) Pharmacological hypogonadotropism can be used to advantage for ovulation induction protocols. In Vickery BH and Lunenfeld B (eds) *GnRH Analogues in Reproduction and Gynecology*, pp 89–100. Dordrecht, Boston, London: Kluwer Academic Publishers.

Birkhäuser MH, Huber PR, Neuenschwander E & Näpflin S (1988) Induktion der Follikelreifung mit 'reinem' FSH beim polyzystischen Ovar Syndrom. *Geburtshilfe und Frauenheilkunde* **4**: 203–284.

Blankstein J, Mashiach S & Lunenfeld B (1986) *Ovulation Induction and In vitro Fertilization*. Chicago, London: Year Book Medical Publishers.

Borth R, Lunenfeld B & Menzi A (1961) Pharmacologic and clinical effects of a gonadotropin preparation from human postmenopausal urine. In Albert A (ed.) *Human Pituitary Gonadotropins*, pp 13–72. Springfield, Illinois: Charles C. Thomas.

Braendle W, Sprotte C & Bettendorf G (1985) Gonadotropinbehandlung bei Ovarial-insuffizienz, Stimulation der Follikelreifung mit humanem urinären FSH. *Geburtshilfe und Frauenheilkunde* **45**: 438–448.

Brzyski R, Muasher SJ, Droesch K, Simonetti S, Jones GS & Rosenwak Z (1988) Follicular atresia associated with concurrent initiation of gonadotropin-releasing hormone agonist and follicle-stimulating hormone for oocyte recruitment. *Fertility and Sterility* **50(6)**: 917–921.

Butt WR (1988) Gonadotropins in the treatment of infertility. *Acta Endocrinologica* **288**: 51–57.

Buvat JM, Buvat-Herbaut M, Marcollin G, Dehaene JL, Verbecq P & Renouard O (1989) Purified follicle-stimulating hormone in polycystic ovary syndrome: slow administration is safer and more effective. *Fertility and Sterility* **52(4)**: 553–559.

Buxton CL & Herrmann W (1961) Induction of ovulation in the human with human gonadotropins. *American Journal of Obstetrics and Gynecology* **81**: 584–590.

Claman P, Seibel MM, McArdle C, Berger MJ & Taymor ML (1986) Comparison of intermediate-dose purified urinary follicle-stimulating hormone with and without human chorionic gonadotropin for ovulation induction in polycystic ovarian disease. *Fertility and Sterility* **46(3)**: 518–521.

Couzinet B, Lestrat N, Brailly S, Forest M & Schaison G (1988) Stimulation of ovarian follicular maturation with pure follicle-stimulating hormone in women with gonadotropin deficiency. *Journal of Clinical Endocrinology and Metabolism* **66(3)**: 552–556.

Crosignani PG, Donini P, Lombroso GC, Dorini S, Caccamao A & Trojsi L (1980) Preparation of a partially desialylated human chorionic gonadotrophin (hCG) and its use for induction of ovulation after ovarian stimulation with human menopausal gonadotrophin. *Acta Endocrinologica* **95**: 232–236.

Crosignani PG, Donini P, Lombroso GC, Donini S, Caccamo A & Trojsi L (1982) Induction of ovulation with desialo-hCG. In Flamigni C & Givens JR (eds) *The Gonadotropins: Basic Science and Clinical Aspects in Females*, Serono Symposium No. 42, pp 451–456. London, New York: Academic Press.

Diczfalusy E, Johannisson E, Tillinger KG & Bettendorf G (1964) Comparison of the clinical and steroid metabolic effect of human pituitary and urinary gonadotrophins in amenorrhoeic women. *Acta Endocrinologica* **45 (supplement 90)**: 35–56.

Donini P (1970) Preparations and biological characteristics of hMG preparations used clinically. In Rosenberg CA & Paulsen E (eds) *The Human Testis*, pp 277–287. New York, London: Plenum.

Donini P & Montezemolo (1949) Gonadotropina preipofisaria e gonadotropina preipofiso-simile umana. *La Rassegna di Clinica Terapia e Scienze Affine* **48**: 143–163.

Donini P, Puzzuoli D, D'Alessio I, Lunenfeld B, Eshkol A & Parlow AF (1966a) Purification and separation of follicle stimulating hormone (FSH) and luteinizing hormone (LH) from human postmenopausal gonadotrophin (hMG). I. Separation of FSH and LH by electrophoresis, chromatography and gel filtration procedures. *Acta Endocrinologica* **52**: 169–185.

Donini P, Puzzuoli D, D'Alessio I, Lunenfeld B, Eshkol A & Parlow AF (1966b) Purification and separation of follicle stimulating hormone (FSH) and luteinizing hormone (LH) from human postmenopausal gonadotrophin (hMG). II. Preparation of biological apparently pure FSH by selective binding of the LH with an anti-HCG serum and subsequent chromatography. *Acta Endocrinologica* **52**: 186–198.

Flamigni C, Venturoli S, Paradisi R, Fabbri R, Porcu E, Magrini O (1985) Use of human urinary follicle-stimulating hormone in infertile women with polycystic ovaries. *The Journal of Reproductive Medicine* **30**: 184–188.

Franks S, Mason HD, Polson DW, Winston RML, Margara R & Reed MJ (1988) Mechanism and management of ovulatory failure in women with polycystic ovary syndrome. *Human Reproduction* **3(4)**: 531–534.

Garcea N, Campo S, Panetta V et al (1985) Induction of ovulation with purified urinary follicle-stimulating hormone in patients with polycystic ovarian syndrome. *American Journal of Obstetrics and Gynecology* **151:** 635–640.

Gemzell C, Diczfalusy E & Tillinger KG (1958) Clinical effect of human pituitary follicle stimulating hormone (FSH). *Journal of Clinical Endocrinology and Metabolism* **18:** 1333–1348.

Givens JR (1984) Polycystic ovaries—a sign, not a diagnosis. *Seminars in Reproductive Endocrinology* **2:** 271–280.

Graesslin D, Weise HC & Braendle W (1973) The microheterogeneity of hCG and its subunits. *FEBS Letters* **31:** 214–217.

Grillo M, Buck S, Freys I & Mettler L (1989) Results of the use of a pure urinary FSH stimulating regime in patients unsuccessfully treated with hMG in an in vitro fertilization program. *Gynecological and Obstetric Investigations* **28:** 169–173.

Hoffman D, Lobo RA, Campeau JD et al (1985) Ovulation induction in clomiphene-resistant anovulatory women: differential follicular response to purified urinary follicle-stimulating hormone (FSH) versus purified urinary FSH and luteinizing hormone. *Journal of Clinical Endocrinology and Metabolism* **60:** 922–927.

Jacobs HS (1987) Polycystic ovaries and polycystic ovary syndrome. *Gynecological Endocrinology* **1:** 113–131.

Jewelewicz R (1973) In Rosemberg E (ed.) *Gonadotropin Therapy in Female Infertility*, general discussion, p 250. Amsterdam: Excerpta Medica.

Jones GS, Acosta AA, Garcia JE, Bernardus RE & Rosenwaks Z (1985) The effect of follicle-stimulating hormone without additional luteinizing hormone on follicular stimulation and oocyte development in normal ovulatory women. *Fertility and Sterility* **43(5):** 696–702.

Lanzone A, Fulghesu AM, Spina MA, Apa R, Minini E & Caruso A (1987) Successful induction of ovulation and conception with combined gonadotropin-releasing hormone agonist plus highly purified follicle-stimulating hormone in patients with polycystic ovarian disease. *Journal of Clinical Endocrinology and Metabolism* **65:** 1253–1258.

Lavy G, Pellicer A, Diamond MP & DeCherney AH (1988) Ovarian stimulation for in vitro fertilization and embryo transfer, human menopausal gonadotropin versus pure human follicle stimulating hormone: a randomized prospective study. *Fertility and Sterility* **50(1):** 74–78.

Lunenfeld B, Menzie A & Volet B (1960) Clinical effects of human post menopausal gonadotrophins. *Acta Endocrinologica* **Supplement 51:** 587.

Murdoch A, White MC, Kendall-Taylor P, Dunlop W & Rose P (1985) Purified FSH in the induction of ovulation in women with PCOS. *Journal of Endocrinology* **Supplement 104:** abstract 40.

Neale Ch & Bettendorf G (1970) Comparison of the results of gonadotropin therapy under various conditions. In Bettendorf G & Insler V (eds) *Clinical Application of Human Gonadotropins*. Workshop Conference, Hamburg, p 21. Stuttgart: Georg Thieme.

Neveu S, Hedon B, Bringer J et al (1987) Ovarian stimulation by a combination of a gonadotropin-releasing hormone agonist and gonadotropins for in vitro-fertilization. *Fertility and Sterility* **47(4):** 639–643.

Palermo R, Amodeo G, Navot D, Rosenwaks Z & Cittadini E (1988) Concomitant gonadotropin-releasing hormone agonist and menotropin treatment for the synchronized induction of multiple follicles. *Fertility and Sterility* **49(2):** 290–295.

Polan ML, Daniele A, Russell JB & DeCherney AH (1986) Ovulation induction with human menopausal gonadotropin compared to human urinary follicle-stimulating hormone results in a significant shift in follicular fluid androgen levels without discernible differences in granulosa-luteal cell function. *Journal of Clinical Endocrinology and Metabolism* **63(6):** 1284–1291.

Quartero HWP, Dixon JE, Westwood O, Hicks B & Chapman MG (1989) Ovulation induction in polycystic ovarian disease by pure FSH (Metrodin)—a comparison between chronic low-dose pulsatile administration and i.m. injections. *Human Reproduction* **4(3):** 247–249.

Remorgida V, Anserini P, Croce S et al (1989) The duration of pituitary suppression by means of intranasal gonadotropin hormone-releasing hormone analogue administration does not influence the ovarian response to gonadotropin stimulation and success rate in a gamete intrafallopian transfer (GIFT) program. *Journal of in vitro Fertilisation and Embryo Transfer* **6(2):** 76–80.

Rosemberg E, Lee SG & Butler PS (1972) Induction of ovulation. In Saxena BB, Beling CG & Gandy HM (eds) *Gonadotropins*, pp 704–729. New York, London, Sydney, Toronto: Wiley Interscience.

Sairam MR & Manjunath P (1985) Hormonal antagonistic properties of chemically deglycosylated human choriogonadotropin. *Journal of Biological Chemistry* **258:** 445–449.

Scoccia B, Blumenthal P, Wagner C, Prins G, Scommegna A & Marut E (1987) Comparison of urinary human follicle-stimulating hormone and human menopausal gonadotropins for ovarian stimulation in an in vitro fertilization program. *Fertility and Sterility* **48(3):** 446–449.

Seibel MM (1984) Toward understanding the pathophysiology and treatment of polycystic ovary disease. *Seminars in Reproductive Endocrinology* **2:** 297–304.

Seibel MM, McArdle C, Smith D & Taymor ML (1985) Ovulation induction in polycystic ovary syndrome with urinary follicle-stimulating hormone or human menopausal gonadotropin. *Fertility and Sterility* **43(5):** 703–708.

Stein IF & Leventhal ML (1935) Amenorrhea associated with bilateral polycystic ovaries. *American Journal of Obstetrics and Gynecology* **29:** 181–191.

Taymor ML (1973) Induction of ovulation with gonadotropins. *Clinical Obstetrics and Gynecology* **16:** 201–220.

Van de Wiele RJ, Bogumil J, Dyrenfurth I et al (1970) Mechanisms regulating the menstrual cycle in women. *Recent Progress in Hormone Research* **26:** 63–103.

van Hall E, Vaitukaitis JL, Ross GF, Hickman JW & Ashwell G (1971) Immunological and biological activity of hCG following progressive desialytion. *Endocrinology* **88:** 456–464.

WHO Scientific Group (1973) *Agents stimulating gonadal function in the human.* World Health Organization Technical Report Series, No. 514.

Zimmermann R, Soor B, Braendle W, Lehmann F, Weise HC & Bettendorf G (1982) Gonadotropin therapy of female infertility. Analysis of results in 416 cases. *Gynecological and Obstetric Investigation* **14:** 1–18.

8

Programming ovulation

R. FRYDMAN

The first births after in vitro fertilization (IVF) were obtained with ova collected in the spontaneous cycle (Steptoe and Edwards, 1978), but the constant availability of the entire IVF team was not well compensated, since only one oocyte was obtained in even the best cases. The development of ovarian stimulation made it possible to have simultaneous growth of several follicles. Ovulation induction with human chorionic gonadotrophin (hCG) allowed oocyte retrieval to be performed approximately 34 h later. The ideal stimulation is that which gives the maximum number of fertilizable oocytes, but without disruption of the luteal phase so as to obtain a high percentage of ongoing pregnancies.

Several therapeutic regimens for follicular stimulation, using varying combinations of gonadotrophins with or without clomiphene citrate, have been proposed (Garcia et al, 1983; Lopata, 1983).

Until now it has been widely believed that IVF success can be maximized by individualized controlled ovarian hyperstimulation regimens tailored to the patient's requirements (Taymor et al, 1985; Yee and Vargyas, 1986). Most protocols for ovarian stimulation for in vitro fertilization and embryo transfer (IVF-ET) or gamete intrafallopian transfer (GIFT) start at the beginning of a natural cycle and may result in the need to do ovum pick-up, fertilization, and gamete or embryo transfer during the weekend. A further disadvantage of classical stimulation treatment is the necessity for fairly intensive monitoring of follicular growth to select the most appropriate time for hCG administration. This considerably disrupts the patient's domestic and professional life, not to speak of the lives of the IVF unit staff. The hormone treatment preceding IVF is stressful to patients and their partners. The treatment is accompanied by daily blood sampling and ultrasonic examination, with all the stress involved in whether or not the follicle stimulation will come up to expectations. Many patients consider this phase stressful for other reasons, too, which may have unfavourable effects on the neuroendocrine system (Kemeter et al, 1986).

An acceptable recovery rate of preovulatory eggs can be obtained by a fixed schedule of ovulation induction and follicular aspiration, based on the ideas of Templeton et al (1984) and Braude et al (1984). The main advantage of this protocol is that treatment need not be matched to the patient's cycle, but the cycle may be adjusted to the patient's and treatment team's time plan. The stimulation treatment, as such, is completely defined and may be carried out by the established specialist or by the general practitioner. Determination of hormones is unnecessary, and patient and partner must appear at the IVF centre only a short time before follicle puncture.

In 1986 we proposed (Frydman et al, 1986a) programmed oocyte retrieval during routine laparoscopy. Fixed-schedule ovulation induction and cryopreservation of the embryos obtained was performed for women undergoing preliminary laparoscopy for infertility investigation before possible inclusion in an in vitro fertilization programme. The cycle before follicular stimulation was modified by a progestogen (P) or an oestrogen–progestogen (EP) contraceptive pill. Ovarian inaccessibility prevented follicular aspiration for four of an original group of 34 patients, but at least one oocyte was obtained from 29 of the remaining 30. Although fewer oocytes were obtained from these patients than from a control group (C) being treated for in vitro fertilization, one or more embryos were obtained from 22 patients of the study group (Table 1). All embryos were frozen, and to date 25 embryos from 17

Table 1. Results per patient for the control group (group C) and the two programme groups (groups P and EP).

	Group C (n = 30)	Group P (n = 13)	Group EP (n = 17)
Follicles per patient	4.77 ± 0.32*−**	3.23 ± 0.28*	2.80 ± 0.36**
Oocytes per patient	3.67 ± 0.37*	2.46 ± 0.31	1.76 ± 0.28*
Embryos per patient	2.23 ± 0.32*	1.30 ± 0.33	0.88 ± 0.17*

* $P < 0.01$.
** $P < 0.001$.

patients have been thawed. Embryos have been placed in 16 of the 17 patients and six pregnancies have been initiated. Three have delivered, one ectopic pregnancy occurred, and two pregnancies were classified as 'chemical'. Programmed oocyte retrieval and embryo cryopreservation resulted in an extra chance of pregnancy for patients undergoing laparoscopy for infertility investigation.

We then proposed to use the programmed oocyte retrieval (POR) for our patients in the IVF programme (Frydman et al, 1986b). We decided to analyse one year's experience with POR and compare the results with those for all cases of classically monitored ovarian stimulation performed during the same time period (Rainhorn et al, 1987). These data add to our previous reports and indicate the practical application of this technique to a large series of unselected patients.

POR was originally proposed to facilitate the process of follicular stimulation for in vitro fertilization. Accumulated experience indicates that this goal has been achieved, since 88% of patients had oocyte retrieval performed on the day determined 2–3 months in advance. Only one blood sample for hormonal assay—oestradiol (E_2) and luteinizing hormone (LH)—was necessary prior to the decision to administer hCG. There was no major disruption of the patient's domestic or professional life prior to her entry into the hospital for oocyte retrieval, and this was achieved without

Table 2. Ovarian response to two regimens of follicular stimulation: comparison between classical and programmed ovarian stimulation.

	Monitored IVF cycles	Programmed IVF cycles
1. E_2 (at the time of hCG injection)	$1781 \pm 46^*$	$954 \pm 46^*$
2. Follicles/AOR	4.95 ± 0.15	4.85 ± 0.23
3. Mature oocytes/AOR	2.74 ± 0.11	2.42 ± 0.13
4. Embryos/AOR	2.07 ± 0.09	1.93 ± 0.11

E_2, oestradiol; IVF, in vitro fertilization; hCG, human chorionic gonadotrophin; AOR, attempts oocyte retrieval.
* $P < 0.01$.

Table 3. Comparison of pregnancy rates after transfer of fresh frozen–thawed embryos.

	Monitored IVF cycles	Programmed IVF cycles
Cycles	356	296
Pregnancies	50	41
Ongoing pregnancies	35	30
Ongoing pregnancies/cycle	9.8% (35/356)	10.1% (30/296)
Ongoing pregnancies/puncture	11.4% (35/308)	12.5% (30/240)
Ongoing pregnancies/ transferred patient	14.6% (35/239)	18.1% (30/165)

IVF, in vitro fertilization.

diminishing the clinical efficacy of the IVF programme (Tables 2 and 3). In addition, POR considerably facilitated administration of the IVF programme. Oocyte retrievals are scheduled for 4 days each week and resources, both human and material, are allocated accordingly.

The technique and results of POR have been reproduced in other IVF centres. A recent report describes a similar method of pretreatment with norethisterone followed by fixed-schedule ovulation induction (Wardle et al, 1986). In that study, as in our previous one (Frydman et al, 1986a), the day of oocyte retrieval was not changed and patients with inadequate follicular maturation on the day scheduled for hCG administration were cancelled. Although their technique differs slightly from ours, the pregnancy rate appears to have been comparable. Others have used a contraceptive pill to modify the date of menstruation for the IVF treatment cycle.

A new fixed schedule of ovarian stimulation for IVF was developed (Kemeter and Feichtinger, 1989), one that is not only simpler and easier for the patients to handle but also gives better fertilization and pregnancy rates. The period and the start of stimulation are shifted by a contraceptive pill so that stimulation is generally started on a Sunday. The patient takes clomiphene (100 mg) for 5 days and prednisolone (7.5 mg) for 30 days to suppress possible exaggerated adrenal androgen secretion and is given 150 IU human menopausal gonadotrophin (hMG) intramuscularly every other day by her doctor at home. From the 8th day of stimulation onward follicular growth is recorded by daily ultrasound at the IVF centre. A dose of 5000 IU hCG is given when the dominant follicle exceeds 18 mm in diameter.

First, unlike us (Frydman et al, 1986b), they give a low standard dose of a combined contraceptive pill rather than progestogen alone during the cycle prior to IVF, to achieve withdrawal bleeding before stimulation with a greater degree of certainty. Second, the interval between the last pill and the first day of stimulation has been increased from 2 to 5 days, so that bleeding will not occur after stopping the pill when stimulation has started and they can assume that most of the steroids of the pill have been excreted.

In the report of Templeton et al (1984) about fixed-schedule ovulation induction, a preference was expressed for progestogens rather than the combined contraceptive pill to modify the preceding cycle, since at least one cleaving egg was obtained from only 38% of patients given the pill as compared to 63% of patients given progestogens. In our series, the percentages of women undergoing follicular aspiration for whom at least one embryo was obtained were similar in both groups (71% in group EP and 77% in group P) (Table 1). The oestrogen–progestogen pill does, however, result in lower levels of serum oestradiol in the preovulatory phase, presumably associated with suppression of the hypothalamic–pituitary–ovarian axis. This reduction is not significant, possibly because of the small number of cases assessed. It is possible that programming of oocyte recovery helps to select a group of 'healthy' oocytes that are able to achieve maturity despite prior suppression of ovarian function. This is suggested by the fact that survival after cryopreservation and thawing of the embryos resulting from insemination of these programmed oocytes is at least equal to the overall survival of frozen–thawed embryos in our unit.

Even though the attainment of artificial cycles, with progestins or with combined oestrogen–progestagen pills followed by stimulation with clomiphene–hMG or gonadotrophins alone, avoids the need for clinical and laboratory staff to be on duty 7 days a week, it does not avoid spontaneous LH surges. In the study by Kemeter and Feichtinger (1989) endogenous LH increases occurred before hCG administration in 20.2% of the women. In our series, treatment was cancelled in 10–20% of stimulated cycles, owing mainly to inadequate responses of the programmed patient and premature LH surges in the monitoring group. Elevated serum E_2 levels are associated with a large number of oocytes collected, and therefore a large number of embryos and a high pregnancy rate (which is related to the number of embryos transferred). Ferraretti (1984) previously noted that the frequency of spontaneous LH surges was increased when the serum E_2 was > 2000 pg/ml. In a recent elegant cross-over study from the Melbourne groups, there was a higher incidence of premature LH surges in association with elevated E_2 levels (Rogers et al, 1986).

For this reason, the recent development of analogues of GnRH appears to be very promising. This treatment avoids premature LH surges (Fleming and Coutts, 1986), increases follicular recruitment and consequently the number of oocytes recovered, and appears to be useful for treating women who have been resistant to conventional methods of stimulation.

Two fundamentally different approaches may be employed when using these agents. The first is based upon achieving a state of complete pituitary suppression before commencing stimulation (Neveu et al, 1987); this takes between 10 and 14 days and is accompanied by low basal levels of E_2 and gonadotrophins. Follicular stimulation is then concurrently carried out with hMG or FSH, and ovulation is induced an average of 21–28 days after the start of analogue treatment. The second method does not depend on an initial phase of down-regulation (Barrière et al, 1987). In this the gonadotrophin flare-up effect after analogue administration is used to promote follicular recruitment, and administration of gonadotrophins is commenced on the third or fourth day of treatment to continue follicular stimulation as the endogenous gonadotrophin levels decline. This method has the advantage of being shorter since ovulation is usually induced by hCG within 11–15 days after initiation of treatment, which is a considerable advantage for the patient. In addition to these two different therapeutic principles, there are various types of analogues and modes of administration.

We compared these two protocols in a randomized study (Frydman et al, 1988). One hundred and eighty-six patients were equally divided between the short and long protocol. No differences were seen in serum E_2 levels, number of mature oocytes or pregnancy rate by transfer. Therefore, we must still determine what clinical indications might favour one or the other regimen for use of GnRH analogs (GnRHa) in IVF. The theoretical advantages of routinely using a GnRHa for IVF are the improvement of the patient's comfort and convenience for the members of the medical team achieved by improving IVF scheduling. With the long protocol, the pituitary suppression is obtained 10–14 days after the beginning of GnRHa, but the ovarian stimulation can be started at that time or a few days later so as to obtain day 10 of the stimulation on a Saturday (Zorn et al, 1987). Normally, hCG is given between days 10 and 13. The majority of the oocyte recoveries will be done from Monday to Thursday, during the week. For the short protocol, investigators are currently involved in trying to associate programmed stimulation and analogue treatment so as to combine the advantages of both therapies.

REFERENCES

Barrière P, Lopes P, Boiffard JP et al (1987) Use of GnRH analogues in ovulation induction for in vitro fertilization: benefit of a short administration regimen. *Journal of In Vitro Fertilization and Embryo Transfer* **4**: 64–65.
Braude PR, Bright MV, Douglas CP et al (1984) A regimen for obtaining mature human oocytes from donors for research into human fertilization in vitro. *Fertility and Sterility* **42**: 34–38.
Ferraretti AP (1984) Serum FSH and LH values in normal women given varying doses of Pergona at varying times in the cycle. In Lovero G (ed.) *Human In Vitro Fertilization and Embryo Development*, pp 116–121. Rome: Bari Congress, Edizioni International.
Fleming R & Coutts JRT (1986) Induction of multiple follicular growth in normally menstruating women with endogenous gonadotropin suppression. *Fertility and Sterility* **45**: 226–230.
Frydman R, Rainhorn JD, Forman RG et al (1986a) Programmed oocyte retrieval during routine laparoscopy and embryo cryopreservation for later transfer. *American Journal of Obstetrics and Gynecology* **55**: 112–117.
Frydman R, Forman RG, Rainhorn JD et al (1986b) A new approach to follicular stimulation for in vitro fertilization: programmed oocyte retrieval. *Fertility and Sterility* **46**: 657–662.
Frydman R, Belaïsch-Allart J, Parneix I et al (1988) Comparison between flare up and down

regulation effects of luteinizing hormone-releasing hormone agonists in an in vitro fertilization program. *Fertility and Sterility* **50(3):** 471–475.

Garcia JE, Jones GS, Acosta AA et al (1983) Human menopausal gonadotropin/human, chorionic gonadotropin follicular maturation for oocyte aspiration: Phase 1, 1981. *Fertility and Sterility* **39:** 174–179.

Kemeter P & Feichtinger W (1989) Experience with a new fixed-stimulation protocol without hormone determinations for programmed oocyte retrieval for in-vitro fertilization. *Human Reproduction* **4 (supplement):** 53–58.

Kemeter P, Eder A & Springer-Kremser (1986) In vitro fertilization patients and the outcome of in vitro fertilization: psychological and psychoendocrinological factors. In Leysen B, Nijs P & Richter D (eds) *Research in Psychosomatic Obstetrics and Gynaecology*, pp 89–101. Leuven-Amersfoort: Acco.

Lopata A (1983) Concepts in human in vitro fertilization and embryo transfer. *Fertility and Sterility* **40:** 289–301.

Neveu S, Hedon B, Bringer J et al (1987) Ovarian stimulation by a combination of gonadotropin-releasing hormone agonist and gonadotropins for in vitro fertilization. *Fertility and Sterility* **47:** 639–643.

Rainhorn JD, Forman RG, Belaïsch-Allart J et al (1987) One year's experience with programmed oocyte retrieval for IVF. *Human Reproduction* **2(6):** 491–494.

Rogers P, Molloy D, Healy D et al (1986) Cross-over trial of superovulation protocols from two major in vitro fertilization centres. *Fertility and Sterility* **46:** 424–431.

Steptoe PC & Edwards RG (1978) Birth after the reimplantation of the human embryo. *Lancet* **ii:** 366.

Taymor MI, Seibel MM, Oskowitz SP et al (1985) In vitro fertilization and embryo transfer. An individualized approach to ovulation induction. *Journal of In Vitro Fertilization and Embryo Transfer* **2:** 162–165.

Templeton A, van Look P, Lumsden MA et al (1984) The recovery of preovulatory oocytes using a fixed schedule of ovulation induction and follicle aspiration. *British Journal of Obstetrics and Gynaecology* **91:** 148.

Wardle PG, Foster PA, Mitchell JD et al (1986) Norethisterone treatment to control timing of the IVF cycle. *Human Reproduction* **1:** 455–457.

Yee B & Vargyas JM (1986) Multiple follicular development utilizing combination of clomiphene citrate and human menopausal gonadotropins. *Clinical Obstetrics and Gynecology* **29:** 141–147.

Zorn JR, Boyer P & Guichard A (1987) Never on Sunday: programming for IVF-ET and GIFT. *Lancet* **i:** 385–386.

9

Induction of ovulation for assisted reproduction programmes

SERGIO OEHNINGER
GARY D. HODGEN

In vitro fertilization and embryo transfer (IVF-ET) and gamete intra-fallopian transfer (GIFT) have become established and successful therapeutic modalities for couples with different aetiologies of infertility. Almost all IVF and GIFT programmes throughout the world use ovarian stimulatory regimens in order to recruit and develop multiple follicles, with an ultimate goal of transferring more than one preovulatory oocyte or embryo. The decision to use enhancement of the natural ovarian/menstrual cycle to attempt collection of several oocytes during each treatment cycle has dramatically increased the ongoing pregnancy rates. Furthermore, the recovery of multiple fertilizable oocytes allows for cryopreservation of extra or surplus

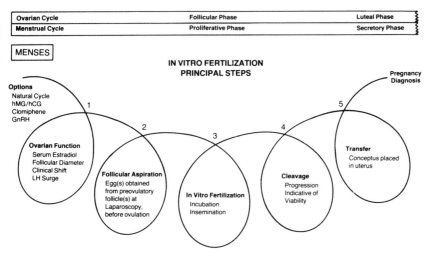

Figure 1. The five principal steps in in vitro fertilization and embryo transfer (IVF/ET) therapy. Hormonal stimulation of the ovarian cycle is of crucial importance for collection of several oocytes of high quality. The success of the first and second steps greatly influences the pregnancy rate after one or more pre-embryos are transferred to the uterus. hMG, human menopausal gonadotrophin; hCG, human chorionic gonadotrophin; GnRH, gonadotrophin-releasing hormone. From Hodgen (1986) with permission.

pre-embryos (or embryos), with the consequent reduction in the risk of multiple pregnancies and improvement in the cumulative pregnancy rate following IVF and GIFT cycles (Figure 1). Here, we will review first the underlying physiological mechanisms in the natural ovarian/menstrual cycle; we will then discuss different strategies designed to override selection of the dominant follicle to facilitate the aspiration of several preovulatory oocytes for IVF-ET and GIFT therapies.

THE NATURAL OVARIAN/MENSTRUAL CYCLE

The specialized investments of the growing preovulatory follicle and its successor, the corpus luteum, establish and maintain the changing hormonal milieu which nurtures the ovum throughout maturation, fertilization, and the initial stages of embryogenesis. Indeed, it is the ovarian cycle which temporarily modulates the hypothalamic–pituitary function through both negative and positive feedback on gonadotrophin release as well as orchestration of uterine proliferative and secretory phases of the menstrual cycle (Hodgen, 1982).

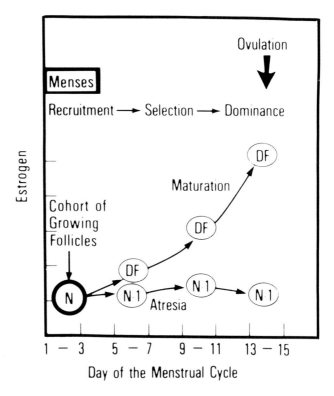

Figure 2. Time course for recruitment, selection, and ovulation of the dominant ovarian follicle with onset of atresia among other follicles of the cohort. From Hodgen (1986) with permission.

Whereas many follicles may begin their developmental course at each ovarian/menstrual cycle, typically only a single follicle sustains its inherent gametogenic potential; all others succumb to atresia, finally having forfeited their latency. The provision of more gonadotrophins during stimulated or induced cycles (clomiphene citrate or human menopausal gonadotrophins) will violate the normal mono-ovular quota. On a controlled basis, this is a desirable effect to recover multiple eggs and facilitate in vitro fertilization. However, the alternative risk is to have impaired (qualitatively) the normality of the growing follicle and the sequelae of the ovarian/menstrual cycle, requisite for establishment of a viable pregnancy.

Normally, within the first half of the follicular phase of the menstrual cycle many follicles begin to develop from either the primary to secondary stage or all the way from primordial to secondary follicles. This process is known as 'recruitment' (diZerega and Hodgen, 1981) (Figure 2). Thus, a cohort of resting follicles begins a well-characterized pattern of growth and development, ultimately providing the species-characteristic ovulatory quota of eggs. This pattern of growth has been termed the 'trajectory of follicle growth' (Schwartz, 1974), gonadotrophins providing the 'thrust' and ovarian factors the 'guidance' along the trajectory (Hodgen, 1986) (Figure 3). Recruitment of primordial follicles is not wholly dependent on gonadotrophins but may be only enhanced by these hormones (Lunenfeld et al, 1976).

Several morphologically indistinct follicular ovarian structures progress prior to cycle days 5–7; loss of any of these follicles will not delay timely ovulation. In contrast, after about cycle day 7, this multi-potentiality is lost;

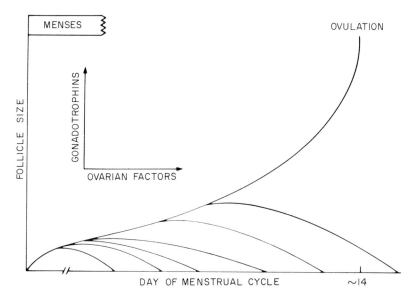

Figure 3. Proposed relationship between gonadotrophins and ovarian factors in regulating maturation or atresia along the so-called trajectory of follicle growth. From Hodgen (1986) with permission.

typically, only one will be capable of proceeding to timely ovulation. This one follicle, destined to ovulate and form the corpus luteum, is termed the 'dominant follicle'. Destruction of the dominant follicle, such as by selective cautery, will result in a frame-shift delay of approximately one follicular phase until the next ovulation (Goodman and Hodgen, 1978a). This time, at which all of the recruited follicles become qualitatively unequal in potential, is the time of 'selection' (Figure 2). That the process of selection is predetermined by some intrinsic aspect of a particular follicle seems unlikely, but once acquired it is certainly not transferable. No other follicles can immediately take its place upon extinction. Upon selection of the single dominant follicle, all others become destined for atresia (Kenigsberg and Hodgen, 1987).

It is accepted that selection is begun and is completed only during the cycle in which ovulation occurs. In contrast, the time of recruitment and thus the total length (duration) of the trajectory are unknown. Based on present evidence, the duration of the trajectory in macaques and women appears to be not less than about 2 weeks. It has been hypothesized that in the physiological setting of the ovarian/menstrual cycle, the folliculogenic actions of gonadotrophins—principally follicle-stimulating hormone (FSH)—are permissive at tonic levels and that the steroidogenic actions of gonadotrophin—principally luteinizing hormone (LH)—are graded. If FSH at tonic levels is actually permissive to folliculogenesis, then graded effects observed may be attributable to supraphysiological (supratonic) levels. Graded actions of gonadotrophins on steroidogenesis (and perhaps on inhibin secretion) are necessary for ovarian mechanisms to control circulatory gonadotrophins near the tonic set-point, so that the mechanisms of follicle selection are effective (Hodgen, 1986).

The dominant follicle and its successor, the corpus luteum, comprise the 'dominant structures' of the ovarian cycle, having remarkable authority over both intraovarian (bilateral) and systemic events regulating folliculogenesis. In the natural cycle, although either ovary may provide the dominant ovary in any given cycle, once the dominant follicle has been selected, the two ovaries are partitioned into those that are gametogenically active and those that are gametogenically inactive. Necessarily, ovarian function is then 'asymmetric'. However, after corpus luteum demise, the follicular apparatus of both ovaries becomes available for recruitment and then the gonads become 'symmetric'; at that time, probably local ovarian factors in conjunction with gonadotrophin actions will initiate a typical follicle trajectory.

The most prominent physiological marker of impending ovulation is the midcycle LH surge. Within the microenvironment of the dominant follicle three major events occur at this time.

1. Resumption of meiosis I. At this time the oocyte resumes nuclear maturation as evidenced by germinal vesicle breakdown, transition from prophase I to metaphase I stage, and extrusion of the first polar body (metaphase II stage). Nuclear maturation occurs probably in synchrony with cytoplasmic and zona pellucida maturation in preparation for fertilization. The intracellular processes which account for

these maturational changes are not yet fully understood but may involve oocyte factors as well as follicular paracrine factors, steroids and gonadotrophin actions.

2. Luteinization. Although there is some increased progesterone secretion prior to the onset of the LH surge, the exposure of the follicle to the midcycle high LH levels magnifies the extent and degree of transformation of the follicular stromal cells from an oestrogen- and protein-secreting apparatus to predominantly steroid secretion (mainly progesterone, oestradiol and androstenedione). That progesterone secretion starts on the absence of perceptible changes in the endogenous LH pulse amplitude, or frequency may implicate an independent intraovarian mechanism that begins to shift ovarian steroidogenesis and/or secretion towards progesterone, even before initiation of the LH surge (Hoff et al, 1983; Collins et al, 1984).

3. Ovulation. The exact mechanism by which follicle rupture occurs and the oocyte surrounded by the cumulus oophorus is released is not completely understood. Gonadotrophins (especially LH) stimulate prostaglandin secretion and plasminogen activator release, as well as mucification of the cumulus; enzymatic digestion of the follicular wall seems to be one of the principal mechanisms leading to ovulation.

At ovulation, the theca cells continue to furnish the angiogenesis factor, ensuring a greater blood supply (mostly low-density lipoproteins) for progesterone biosynthesis and secretion by the corpus luteum. The luteinized theca cells continue to respond to the LH pulse with both oestradiol (E_2) and progesterone synthesis and secretion. They continue to multiply and divide, and if pregnancy ensues these cells respond to human chorionic gonadotrophin (hCG) stimulation from the conceptus and compose the corpus luteum of pregnancy. Studies in monkeys (Healy et al, 1984) and women (Filicori et al, 1984) have demonstrated that progesterone from the corpus luteum is secreted in a pulsatile fashion. The pulses are most frequent in the early and mid-luteal phase when progesterone secretion is at its zenith; luteinized theca cells may be responsible for this pulsatile secretion (Alila and Hansel, 1984). On the other hand, the luteinized granulosa cells do not luteinize LH receptors, but continue to translate and secrete progesterone during a 10-day span, presumably due to a stable messenger. These cells secrete progesterone for 10 days, at which time steroidogenesis ceases. Thus, as the measurable LH pulses decrease at the end of the luteal phase, and in the absence of pregnancy and hCG production, the LH stimulation to the theca cells decreases, and progesterone and E_2 production decrease. Presumably, the effects of oxytocin and prostaglandin synthesized by the granulosa cells are maximized, leading to vasoconstriction and necrosis of the luteinized theca cells, inducing corpus luteum demise by day 14 in the absence of pregnancy.

The normal process of selection of the dominant follicle leading to ovulation and luteal phase function in the natural cycle can be overridden by the presence of supraphysiological gonadotrophin stimulation of the ovary. Typically, exogenous gonadotrophin therapy allows several recruited fol-

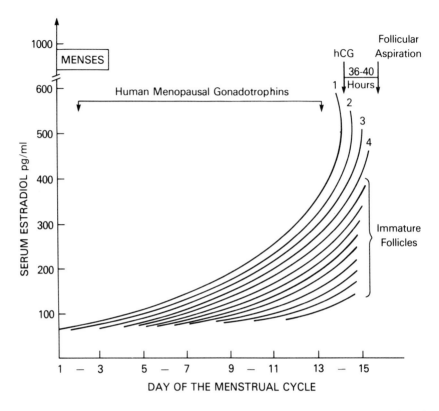

Figure 4. Relation of serum LH to E_2 in 16 human menopausal gonadotrophin (hMG)-stimulated cycles followed by hCG ovulation induction. Human menopausal gonadotrophin (hMG)-stimulated follicular maturation overrides selection of a single follicle in the natural cycle. Note that only a few follicles can be regarded as quasisynchronous. If human chorionic gonadotrophin (hCG) is given too late, advanced follicles may yield postmature eggs of low viable potential. From Hodgen (1986) with permission.

licles to avert atresia; although their development is not perfectly synchronous, a few are likely to be mature enough for ovulation, fertilization and implantation to ensue (Figure 4). As we will see next, this supraphysiological stimulation is desirable for enhanced oocyte recovery for IVF-ET and GIFT programmes. Luteal steroidogenesis in the stimulated cycle cannot be assessed by a comparison with luteal steroidogenesis in the natural cycle. The oestrogen/progesterone ratio is an important determinant of the endometrial response pattern. Thus, the adequate support of the luteal function and pregnancy with progesterone may overcome a possible excessive E_2 stimulation which can occur with supraphysiological gonadotrophin levels and may ensure that the endometrial pattern is adequate and conducive to normal implantation (Jones, 1986).

GONADOTROPHIC STIMULATION OF THE OVARIAN CYCLE: RECRUITMENT OF MULTIPLE FERTILIZABLE EGGS FOR ASSISTED REPRODUCTION

Although Steptoe and Edwards (1978) used the natural cycle that led to their first successful birth, it was soon realized that this method had many disadvantages. Only one preovulatory oocyte could be recovered at midcycle. Extensive monitoring of the natural cycle for the detection of the simultaneous LH surge, a process that involved frequent sampling of blood or urine for measurement of LH, was required. The timing of laparoscopy, which was scheduled 25–29 h after the initiation of the LH surge, could occur at odd hours that were inconvenient not only for the surgical team but for the embryology laboratory as well. This proved to be highly impractical for any programme dealing with a sizeable number of patients, and above all, resulted in low success rates due to the retrieval and transfer of only one successfully fertilized preovulatory oocyte. Because of the above reasons, the natural cycle was soon abandoned by most programmes (Rosenwaks et al, 1987).

The Norfolk programme has primarily utilized various gonadotrophins for ovarian stimulation in assisted reproduction. It was elected to use gonadotrophins in preference to clomiphene citrate (CC) for multiple follicular development because it was anticipated that in a normal cycle the ovarian response would be more dependable with gonadotrophins than with CC. At the same time, the Australian experience (Johnston et al, 1981) indicated a high cycle cancellation rate prior to laparoscopy in CC-stimulated cycles due to poor ovarian response. Prior experience also indicated that the pregnancy rate was higher with human menopausal gonadotrophin (hMG; Pergonal, Serono Laboratories Inc., Randolph, MA) than with CC when used for ovulation induction in anovulatory patients. The anti-oestrogenic effects of CC on the cervical mucus (significant for the assessment of the biological oestrogenic shift), possibly on the oocyte and follicular apparatus, and on the endometrium, were of concern.

The goal of recruitment and development of multiple follicles was readily accomplished with the use of hMG alone, hMG in combination with pure FSH (Metrodin, Serono Laboratories Inc., Randolph, MA), or with pure FSH alone (Rosenwaks and Muasher, 1987). Gonadotrophin stimulation was begun early on in the follicular phase to allow for recruitment of multiple follicles before the selection of the dominant follicle. The retrieval of multiple mature oocytes was considered desirable as initial results showed that increasing the number of concepti transferred resulted in an improved pregnancy rate. In all gonadotrophin protocols used in Norfolk the dose of gonadotrophin has been highest on days 3 and 4 of the menstrual cycle and then tapered down for the remainder of the follicular phase. This approach mimics the physiological conditions during the natural ovarian/menstrual cycle when in the early follicular phase relatively high levels of FSH recruit follicles from the 'gonadotrophin-sensitive' pool. Moreover, Abbasi et al (1987) have shown that in the primate model (cynomolgus monkey) a 'step-down' protocol may lead to more synchronized follicular maturation

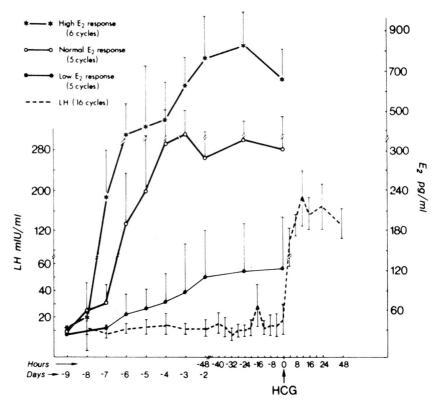

Figure 5. Oestradiol (E_2) response patterns to the two human menopausal gonadotrophin (hMG) protocol. Note: the endogenous luteinizing hormone (LH) surge is suppressed in all patients despite oestradiol levels which exceed the usual midcycle levels. From Ferraretti et al (1983) with permission.

than a 'step-up' dose regimen, resulting in a narrower versus wider, respectively, 'ovulatory window'.

The majority of patients undergoing IVF/GIFT are usually normal individuals with normal feedback mechanisms, who therefore respond to gonadotrophin stimulation differently from patients having ovulation induction with obviously abnormal feedback mechanisms. Since follicular growth was assumed to parallel oocyte maturation, serum E_2 levels and the biological response to E_2 by the peripheral end organs (maturation of vaginal cells and mucus score) were used as a measure of the follicular secretory function; the anatomical growth and number of follicles stimulated was monitored by ultrasound. It was observed that in these normally cycling women there was a striking repetitiveness of the peripheral E_2 response to gonadotrophins for each individual from cycle to cycle if given an identical stimulation (Jones, 1984). This repetitiveness allows one to adjust stimulation for a more successful pattern in subsequent cycles. Likewise, three types of peripheral E_2 responses were recognized: low, intermediate, and high (Ferrareti et al, 1983) (Figure 5). These categories relate to the serum E_2 values in relation to the peripheral oestradiol end-organ responses. The numbers of follicles stimulated or seen on ultrasound and confirmed by follicular aspiration are not reflected as a multiple of the serum E_2 values, although as the number of follicles increases so does the serum oestradiol. In contrast, serum progesterone does not increase in relation to the number of follicles stimulated (Jones, 1984).

As a rule, patients are given 10000 units of hCG as a surrogate LH surge, 50–52 h after the last dose of hMG (or FSH in 'pure' FSH protocols), and oocyte harvest takes place 35–36 h after hCG injection. This 'coasting period' of 50 h (long interval) has been estimated to be necessary to achieve final follicular-oocyte maturation. The criteria for hMG discontinuation and hCG administration depend upon the E_2 response pattern, peripheral end-organ biological shift and follicle size as evaluated by ultrasound; slightly different guidelines are followed when combinations of FSH and hMG are used (Rosenwaks et al, 1987). However, if there is evidence that the follicles are responding to gonadotrophins rapidly, suggesting imminent oocyte maturity, a short interval between the discontinuation of hMG and hCG administration is utilized. These criteria include a rapid increase in follicular size, a doubling of the serum E_2 level, or a plateau of the E_2 level during the last 24 h of stimulation.

Stimulation with 300 IU of FSH alone or 150 IU of FSH in combination with 150 IU of LH on days 3 and 4 of the cycle (four FSH or two FSH/two hMG) results in a higher steroidogenic response than when only two ampoules of hMG are administered continuously. Whereas the height of the E_2 response to gonadotrophin is related to the number of developing follicles and to the patient's follicular endowment, it is the terminal E_2 response pattern to gonadotrophin which reflects granulosa cell health (maturity) and oocyte viability (Jones et al, 1983) (Figure 6). A continued rise in serum E_2 levels during hMG administration, during the coasting period, and after hCG administration (pattern A) is associated with the highest number of preovulatory oocytes retrieved and transferred, as well as the highest pregnancy rate per cycle.

Aberrant responses to gonadotrophins are observed in some groups of patients. Patients with ultrasonagraphic and/or endocrinological findings of polycystic ovarian syndrome (PCO) tend to produce a large number of oocytes after gonadotrophin stimulation. However, following the standard criteria for stimulation discontinuation and hCG administration, it was observed that most of these oocytes tended to be immature or postmature and atretic. On the other hand, patients who do not respond with an expected increase in the serum E_2 level have been seen in all categories of stimulation protocols ('poor responders').

The work of Muasher et al (1988) has contributed to our understanding of these different responses to gonadotrophin stimulation. These authors have shown that basal serum FSH and LH values on cycle day 3 are helpful in identifying different populations of IVF patients, who tend to behave differently in terms of E_2 response, oocytes obtained and transferred, and pregnancy rates. Interestingly, a gonadotrophin-releasing hormone

(GnRH) test performed on cycle day 3 corroborated the results, but did not add to the information gained by dosification of basal serum gonadotrophin levels. Patients with a higher basal LH:FSH had the highest increase in serum E_2 during stimulation, the highest number of preovulatory oocytes aspirated, and a pregnancy rate comparable with an FSH:LH of 1:1. In our experience, patients with high basal LH:FSH (PCO-like or multifollicular ovarian response; Romeu et al, 1987) benefit from lower-dose gonadotro-

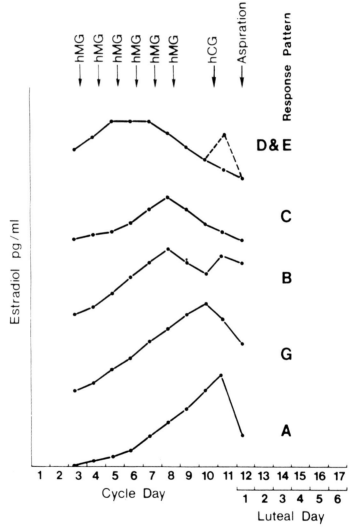

Figure 6. Diagrammatic representation of the various oestradiol (E_2) patterns of response together with the number of cases in each pattern and the pregnancy rate by pattern. hMG, human menopausal gonadotrophin; hCG, human chorionic gonadotrophin. From Rosenwaks and Muasher (1986) with permission.

phin stimulation regimes (two ampoules of FSH daily) rather than higher-dose conventional (two FSH/two hMG or four FSH) regimens. As will be discussed later, these patients also benefit significantly when gonadotrophin stimulation is performed concomitantly with the use of a GnRH agonist (GnRHa).

On the other hand, patients with elevated basal FSH levels or higher FSH:LH ratios respond poorly to stimulation in terms of peripheral E_2, oocytes obtained, and pregnancy rates. These patients belong to the group of 'perimenopausal' patients. The finding has nothing to do with the patient's age and may be more closely related to the numbers of operative procedures which she has had (ovarian) or perhaps to her own inherent follicular pool. These women are normally menstruating and ovulating regularly (Jones, 1985). However, as described by Sherman and Korneman (1975), they may have a short follicular phase with moderately low E_2 levels. Thus, cycle day 3 serum FSH levels are predictive of IVF outcome (Scott et al, 1989) (Table 1). Furthermore, two basal FSH values (from two different cycles) which are in agreement may be used to counsel patients regarding their performance during gonadotrophin stimulation; if wide intercycle variations in basal FSH levels are observed, the patients will probably behave as 'poor responders' (Scott et al, 1990).

Table 1. Pregnancy rates with in vitro fertilization based on basal day 3 follicle-stimulating hormone (FSH) concentrations.

Basal FSH (mIU/ml)	No.	Pregnant n (%)	Ongoing n (%)	Miscarried n (%)
< 15	541	130 (24.0)*	92 (17.0)†	38 (29.2)
15 to 24.9	161	22 (13.6)	15 (9.3)	7 (31.8)
≥ 25	56	6 (10.7)	2 (3.6)	4 (66.6)

*FSH < 15 mIU/ml > FSH 15–24.9 mIU/ml and FSH ≥ 25 mIU/ml; $P < 0.01$.
†FSH < 15 mIU/ml > FSH 15–24.9 mIU/ml > FSH ≥ 25 mIU/ml; $P < 0.01$.
From Scott et al (1989b) with permission.

A 'golden standard' of the Norfolk programme has been the adjustment and individualization of gonadotrophin therapy according to the patient's characteristics and response. One should keep in mind that the administration of a high dosage of hMG or FSH may induce the development of many follicles, but if stimulation is excessive or too short or prolonged, immature and/or postmature eggs may be obtained with subsequent failed or abnormal fertilization and cleavage and possibly reduced embryo quality. The remarkable results achieved in Norfolk can probably be attributed, at least in part, to the relatively moderate ovarian hyperstimulation used in these protocols, as compared to the marked hyperstimulation used by others (Blankstein et al, 1986). This also explains why the incidence of the severe, sometimes dramatic, ovarian hyperstimulation syndrome has been kept to a minimum.

Cycle cancellation in IVF is defined as the interruption of a treatment attempt after admission and before oocyte retrieval. The cancellation rate is an index of the complexity of the population and of the success in predicting, diagnosing and correcting its problems. In a large number of IVF cycles studied in the Norfolk programme, the cancellation rate was 4.6% per patient and 17.9% per cycle (Acosta et al, 1989). The most common causes of cancellation were (1) absent or poor response to stimulation (53.2%); (2)

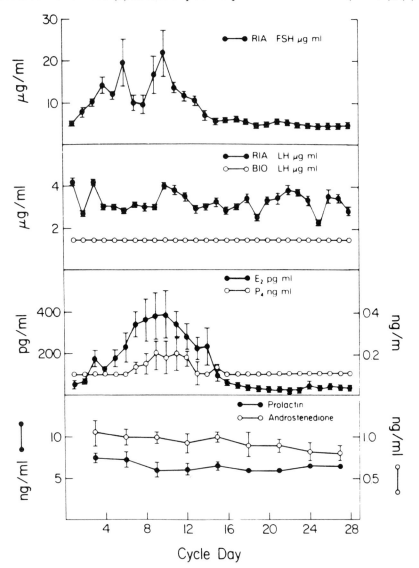

Figure 7. Composite patterns (mean ± SE) of serum follicle-stimulating hormone (FSH), luteinizing hormone (LH), oestradiol (E_2), progesterone (P_4), androstenedione, and prolactin in five intact monkeys treated with FSH (25 or 50 IU daily on cycle days 1–12). Note the failure of oestrogen-positive feedback for the LH surge. Typically, FSH doses of 12.5 IU or less daily did not produce ovarian hyperstimulation. BIO, bio-assayable; RIA, radio-immunoassayable. From Hodgen (1986) with permission.

abnormal terminal E_2 patterns and premature LH surges (17.2%); and (3) ovarian cyst (8.9%). Overall, patients with multiple treatment cycles having had at least one cycle cancelled had a significantly lower term pregnancy rate than the general IVF population.

During the past years, mounting physiological evidence has indicated that the ovaries of pigs, monkeys and women produce a non-steroidal substance that inhibits the surge mode of LH and FSH secretion otherwise induced by either oestradiol or GnRH (Schenken and Hodgen, 1983; Littman and Hodgen, 1984; Schenken et al, 1984; Sopelak and Hodgen, 1983). This putative substance has been called gonadotrophin surge-inhibiting factor (GnSIF) (Danforth et al, 1989). Its activity is distinct from that of inhibin, which selectively suppresses pituitary release of FSH.

The first inkling that GnSIF might exist occurred in 1978 when it was noted that exogenous administration of gonadotrophins to cynomolgus monkeys resulted in persistently high levels of E_2; however, no LH surges occurred (Goodman and Hodgen, 1978b) (Figure 7). Since then, numerous investigators have observed that administration of hMG to endocrino-logically normal women or monkeys is frequently associated with an absence of an LH surge, despite high levels of E_2 (Hodgen, 1982; Ferrareti et al, 1983). The presence of GnSIF in follicular fluid was supported by evidence that coadministration of purified follicular fluid with exogenous oestradiol to normal cycling monkeys resulted in the blockade of the expected midcycle-type gonadotrophin surges (Hodgen et al, 1980). To date, there is limited evidence that GnSIF and inhibin are distinct molecular entities with different physical characteristics and differential effects on pituitary gonadotrophin secretion. However, until GnSIF is isolated, purified to homogeneity, and its exact molecular structure determined, the possibility should also be considered that GnSIF activity is simply an expression of one of the several molecular members of the inhibin family if not inhibin itself.

The occurrence of a spontaneous endogenous LH surge as a complication of IVF/GIFT cycles has been reported accompanying CC stimulation (Edwards et al, 1984) and also gonadotrophin stimulation, although with a decreased frequency (Jones et al, 1982). Messinis et al (1986) found that the endogenous LH surge associated with superovulation was attenuated by factors related to the degree of hyperstimulation. Droesch et al (1988) evaluated IVF results in patients with a spontaneous LH surge undergoing gonadotrophin stimulation at the Norfolk programme. The mean age of patients exhibiting an LH surge was slightly, although significantly, higher compared to the control (overall) IVF population. There was no significant difference in the type of stimulation used between the two groups. Mean baseline E_2, mean E_2 on the day of LH surge or hCG administration, and mean day of LH surge or hCG administration did not differ between these two groups. However, the mean number of preovulatory oocytes retrieved and transferred was significantly less in cycles complicated by an LH surge. Interestingly, the mean number of mature oocytes transferred was higher when the hCG-oocyte retrieval interval was > 35 h, compared with < 24 h. In cycles with an hCG-retrieval interval of < 24 h, the percentage of pre-ovulatory oocytes was higher when serum E_2 decreased by $> 15\%$ on the morning after hCG administration compared with a plateau or an increase in serum E_2. Thus, the timing of oocyte retrieval after the occurrence of a spontaneous LH surge should consider the hCG-retrieval interval and changes in E_2 levels after hCG administration. These guidelines may avoid cancellation for many patients.

With regard to hCG administration to replace the blocked LH surge, Williams and Hodgen (1980) had shown disparate effects of hCG during the late follicular phase of the primate ovarian cycle. More specifically, if the E_2-induced surges of FSH and LH had been initiated, ovarian function was unaffected by hCG. By contrast, hCG given before incipient gonadotrophin surges resulted in anovulation lasting 4–6 weeks and sometimes disruption of the tonic FSH secretion. These findings may indicate some potential risks of premature administration of hCG to women during induced follicular maturation. Inappropriately timed (precocious) administration of hCG may actually preclude the objective, namely to provide fertilizable oocytes and a milieu in which to mature the pre-embryo(s) through a normal luteal phase, while achieving a fertile menstrual cycle.

As mentioned before, hMG treatment will sustain the concurrent development of many follicles for a limited interval. Even so, only a few quasisynchronous follicles can be harvested together by follicular aspiration some 32–36 h after hCG injection. If hCG is given too late, one or more of the more advanced follicles may yield postmature (fragmented or fractured zonae) eggs of low potential viability; conversely, if hCG is given too soon, the follicles and oocytes may be immature (Hodgen, 1986).

The importance of adequate luteal-phase serum levels of E_2 and progesterone for early pregnancy maintenance is well known. An optimal peri-implantation hormonal milieu reflects a healthy embryo and a responsive corpus luteum, and supports the endometrial environment for further growth and development of the conceptus. The luteal phase of IVF-ET/GIFT cycles has come under great scrutiny as the cause for the discrepancy between fertilization rates (80–90%) and pregnancy rates (~20%) is sought. IVF manipulations may compromise this critical period through (1) the endocrine sequelae of ovulation induction regimens employed, specifically the known contraceptive actions of elevated luteal-phase E_2 levels; (2) the potentially damaging impact of ovum retrieval on granulosa cell function (Hodgen, 1982); and (3) the sequelae of aberrant in vitro embryogenesis (Hutchinson-Williams et al, 1989).

Efforts to improve endometrial receptivity and pregnancy maintenance during IVF cycles have not resulted in any generally accepted therapeutic regimen. Because the hormonal profiles of conception cycles are characterized by sustained luteal-phase progesterone secretion, the use of supplemental progesterone has been advocated (Jones et al, 1982). However, reports of Trounson et al (1986) and Leeton et al (1985) did not demonstrate a significant improvement in the outcome of IVF/ET in controlled trials employing such support. A number of studies investigating the efficacy of a variety of regimens, including hCG supplementation, have been published (Casper, 1983; Mahadevan, 1985; Buvat et al, 1988). Nevertheless, there is no consensus regarding the impact of hCG support. Based on the present evidence, the Norfolk programme (Jones et al, 1982; Jones, 1986) and others (Hutchinson-Williams et al, 1989) advocate the use of progesterone supplementation to 'support' corpus luteum function in gonadotrophin-stimulated IVF-ET and GIFT cycles. The classic studies of Csapo, examining pregnancy maintenance following luteectomy or oophorectomy in women, have shown that the luteal–placental shift occurs at approximately 8 weeks after the last menstrual period (Csapo et al, 1972). We routinely continue progesterone support a few weeks beyond luteal–placental shift in IVF cycles (Jones, 1986).

CLOMIPHENE CITRATE

Although the precise mechanisms of action of CC have not been fully elucidated, more than 20 years of experience have shown it to be an effective, low-toxicity, and safe agent for ovulation induction in women with endogenous oestrogens in or near the normal range (Adashi, 1984). This later criterion is usually fulfilled in patients with sufficient endometrial proliferation to manifest withdrawal bleeding after progestins. This finding correlates with tonic peripheral E_2 of approximately 40 pg/ml or greater (Kenigsberg and Hodgen, 1987). CC is an anti-oestrogen (weak oestrogen) that reduces endogenous oestrogen-negative feedback to the pituitary, causing augmented FSH and LH secretion. Dogma has it that resultant elevated gonadotrophins enhance ovarian stimulation to the point that ovulatory cycles are produced in the previously oligo-ovulatory or acyclic individual. There may also be important intraovarian actions of CC, including enhancement of aromatase activity.

CC used alone, or usually in combination with hMG, is one of the most common stimulants used for induction of multiple follicular development in assisted reproduction. Among the advantages for its use are decreased expense, less extensive monitoring than that required with gonadotrophins, and lower risk of severe hyperstimulation. Among its disadvantages are the recruitment of fewer follicles when used alone, the anti-oestrogenic effect on cervical mucus and endometrium, and higher incidence of cancellation prior to oocyte retrieval due to either poor E_2 response or spontaneous LH surge (Rosenwaks et al, 1987). Marut and Hodgen (1982) have stressed the vulnerability of normal follicular maturation to the attenuating (anti-oestrogen) effects of high-dose CC treatment in primates, whereby ovarian refractoriness and latent luteal irregularities may impair fecundity despite transient augmentation of pituitary gonadotrophin secretion.

All combination therapy protocols for IVF have described sequential regimens in which CC is followed by hMG, followed by hCG. Discrepancies between the different treatment protocols concern the dosage of CC and hMG, the day of commencement of CC and/or hMG, and whether the hMG treatment is continuous or interrupted.

In most sequential treatment regimens, the dose of CC varies between 50 and 150 mg/day. The day for starting CC is either arbitrarily fixed for the third or fifth day or is individualized to the patient's endogenous cycle, being started on the fifth day of the cycle if the cycle length exceeds 26 days and on the third day if the cycle is shorter. The duration of CC treatment varies from 4 to 7 days. Similarly, hMG, at a dose of 75–300 IU/day is started either on the day when CC is discontinued or arbitrarily on the seventh or eighth day. The hMG is discontinued when the leading follicle is 18 mm or greater (slightly larger size in comparison with pure gonadotrophin stimulation), and/or a pattern of rising E_2 is obtained. The hCG is usually administered 32–56 h after the last dose of hMG (Lopata, 1983; Feichtinger and Kemeter, 1984). With the sequential use of CC and hMG, several IVF/GIFT programmes have achieved results similar to those using gonadotrophins alone.

Several conclusions may be drawn from the experience to date with the already discussed methods of ovarian stimulation. Primarily, lower doses of medication, when used appropriately, may result in a more favourable outcome. Most significant, it seems to be beneficial to tailor the dosages and timing of drug administration to the patient's individual response to medication (Rosenwaks et al, 1987; Yee and Vargyas, 1986).

PHYSIOLOGICAL BASIS FOR THE CLINICAL APPLICATIONS OF GnRH AGONISTS AND ANTAGONISTS

Because ovarian stimulation therapy is difficult to manage, in part due to the marked individual variability in response to exogenous agents, a major challenge in reproductive endocrinology has been to develop an ovarian stimulation protocol that would 'ideally' synchronize the development of a cohort of follicles. From the experience gained after the advent of IVF, it is now appreciated that although endocrinologically normal women show an inherent variability to gonadotrophin stimulation, individual response types tend toward a consistent pattern from cycle to cycle, thus suggesting a constancy of physiological status, as opposed to a stochastic response (Kenigsberg et al, 1984a).

In 1971, two research teams first announced the structure and chemical synthesis of GnRH (Ammos et al, 1971; Matsuo et al, 1971). The physiological and therapeutic potency of GnRH prompted efforts to synthesize long-acting and potent agonistic and antagonist analogues. In the past 15 years, more than 2000 GnRH analogues have been synthesized (Karten and Rivier, 1986), representing the effort of many research laboratories and pharmaceutical companies.

GnRH antagonists were the first subclass of analogues to be synthesized and biologically evaluated. The rationale for their development came with the recognition that they might represent a new non-steroidal method of contraception. GnRH antagonists function by binding to the GnRH receptor in the pituitary, thereby preventing the release of FSH and LH (Andreyko et al, 1987). Thus, ovulation would be blocked. However, efforts to synthesize potent and clinically useful antagonists have been partially less rewarding than expected earlier. The effectiveness of these early antagonistic analogues was diminished by a low agonistic potential. In addition, most potent antagonists stimulate histamine release, and initial efforts to curtail this effect had to precede clinical trials.

The original incentive for the development of the analogues was that they could eventually be used for the treatment of anovulation. With the half-life of GnRH being only 4–8 min, longer-acting and more potent agonists were thought to be necessary for practical clinical utility. However, the potent agonists, or superagonists, were found to have paradoxical antireproductive effects (Andreyko et al, 1987). They stimulate the release of LH and FSH initially, but continuous activation of pituitary GnRH receptors eventually leads to desensitization of GnRH receptors on gonadotrophs and decreased gonadotrophin secretion (Rabin and McNeil, 1980). Promising clinical applications have provided further incentive to continue to improve the analogue preparations. In the case of enhanced receptor binding with relative resistance to degradation, analogues were obtained that, by virtue of their enhanced potency, caused down-regulation even at low and infrequent doses (agonists). By substitution at the biologically active centre (positions 2 and 3 of the original GnRH decapeptide molecule), an analogue could be produced that bound ardently to GnRH receptors without any detectable promotion of LH and FSH secretion (antagonist). The net result of both types of analogues was an inhibition of GnRH action on the hypophysis; however, GnRH agonists had a transient 2–3-week episodically stimulatory phase prior to achieving full down-regulation. In contrast, GnRH antagonists almost immediately (within 2–3 days) eliminated all measurable LH and FSH (Schally et al, 1980).

With this background, ways of reducing individual variability of responses to gonadotrophin therapy based on understanding the physiological origin(s) of that variability were sought. Kenigsberg et al (1984b) approached this issue through two main objectives: (1) to identify the source of individual variability in the hypothalamic–pituitary ovarian axis, and (2) to

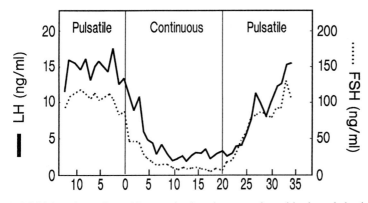

Figure 8. Inhibition of gonadotrophin secretion in a rhesus monkey with a hypothalamic lesion when an intermittent gonadotrophin-releasing hormone (GnRH) replacement regimen (1 μg/min for 6 min every hour) was replaced by a continuous infusion of the decapeptide beginning on day 0. This inhibition was gradually reversed when the pulsatile mode of GnRH administration was reinstituted on day 20. The small vertical lines below some data points indicate levels below the sensitivity of the assay. LH, luteinizing hormone; FSH, follicle-stimulating hormone. (From Belchetz et al, 1978 with permission.)

study the differential action of FSH treatment alone versus FSH/LH therapy in the ovary. They reasoned that by eliminating endogenous pituitary output of gonadotrophin ('medical hypophysectomy'), as well as ovarian feedback influencing hypothalamic–pituitary functions, ovarian response to exogenous gonadotrophins could be more clearly distinguished. The developments on the essential nature of appropriate pulsatile GnRH secretion (to achieve ovulation induction) contributed the basis for this approach (Knobil, 1980; Figure 8). Thank goodness endocrinology is such a simple science (Hodgen, 1989). There are, after all, only three hormonal conditions: (1) too much, (2) too little, and (3) just right (Hodgen, 1987). Indeed, GnRH agonists are powerful therapeutic agents that work because too much stimulation of the GnRH receptor system in the anterior pituitary causes too

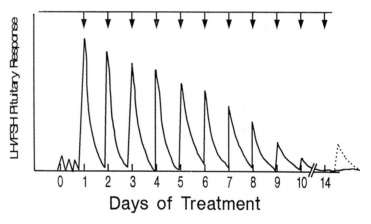

Figure 9. Schematic of gonadotrophin-releasing hormone (GnRH) agonist-induced down-regulation of pituitary gonadotrophins. LH, luteinizing hormone; FSH, follicle-stimulating hormone. From Hodgen (1989) with permission.

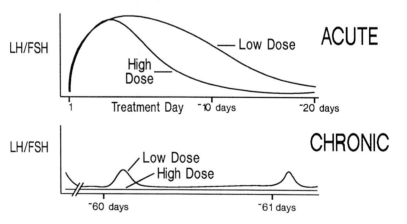

Figure 10. Gonadotrophin-releasing hormone (GnRH) agonists: daily down-regulation of the pituitary gonadotrophs. LH/FSH, luteinizing hormone/follicle-stimulating hormone. From Hodgen (1989) with permission.

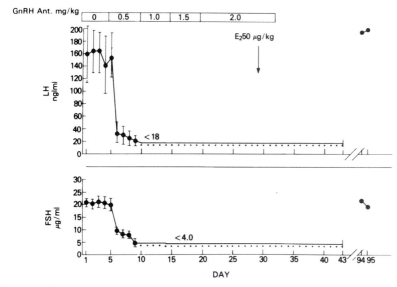

Figure 11. Gonadotrophin-releasing hormone (GnRH) antagonist suppresses follicle-stimulating hormone (FSH) and luteinizing hormone (LH) levels in serum to below limits of assay detection. Long-term ovariectomized monkeys did not respond to an oestrogen challenge test. Note the full recovery of gonadotrophin secretion by 2 months after cessation of treatment. E_2, oestradiol. From Kenigsberg (1984b) with permission.

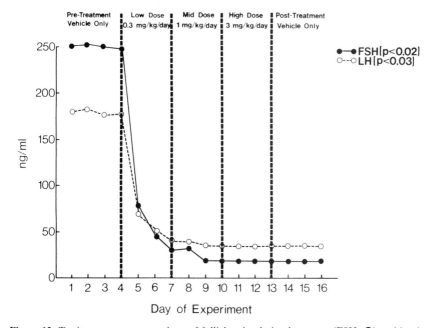

Figure 12. Tonic serum concentrations of follicle-stimulating hormone (FSH; ●) and luteinizing hormone (LH; ○) before, during and after gonadotrophin-releasing hormone (GnRH) antagonist treatment. Each point represents the mean of four animals. The decrease in serum FSH and LH throughout the study was significant ($P < 0.05$). From Chillik et al (1987) with permission.

little gonadotrophin secretion which, in turn, arrests both steroidogenic and gametogenic gonadal functions. GnRH agonists induce a pharmacological state resembling the prepubertal pituitary–gonadal axis (Figure 9). Seemingly, this induced hypopituitary (gonadotrophs) hypogonadal condition, achieved within about 2 weeks of initiating treatment, can be sustained for a month or years, both with acute and chronic administration regimens (Figure 10). Moreover, these compounds have direct effects on gonadal structure, but the absence of cellular changes and lesions on the human testis has been reassuring to clinicians and scientists (Hodgen, 1987).

Kenigsberg et al (1984a, 1984b) individually conducted a series of experiments in the cycling cynomolgus monkey using the previously developed GnRH antagonistic analogues (Figure 11). Due in large measure to the persistent endeavours of the Contraceptive Development Branch, National Institute of Child Health and Human Development (NICHHD) and certain pharmaceutical companies, peptide chemists and biologists have continued in their search for high-potency GnRH antagonists possessing marked reduction in allergenicity.

GnRH antagonists inhibit gonadotrophin secretion presumably by competing with GnRH for its receptor on the gonadotrophs. Most studies examining the effects of GnRH antagonists have revealed a rapid (within minutes) inhibition of LH/FSH secretion which typically lasts 1–4 days (Hodgen, 1989; Figure 12).

'First-generation' GnRH antagonists (GnRHant) inhibit gonadotrophin release and gonadal function; however, these compounds induce transient systemic oedema and inflammation at the injection site, characterized as an allergic response associated with histamine release. Whereas 'second-generation' GnRHant, such as Nal-Glu-GnRHant, retain ovulation inhibition potency and have markedly less in vitro histamine-releasing activity, local allergic response in some human subjects remains a concern. Thus, safety needs have led to a search for a 'third-generation' GnRHant having negligible histamine-release properties while retaining the ability to effectively inhibit gonadotrophin secretion. Recently, Leal et al (1988) reported primate data demonstrating unexpectedly prolonged inhibition of LH and FSH secretion after either subcutaneous or intravenous administration of a 'third-generation' GnRHant (Figures 13 and 14).

The dose–response effects of a single administration of Nal-Lys-GnRHant on serum LH and FSH concentrations were compared to the effects of Nal-Glu-GnRHant in monkeys. Twenty ovariectomized monkeys were divided into four subcutaneous treatment groups: (1) 1.0 mg/kg Nal-Glu-GnRHant, or Nal-Lys-GnRHant at (2) 0.3, (3) 1.0, or (4) 3.0 mg/kg. Each monkey received vehicle (propylene glycol/water, 1:1) on day 0, followed by an antagonistic preparation on day 11. Serum LH and FSH were measured by radio-immunoassay (RIA); serum LH was also measured by in vitro bio-assay. The short-term effects were similar among the four treatment groups. Typically, serum LH declined ($P < 0.05$) within 4–8 h, achieving maximal reduction by 24 h. Serum FSH levels declined more slowly, but were significantly reduced by 24 h ($P < 0.05$). Recovery during the study interval to pretreatment control values occurred in only two

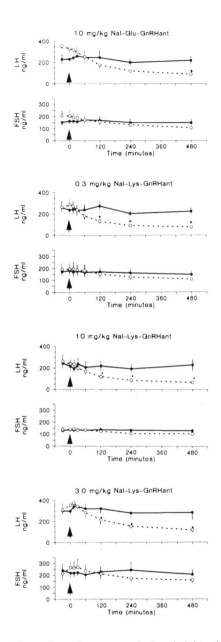

Figure 13. Short-term effects of a subcutaneous single administration of gonadotrophin-releasing hormone antagonists Nal-Glu-GnRHant or Nal-Lys-GnRHant on mean (± SE) serum luteinizing hormone (LH) and follicle-stimulating hormone (FSH) concentrations in ovariectomized monkeys. The arrows indicate the time of injection of vehicle (●) or GnRH antagonist (○). The asterisks indicate significant differences from corresponding controls (P < 0.05). (For SI units, ng/ml = μg/litre.) From Leal et al (1988) with permission.

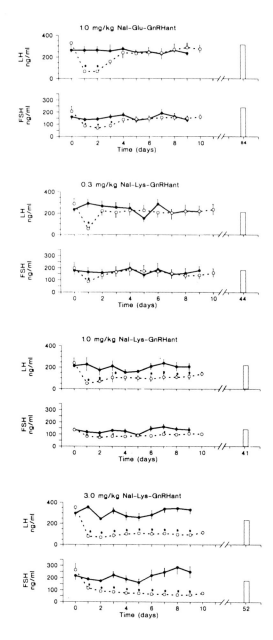

Figure 14. Long-term effects of a subcutaneous single administration of gonadotrophin-releasing hormone (GnRH) antagonists on mean (± SE) serum luteinizing hormone (LH) and follicle-stimulating hormone (FSH) concentrations in ovariectomized monkeys. Injection of vehicle (●), or GnRH antagonist (○), were made on day 0. The asterisks indicate significant differences from corresponding controls ($P < 0.05$). (For SI units, ng/ml = µg/litre.) From Leal et al (1988) with permission.

groups: (1) Nal-Glu-GnRHant (1.0 mg/kg) by day 4 post-treatment, and (2) Nal-Lys-GnRHant (0.3 mg/kg) by day 2 post-treatment. Monkeys receiving 1.0 or 3.0 mg/kg Nal-Lys-GnRHant had a prolonged inhibition of serum LH and FSH levels. In all animals, serum FSH and LH returned to control levels within 2 months. The duration of gonadotrophin inhibition was also prolonged when the Nal-Lys-GnRHant was administered intravenously. In contrast, Nal-Glu-GnRHant reduced serum LH and FSH for 3 days or less in all monkeys. The serum bio-assayable LH levels paralleled those of immunoassayable LH. The prolonged inhibition of gonadotrophin secretion following Nal-Lys-GnRHant distinguishes its action from those of previous GnRH antagonists and makes this compound of great interest for clinical investigations (Figures 15 and 16).

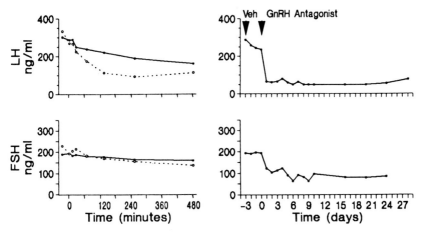

Figure 15. Short-term (left) and long-term (right) effects of a single administration of vehicle (veh; ○) or the gonadotrophin-releasing hormone antagonist Nal-Lys-GnRHant (3.0 mg/kg; ●) injected intravenously into an ovariectomized monkey. LH, luteinizing hormone; FSH, follicle-stimulating hormone. (For SI units, ng/ml = μg/litre.) From Leal et al (1988) with permission.

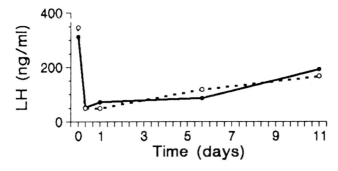

Figure 16. Patterns of bio-assayable (●) and immunoassayable (○) serum luteinizing hormone (LH) in a monkey given 3.0 mg/kg Nal-Lys-GnRHant subcutaneously. (For SI units, ng/ml = μg/litre.) From Leal et al (1988) with permission.

These results demonstrated an unexpectedly prolonged duration of action of Nal-Lys-GnRHant at subcutaneous doses of 1.0 or 3.0 mg/kg. Since intravenous administration induced a similar lengthy duration of gonadotrophin inhibition, a depot effect at the site of subcutaneous injection could not explain these findings. Nal-Glu-GnRHant had no such prolonged effects. Possible explanations for these results include: (1) the Nal-Lys-GnRHant may be sequestered in peripheral tissues and slowly released; (2) it may be highly resistant to enzymatic degradation and thereby recycled extensively in the circulation; and (3) this antagonist may have a noxious effect on anterior putuitary gondotrophs or hypothalamic function. In fact, whether the mechanisms of action involves hypothalamic or pituitary sites of action, or both, is unknown. However, it does not appear to act by altering the biological activity of the secreted LH.

Ljungquist et al (1987) had reported that the Nal-Lys compound is virtually free of the histamine-release side-effects that have limited the clinical utility of some 'first-' and 'second-generation' compounds. Together, these observations have intensified interest in advancing Antide into clinical trials. As noted in our initial report, the duration of inhibition of gonadotrophin secretion was markedly dose-dependent. Ultimate restoration of FSH/LH to pretreatment levels did occur, although the limited study design did not allow complete characterization of the recrudescence of tonic gonadotrophin secretion (Leal et al, 1989).

A second study was undertaken to compare Nal-Lys-GnRHant with Nal-Glu-GnRHant, specifically addressing the chronic impact of multiple doses on the duration of inhibition of FSH/LH secretion and the recrudescence of gonadotrophin secretion. In addition, acute LH secretory responses to intravenous boluses of GnRH before and during GnRHant-induced suppression of tonic FSH/LH secretion were characterized (Chillik et al, 1987; Danforth et al, 1990a).

This study was designed to extend evaluation of the long-acting effects of a 'third-generation' GnRH antagonist (Nal-Glu-GnRHant, Antide) on gonadotrophin secretion in ovariectomized (OVX) monkeys, with special attention to recrudescence of pitiutary gonadotrophin secretion after multiple-dose treatments, as well as pituitary secretory responsiveness to GnRH. Cynomolgus monkeys were randomly divided into four treatment groups: (1) Nal-Glu-GnRHant, 1.0 mg/kg per day, a 'second-generation' compound used as a basis for comparison, or (2) Nal-Lys-GnRHant at 0.3 mg/kg per day, (3) 1.0 mg/kg per day, and (4) 3.0 mg/kg per day. All eight monkeys received six consecutive daily subcutaneous injections of vehicle (propylene glycol:water, 1:1) on study days 1–6, and one of the GnRHants on study days 18–23. Blood samples were collected for 43 consecutive days and intermittently thereafter up to 100 days post-treatment. Serial GnRH stimulation tests (10 µg/kg, intravenous) were performed every 6 days. In all GnRHant treatment groups significant reductions in circulating gonadotrophin levels were seen in LH ($P<0.001$) and FSH ($P<0.005$) within 24 h after the first injection of GnRHant.

The duration of FSH/LH inhibition by Nal-Lys-GnRHant was dose-dependent, as well as being much longer than for Nal-Glu-GnRHant;

however, full recrudescence of gonadotrophin secretion, albeit gradual, did occur. The acute LH secretory response to serial intravenous boluses of GnRH, in the face of GnRHant-induced suppression of gonadotrophin secretion, was transiently accelerated and biologically active. Thereafter, the state of FSH/LH inhibition was resumed chronically. Thus, treatment with Nal-Lys-GnRHant produced profound long-term inhibition of tonic gonadotrophin levels, yet hyper-responsiveness to exogenous GnRH administration was maintained throughout.

Recently, Danforth et al (1990b) have shown that the prolonged duration of gonadotrophin inhibition by Antide seems to derive from the long circulating half-life of this molecule. In turn, this extended action of Antide may be manifest by binding to serum protein(s) that serves as a built-in peripheral depot release mechanism.

These findings encourage a hastening of efforts to reach clinical trials for Antide early on because: (1) it apparently has intrinsically negligible allergenic side-effects; (2) it promises immediacy of inhibition of pituitary gonadotrophin secretion, without the delay of a GnRH agonist-like paradoxical 'flare' effect, leading to the down-regulation mode of action; (3) it seems to possess a dose-dependent versatility where either acute or chronic regimens may be tailored to specific clinical indications; and (4) its mechanism of action, although not fully elucidated, is conveniently reversible by intravenous administration of GnRH. Current research imperatives include physiological characterization of Nal-Lys-GnRHant action in gonadally intact adult conditions, as well as development of appropriate assays to describe the pharmacokinetics of Antide.

CLINICAL RESULTS WITH THE CONCOMITANT USE OF GnRH AGONISTS AND GONADOTROPHINS FOR THE SYNCHRONIZED INDUCTION OF MULTIPLE FOLLICLES IN ASSISTED REPRODUCTION

GnRH agonists (GnRHa) have now been extensively used in clinical programmes for assisted reproduction. As discussed above, fluctuating gonadotrophin concentrations and premature LH surge can be associated with abnormal E_2 pattern responses in stimulated cycles. Premature luteinization and breakdown of follicular development can occur, with adverse effects on functional viability of the oocytes. Premature progesterone secretion also may adversely effect endometrial maturation, leading to asynchrony with ovarian function.

GnRH agonists have thus been used in our effort to overcome inappropriate or untimely interference from the pituitary–ovarian dynamics. The most-used protocol has consisted in the administration of the GnRHa during the preceding mid-luteal phase (days 21–23) to achieve a 'medical hypophysectomy'. At least two different preparations have been individually tried: (1) Buserelin (Hoechst Pharmaceuticals, West Germany) administered intranasally at a dose of $100\,\mu g$ every 5 h (Porter et al, 1984; Palermo et al, 1988) or subcutaneously at a dose of $0.3\,ml$ twice daily (Neveu et al,

Table 2. Characteristics of cycles with and without gonadotrophin-releasing hormone agonist (GnRHa) therapy related to patient classification.

	Cycles with elevated LH/FSH (n=9) (mean ± SD)		Cycles with normal FSH/LH and history of LH surges (n=7) (mean ± DS)		Cycles with elevated FSH/LH and low response to gonadotrophins (n=8) (mean ± SD)	
	GnRHa	Control	GnRHa	Control	GnRHa	Control
LH ± SD on day 3	23.96 ± 27.7	16.3 ± 9.17	12.12 ± 1.68	12.1 ± 5.2	20.27 ± 11.96	15.7 ± 4.48
FSH ± SD on day 3	7.16 ± 5.08	9.2 ± 3.29	7.37 ± 6.41	10.0 ± 3.04	8.14 ± 2.99	22.9 ± 6.72
Number ± SD of amps						
FSH	9.13 ± 1.55†	5.11 ± 3.33	9.14 ± 3.34†	4.86 ± 1.21	12.57 ± 1.99*	6.38 ± 2.97
hMG	13.78 ± 0.97*	9.63 ± 0.55	18.86 ± 7.65†	10.0 ± 1.91	22.29 ± 7.87†	11.86 ± 1.46
Day of hCG ± SD	10.44 ± 0.53†	9.0 ± 0.87	11.57 ± 1.27*	8.57 ± 1.28	11.71 ± 0.95*	9.33 ± 0.74
E_2 ± SD on day of hCG	758.7 ± 323.7	896.3 ± 555.9	605.1 ± 239.8	797.3 ± 211.8	271.0 ± 52.5	469.0 ± 210.8
P ± SD on day of hCG	0.57 ± 0.34	1.05 ± 0.31	0.57 ± 0.18	1.07 ± 0.73	0.74 ± 0.34	1.38 ± 0.72
LH ± SD on day of hCG	16.54 ± 1.48	49.05 ± 34.05	12.97 ± 0.65†	61.16 ± 47.65	16.20 ± 3.87	32.60 ± 13.68

SD, standard deviation; LH, luteinizing hormone; FSH, follicle-stimulating hormone; hCG, human chorionic gonadotrophin; hMG, human menopausal gonadotrophin; E_2, oestradiol; P, progesterone.
* $P < 0.001$.
† $P < 0.05$. From Droesch et al (1989) with permission.

1987), and (2) leuprolide acetate (Lupron, Tap Pharmaceuticals, North Chicago, Illinois, USA) at a dose of 1.0 mg subcutaneously (Meldrum et al, 1989; Droesch et al, 1989). Under this regimen, patients usually have a menstrual bleeding 7–12 days after initiation of the agonist. Gonadotrophin stimulation is started on day 3 of the menstrual cycle and GnRHa administration is continued until the day of hCG injection.

Results using the luteal-phase schedule of GnRHa and gonadotrophin therapy have been almost universally remarkable. As anticipated, the cancellation rate has been significantly lower when compared with non-GnRHa cycles. Additionally, the number of follicles aspirated and the number of preovulatory oocytes aspirated and transferred has also been significantly improved, thus improving pregnancy rates. Pituitary suppression with GnRHa also suppresses the circulatory concentrations of bio-active LH, thus preventing premature LH release and undesirable effects of excessive LH on oocyte quality (Meldrum et al, 1984, 1989). Even 'poor responders' have been claimed to benefit from this therapy (Serafini et al, 1988), and for this reason routine pituitary suppression with GnRHa before ovarian stimulation for oocyte retrieval in all patients has been suggested (Meldrum et al, 1989).

The initial Norfolk experience with the luteal phase GnRHa protocol (long protocol) also supported the value of pituitary suppression prior to gonadotrophin stimulation for IVF (Droesch et al, 1989; Table 2). This has been corroborated for 'normal' and 'high' responders (or patients with a normal LH: FSH and higher LH: FSH ratios). In these patients, results have been consistently favourable in terms of fertilization rates, number of preovulatory oocytes recovered and transferred, and ongoing pregnancy rates (Droesch et al, 1989; Edelstein et al, 1990a; Brzyski et al, 1989b). The impact of GnRHa treatment also seems to be reflected in a higher progesterone production during the luteal phase (Brzyski et al, 1989). Moreover, in patients pretreated with GnRHa (with normal or high basal LH: FSH ratio), stimulation with pure hMG or pure FSH for IVF resulted in similar favourable cycle characteristics and pregnancy outcome (Edelstein et al, 1990b). In addition, patients with endometriosis (previously shown to constitute an endocrinologically homogeneous group) also benefited from the use of GnRHa concomitantly with gonadotrophin stimulation for IVF (Oehninger et al, 1988, 1989).

However, 'low responders' (or patients with high basal FSH: LH ratio) required the most and longest stimulation, using a significantly higher number of gonadotrophin ampoules (thus requiring a higher expense) and having a lower pregnancy outcome (Droesch et al, 1989; Table 2). If the disorder in the low-responder patients is at the ovarian level (diminished ovarian reserve) then GnRHa therapy may not improve stimulation in this group. In an effort to enhance results in low responders, two other approaches have been elaborated. First, high doses of FSH (six ampoules) were tried on cycle day 1 or 2, under the rationale that such earlier stimulation would result in the recruitment of a larger cohort of follicles and thus improvement of outcome. Preliminary results using such an approach have not been gratifying (Karande et al, 1990). Second, we are now evaluating the use of GnRHa starting on day 2 of the menstrual cycle, while gonadotrophins are begun on day 4 or 5. This is a modification of the 'flare-up' technique (discussed below), and of the protocol designed by Sandler et al (1989) who used a very low dose of leuprolide during the follicular phase to enhance follicular recruitment and to prevent premature luteinization. The protocol consists of 1 mg of leuprolide acetate per day, starting FSH or hMG (or a combination of both) on cycle day 4. Two different groups of responses seem to occur: (1) some patients have a rapid pituitary down-regulation after the initial agonistic effect, and show low E_2 levels on day 5, when gonadotrophin stimulation is begun; and (2) others show the agonistic effect not followed by E_2 suppression. In ongoing studies we are evaluating the advantages and disadvantages of these different response patterns.

In the short GnRHa protocol exogenous stimulation begins at the same time or shortly after GnRH agonist administration, benefiting from the so-called gonadotrophin 'flare-up' (Barriere et al, 1987; Frydman et al, 1987). Although these authors have claimed good clinical results and the benefits of patient convenience, cost and side-effects with this short protocol, Brzyski et al (1988) have reported a poor outcome with the concurrent use of pituitary suppression and gonadotrophin stimulation in low-responder patients. More atretic oocytes and fewer preovulatory eggs were retrieved in these cases, suggesting that the high LH–progesterone environment generated from initial stimulation may be detrimental to normal oocyte development. Therefore, efforts towards improving the outcome in the low-responder patients through the design of newer and more efficient strategies are warranted.

SUMMARY

The decision to use enhancement of the natural ovarian/menstrual cycle to attempt collection of several oocytes during IVF and GIFT cycles has dramatically increased the pregnancy rates. Furthermore, the recovery of multiple fertilizable oocytes allows for cryopreservation of extra or surplus pre-embryos (or embryos), with the consequent reduction in the risk of multiple pregnancies and the improvement of the cumulative pregnancy rate following IVF and GIFT cycles. Here, we have reviewed the underlying physiological mechanisms in the natural ovarian-menstrual cycle. Subsequently, we have analysed the more frequently utilized ovarian stimulatory regimens with special emphasis on the use of gonadotrophins. Several conclusions may be drawn from the experience to date with these methods of ovarian stimulation. Primarily, lower doses of medication, when used appropriately, may result in a more favourable outcome. Most significant, it seems to be beneficial to tailor the dosages and timing of drug administration to the patient's individual response to medication. Because ovarian stimulation therapy is difficult to manage, a major challenge in reproductive endocrinology has been to develop stimulation protocols that would 'ideally' synchronize the development of a cohort of follicles. The development of GnRH analogues (agonists and antagonists) and the experience (both in women and macaques) gained so far when these drugs are used in combination with gonadotrophins, have helped both in the understanding of the underlying physiology and in the improvement of clinical results.

Acknowledgements

We would like to acknowledge the contributions of the entire clinical and basic research staff of The Jones Institute for Reproductive Medicine; we are also extremely grateful to Ms Dara Willett Leary for her preparation of the manuscript.

REFERENCES

Abbasi R, Kenigsberg D, Danforth D, Falk RJ & Hodgen GD (1987) Cumulative ovulation rate in human menopausal/human chorionic gonadotropin-treated monkeys: 'step-up' versus 'step-down' dose regimens. *Fertility and Sterility* **47:** 1019–1024.

Acosta AA, Oehninger S, Muasher SJ, Valdes H & Jones D (1989) Treatment cycle cancellation in the Norfolk IVF Program: critical analysis and prognostic significance. *Abstracts of the VII World Congress in in vitro fertilization and alternate assisted reproduction*, Jerusalem, p 6.

Adashi EY (1984) Clomiphene citrate: mechanism(s) and site(s) of action—a hypothesis revised. *Fertility and Sterility* **42:** 331–344.

Alila HW & Hansel W (1984) Origin of different cell types in the bovine corpus luteum as characterized by specific monoclonal antibodies. *Biology of Reproduction* **31:** 1015–1025.

Ammos M, Burges R, Blackwell R et al (1971) Purification, amino acid composition and n-terminus of the hypothalamic luteinizing hormone releasing hormone factor (LRF) of ovine origin. *Biochemical and Biophysical Research Communications* **44:** 205–210.

Andrey JL, Marshall L, Dumeric D & Jaffe RB (1987) Therapeutic uses of gonadotropin-releasing hormone analogs. *Obstetrical and Gynecological Survey* **42:** 1–21.

Barriere P, Lopes P, Boiffard JP et al (1987) Use of GnRH analogues in ovulation induction for IVF: benefit of a short administration regimen. *Journal of In Vitro Fertility and Embryo Transfer* **4:** 64–65.

Belchetz PE, Plant TM, Nakai Y et al (1978) Hypophysical responses to continuous and intermittent delivery of hypothalamic gonadotropin releasing hormone. *Science* **2:** 631–633.

Blankstein J, Mashiach S & Lunenfeld B (1986) Ovulation induction and in vitro fertilization. In Blankstein J, Mashiach S & Lunenfeld B (eds) *In Vitro Fertilization and Embryo Transfer*, pp 155–200. Chicago: Year Book Medical Publishers.

Brzyski RG, Muasher SJ, Doesch K, Simonetti S, Jones GS & Rosenwaks Z (1988) Follicular atresia associated with concurrent initiation of GnRHa and FSH for oocyte recruitment. *Fertility and Sterility* **50:** 917–921.

Brzyski RG, Jones GS, Oehninger S, Acosta AA, Kruithoff C & Muasher SJ (1989a) Impact of leuprolide acetate on follicular response and/or outcome in in vitro fertilization patients with normal serum gonadotropin levels. *Journal of In Vitro Fertilization and Embryo Transfer* **6:** 290–293.

Brzyski RG, Jones GS, Jones HW Jr, Oehninger S & Muasher SJ (1989b) Improved luteal phase progesterone production following pituitary suppression with leuprolide acetate prior to follicular stimulation for IVF. *Abstracts of the 65th Annual Meeting of the American Fertility Society*, San Francisco, CA, p 92.

Buvat J, Marcolin G, Herbaut JC, Dehaene JL, Verberg P & Fourlinnie JC (1988) A randomized trial of hCG support following IVF/ET. *Fertility and Sterility* **49:** 458–461.

Casper RF, Wilson E, Collins JA, Brown SE & Parker JA (1983) Enhancement of human implantation by exogenous hCG. *Lancet* **ii:** 1191.

Chillik CF, Itskovitz J, Hahn D, McGuire JL, Danforth DR & Hodgen GD (1987) Characterizing pituitary response to a GnRH antagonist in monkeys: tonic FSH/LH hormone secretion versus acute GnRH challenge tests before, during and after treatment. *Fertility and Sterility* **48:** 480–485.

Collins RL, Williams RF & Hodgen GD (1984) Endocrine consequences of prolonged ovarian hyperstimulation: hyperprolactinemia, follicular atresia and premature luteinization. *Fertility and Sterility* **42:** 436–445.

Csapo AL, Pulkkinan MO & Ruttner B (1972) The significance of human corpus luteum in pregnancy maintenance. *American Journal of Obstetrics and Gynecology* **112:** 1061–1067.

Danforth DR, Sinosich MJ, Anderson T, Cheng CY, Bondin W & Hodgen GD (1989) Identification of gonadotropin surge inhibiting factor (GnSIF) in follicular fluid and its differentiation from inhibin. *Biology of Reproduction* **37:** 1075–1082.

Danforth DR, Williams RF, Gordon K & Hodgen GD (1990a) Development of an in vitro bioassay for GnRH antagonists: measurement of circulating Nal-Lys GnRH antagonist levels to examine the mechanism of its long action. *Biology of Reproduction* (in press).

Danforth DR, Gordon K, Leal J, Williams RF & Hodgen GD (1990b) Extended presence of Antide (Nal-Lys GnRH antagonist) in circulation; prolonged duration of gonadotropin inhibition may derive from Antide binding to serum proteins. *Journal of Clinical Endocrinology and Metabolism* **70:** 554–556.

diZerega GS & Hodgen GD (1981) Folliculogenesis in the primate ovarian cycle. *Endocrine Reviews* **2:** 27–49.

Droesch K, Muasher SJ, Kreiner D, Jones GS, Acosta AA & Rosenwaks Z (1988) Timing of oocyte retrieval in cycles with a spontaneous LH surge in a large IVF Program. *Fertility and Sterility* **50:** 451–456.

Droesch K, Muasher SJ, Brzyski R et al (1989) Value of suppression with a GnRH agonist prior to gonadotropin stimulation for IVF. *Fertility and Sterility* **51:** 292–297.

Edelstein M, Brzyski RG, Jones GS, Oehninger S, Sieg S & Muasher SJ (1990a) Ovarian stimulation for IVF using pure FSH with and without GnRHa in high responder patients. *Journal of In Vitro Fertilization and Embryo Transfer* (in press).

Edelstein M, Brzyski RG, Scott R et al (1990b) Equivalency of hMG and FSH for various stimulation for IVF after GnRH agonist suppression. *Fertility and Sterility* (in press).

Edwards RG, Fishel SB, Cohen J et al (1984) Factors influencing the success of IVF for alleviating human infertility. *Journal of In Vitro Fertilization and Embryo Transfer* **1:** 3–23.

Feichtinger W & Kemeter P (1984) IVF as an outpatient procedure. *Abstracts of the III World Congress of IVF/ET, Helsinki* **1:** 108.

Ferrareti AP, Garcia JE, Acosta AA & Jones GS (1983) Serum luteinizing hormone during ovulation induction with human menopausal gonadotropin for in vitro fertilization in normally menstruating women. *Fertility and Sterility* **40:** 742–747.

Filicori M, Butler JT & Crowley WF (1984) Neuroendocrine regulation of the corpus luteum in the human: evidence for pulsatile progesterone secretion. *Journal of Clinical Investigation* **73:** 1638–1647.

Frydman R, Belaisch-Allart J, Parneix I, Forman R, Hazout A & Testart J (1987) Comparison between flare up and down regulation effects of GnRH agonists in an IVF program. *Fertility and Sterility* **50:** 471–475.

Goodman AL & Hodgen GD (1978a) Between ovary interaction in the regulation of follicular growth, corpus luteum function, and gonadotropin secretion in the primate ovarian cycle. I. Effects of follicle cautery and hemiovariectomy during the follicular phase in cynomolgus monkeys. *Endocrinology* **104:** 1310–1316.

Goodman AL & Hodgen GD (1978b) Postpartum patterns of circulating FSH, LH, prolactin, estradiol and progesterone in nonsuckling cynomolgus monkeys. *Steroids* **31:** 731–744.

Healy DL, Schenken RS, Lynch A, Williams RF & Hodge GD (1984) Pulsatile progesterone secretion: its relevance to clinical evaluation of corpus luteum function. *Fertility and Sterility* **41:** 114–121.

Hodgen GD (1982) The dominant ovarian follicle. *Fertility and Sterility* **38:** 281–300.

Hodgen GD (1986) Physiology of follicular maturation. In Jones HW Jr, Jones GS, Hodgen GD & Rosenwaks Z (eds) *In Vitro Fertilization, Norfolk*, pp 8–29. Baltimore: Williams and Wilkins.

Hodgen GD (1987) On the management of orchids by gonadotropin hormone agonist therapy. *Fertility and Sterility* **48:** 914–915.

Hodgen GD (1989) General applications of GnRH agonists in gynecology: past, present and future. *Obstetrical and Gynecological Survey* **44:** 293–296.

Hodgen GD, Channing C, Anderson L, Gagliano P, Turner C & Stouffer R (1980) On the regulation of FSH secretion in the primate hypothalamic–pituitary–ovarian axis. *Proceedings of the 6th International Congress of Endocrinology*, Amsterdam, p 263.

Hoff JD, Quigley ME & Yen SSC (1983) Hormonal dynamics at midcycle: a reevaluation. *Journal of Clinical Endocrinology and Metabolism* **57**: 792–796.

Hutchinson-Williams K, Lunenfeld B, Diamond MP, Lavy G, Boyers SP & DeCherncy AH (1989) Human chorionic gonadotropin, estradiol and progesterone profiles in conception and nonconception cycles in an in vitro fertilization program. *Fertility and Sterility* **52**: 441–445.

Johnston I, Lopata A, Speiro A et al (1981) *In Vitro* fertilization: the challenge of the eighties. *Fertility and Sterility* **36**: 699–706.

Jones GS (1984) Update on in vitro fertilization. *Endocrine Reviews* **5**: 62–75.

Jones GS (1985) Use of purified gonadotropins for ovarian stimulation in IVF. *Clinical Obstetrics and Gynecology* **12**: 775–784.

Jones GS (1986) Luteal phase in a program for in vitro fertilization. In Jones HW Jr, Jones GS, Hodgen GD & Rosenwaks Z (eds) *In Vitro Fertilization, Norfolk*, pp 221–232. Baltimore: Williams and Wilkins.

Jones HW Jr, Jones GS, Andrews MC et al (1982) The program for IVF at Norfolk. *Fertility and Sterility* **38**: 14–21.

Jones HW Jr, Acosta AA, Andrews MC et al (1983) The importance of the follicular phase to success and failure in in vitro fertilization. *Fertility and Sterility* **40**: 317–321.

Karande VC, Jones GS, Veeck LL & Muasher SJ (1990) High-dose FSH stimulation at the onset of the menstrual cycle does not suppress the IVF outcome in low-responder patients. *Fertility and Sterility* (in press).

Karten MJ & Rivier JE (1986) Gonadotropin-releasing hormone analog design. Structure–function studies toward the development of agonists and antagonist: rationale and perspective. *Endocrine Reviews* **7**: 44–73.

Kenigsberg D & Hodgen GD (1987) Physiology of the menstrual cycle and ovarian function: clinical correlates and implications. In Rosenwaks Z, Benjamin F & Stone ML (eds) *Gynecology: Principles and Practice*, pp 11–36. New York: Macmillan.

Kenigsberg D, Littman BA, Williams RF & Hodgen GD (1984a) Medical hypophysectomy: II. Variability of ovarian response to gonadotropin therapy. *Fertility and Sterility* **42**: 116–126.

Kenigsberg D, Littman BA & Hodgen GD (1984b) Medical hypophysectomy: I. Dose–response using a gonadotropin-releasing hormone antagonist. *Fertility and Sterility* **42**: 112–115.

Knobil E (1980) The neuroendocrine control of the menstrual cycle. *Recent Progress in Hormone Research* **38**: 257–323.

Leal J, Williams R, Danforth DR, Gordon K & Hodgen GD (1988) Prolonged duration of gonadotropin inhibition by a third generation GnRH antagonist. *Journal of Clinical Endocrinology and Metabolism* **67**: 1325–1327.

Leal J, Williams RF, Danforth DR et al (1989) Probing studies on multiple dose effects of Antide (NAL-Lys) GnRH antagonist in ovariectomized monkeys. *Contraception* **40**: 623–633.

Leeton J, Trounson A & Jessup D (1985) Support of the luteal phase in IVF programs and results of a controlled trial with intramuscular proluton. *Journal of In Vitro Fertilization and Embryo Transfer* **2**: 166–169.

Littman BA & Hodgen GD (1984) Human menopausal gonadotropin stimulation in monkeys: blockade of the LH surge by a highly transient ovarian factor. *Fertility and Sterility* **41**: 108–113.

Ljungquist A, Feng DM, Tang PF et al (1987) Design, synthesis and bioassays of antagonists of LHRH which have high antiovulatory activity and release negligible histamine. *Biochemical and Biophysical Research Communications* **148**: 849–856.

Lopata A (1983) Concepts in human IVF and embryo transfer. *Fertility and Sterility* **40**: 289–301.

Lunenfeld B, Kraiem Z & Eshkol A (1976) Structure and function of the growing follicle. *Clinical Obstetrics and Gynecology* **3**: 27–39.

Mahadevan MM, Leader A & Tailor RJ (1985) Effects of low dose hCG on corpus luteum function after embryo transfer. *Journal of In Vitro Fertilization and Embryo Transfer* **2**: 190–194.

Marut EL & Hodgen GD (1982) Antiestrogenic action of high-dose clomiphene in primates: pituitary augmentation but with ovarian attenuation. *Fertility and Sterility* **38**: 100–104.

Matsuo H, Baba Y & Naur R et al (1971) Structure of the porcine LH and FSH-releasing hormone. The proposed amino acid reference. *Biochemical and Biophysical Research Communications* **43**: 1334–1339.

Meldrum DR, Wisot A, Hamilton F, Gutlay AL, Kempton W & Huynh D (1989) Routine pituitary suppression with leuprolide before ovarian stimulation for oocyte retrieval. *Fertility and Sterility* **51**: 455–459.

Meldrum DR, Tsao Z, Monroe SE et al (1984b) Stimulation of LH fragments with reduced bioactivity following GnRH agonist administration in women. *Journal of Clinical Endocrinology and Metabolism* **58**: 755–757.

Messinis IE, Templeton A & Baird DT (1986) Relationships between the characteristics of endogenous LH surge and the degree of ovarian hyperstimulation during superovulation induction in women. *Clinical Endocrinology* **25**: 393–400.

Muasher SJ, Oehninger S, Simonetti S et al (1988) The value of basal and/or stimulated serum gonadotropin levels in prediction of stimulation response and in vitro fertilization outcome. *Fertility and Sterility* **50**: 298–307.

Neveu S, Hedon B, Binger J et al (1987) Ovarian stimulation by a combination of a GnRH agonist and gonadotropin for IVF. *Fertility and Sterility* **47**: 639–643.

Oehninger S, Acosta AA, Kreiner D, Muasher SJ, Jones HW Jr & Rosenwaks Z (1988) In vitro fertilization and embryo transfer: an established and successful therapy for endometriosis. *Journal of In Vitro Fertilization and Embryo Transfer* **5**: 249–256.

Oehninger S, Brzyski RG, Muasher SJ, Acosta AA & Jones GS (1989) In vitro fertilization and embryo transfer in patients with endometriosis: impact of a gonadotropin releasing hormone agonist. *Human Reproduction* **4**: 541–544.

Palermo R, Amodeo G, Navot D, Rosenwaks Z & Cittadini E (1988) Concomitant GnRH agonist and gonadotropin treatment for the synchronized induction of multiple follicles. *Fertility and Sterility* **49**: 290–295.

Porter RN, Smith W, Craft IL, Abdulwakid NA & Jacobs HS (1984) Induction of ovulation for IVF using Buserelin and gonadotropins. *Lancet* **ii:** 1284.

Rabin D & McNeil LW (1980) Pituitary and gonadal desensitization of the continuous LH-RH infusion in normal females. *Journal of Clinical Endocrinology and Metabolism* **51**: 873–876.

Romeu A, Muasher SJ, Acosta AA, Liu HC & Rosenwaks Z (1987) Hormonal and follicular behavior of patients displaying multifollicular ovarian response (MOR) when undergoing IVF with different stimulation protocols. *Abstracts of the VI World Congress on IVF/ET*, Norfolk, Virginia, p 29.

Rosenwaks Z & Muasher SJ (1987) Recruitment of fertilizable eggs. In Jones HW Jr, Jones GS, Hodgen GD & Rosenwaks Z (eds) *In Vitro Fertilization, Norfolk*, pp 30–51. Baltimore: Williams and Wilkins.

Rosenwaks Z, Muasher SJ & Acosta AA (1987) Use of hMG and/or FSH for multiple follicle development. *Clinical Obstetrics and Gynecology* **29**: 148–157.

Sandler B, Fox J, Barrisi J, Williams M, Broufeld L & Navot D (1989) Very low dose lupron enhances follicular recruitment and prevents premature luteinization in controlled ovarian hyperstimulation. *Abstracts of the 36th Annual Meeting of the Society for Gynecological Investigation*, San Diego, California, p 306.

Schally AV, Arimura A & Coy DH (1980) Recent approaches to fertility control based on derivatives of LHRH. *Vitamins and Hormones* **38**: 257–323.

Schenken RS & Hodgen GD (1983) FSH induced ovarian hyperstimulation in monkeys: blockade of the LH surge. *Journal of Clinical Endocrinology and Metabolism* **57**: 50–55.

Schenken RS, Anderson WH & Hodgen GD (1984) FSH increases ovarian vein nonsteroidal function with gonadotropin-inhibiting activity. *Fertility and Sterility* **42**: 785–790.

Schwartz NB (1974) The role of FSH and LH and of their antibodies on follicle growth and on ovulation. *Biology of Reproduction* **10**: 236–272.

Scott R, Toner JP, Muasher S, Oehninger S, Robinson S & Rosenwaks Z (1989) FSH levels on cycle day 3 are predictive of in vitro fertilization outcome. *Fertility and Sterility* **51**: 651–654.

Scott R, Hofmann G, Oehninger S & Muasher SJ (1990) Intercycle variability of day 3 FSH levels and its effect on stimulation quality in in vitro fertilization. *Fertility and Sterility* (in press).

Serafini P, Stone B, Kerin J, Batzofin J, Quinn P & Marrs RP (1988) An alternate approach to controlled ovarian hyperstimulation in 'poor responders': pretreatment with a gonadotropin-releasing hormone analog. *Fertility and Sterility* **49:** 90–95.

Sherman BM & Korneman SG (1975) Hormonal characteristics of the human menstrual cycle throughout reproductive life. *Journal of Clinical Investigation* **55:** 669–706.

Sopelak VM & Hodgen GD (1983) Blockade of the estrogen-induced LH surge in monkeys: a non-steroidal, antigenic factor in porcine follicular fluid. *Fertility and Sterility* **41:** 108–113.

Steptoe PC & Edwards RG (1978) Birth after reimplantation of human embryo. *Lancet* **ii:** 366.

Trounson A, Howlett D, Rogers P & Hoppen HO (1986) The effect of progesterone supplementation around the time of oocyte recovery in patients superovulated for IVF. *Fertility and Sterility* **45:** 532–535.

Williams RF & Hodgen GD (1980) Disparate effects of hCG during the later follicular phase in monkeys: normal ovulation, follicular atresia, ovarian acyclicity, and hypersecretion of follicle-stimulating hormone. *Fertility and Sterility* **33:** 64–68.

Yee B & Vangyas JM (1986) Multiple follicle development utilizing combinations of clomiphene citrate and human menopausal gonadotropin. *Clinical Obstetrics and Gynecology* **29:** 141–147.

10

The use of GnRH agonists with hMG for induction or stimulation of ovulation

B. HEDON
J. BRINGER
F. ARNAL
C. HUMEAU
P. BOULOT
F. AUDIBERT
P. BENOS
S. NEVEU
P. MARES
F. LAFFARGUE
J. L. VIALA

To induce ovulation is to provoke follicular maturation and rupture in a patient who would not otherwise ovulate. To stimulate ovulation is to interfere with normal physiological ovarian regulation in order to intensify ovulatory phenomena. In the first case there is a pathological condition which prevents the patient from ovulating spontaneously, and drugs are used to try to correct this condition or to activate the ovary which would otherwise remain quiescent. The aim is to obtain maturation of one follicle which will release one oocyte ready to be fertilized. In the second case, the aim is to obtain several mature oocytes for in vitro fertilization. Both techniques use the same drugs in various regimens. Gonadotrophin-releasing hormone (GnRH) agonists have also been used, but their effects vary widely depending on whether the need is to induce or to stimulate ovulation.

GnRH agonists can create a state of reversible medical hypophysectomy, suppressing the greatest part of endogenous follicle-stimulating hormone (FSH) and luteinizing hormone (LH) secretion (Kenigsberg et al, 1984; Fraser and Sandow, 1985; Monroe et al, 1985). Their use, together with direct stimulation of the ovary by gonadotrophins, makes it possible to conduct follicular and oocyte maturation under exogenous influence only, with no risk of interference from possibly detrimental endogenous phenomena.

Baillière's Clinical Obstetrics and Gynaecology—
Vol. 4, No. 3, September 1990
ISBN 0–7020–1478–8

575

GnRH agonists and ovarian stimulation

Patients undergoing in vitro fertilization and embryo transfer (IVF-ET) or other related fertility-promoting procedures usually have no ovulatory defect and presumably a normally functioning hypothalamo–hypophyseal–ovarian axis. But, surprisingly enough, many cycles of ovarian stimulation have to be cancelled because of an inadequate ovarian response, including absence of follicular growth, follicular atresia, inadequate endogenous LH surge or excessive ovarian responses.

There is some concern about the responsibility of steady and high levels of LH which have been found more frequently during the folliculogenic phase of such cycles (Howles et al, 1986). Moreover, the end result of the IVF procedure seems to be correlated with the level of LH during the days preceding the human chorionic gonadotrophin (hCG) trigger prior to oocyte retrieval. Oocytes obtained from the preovulatory follicles of women with elevated LH levels have impaired fertilizability, and the embryos that result are less likely to implant successfully (Stanger and Yovich, 1985).

For these reasons, use of GnRH agonists has been advocated to prevent any inadequate LH surges before hCG administration and to decrease as much as possible steady and high levels of LH during folliculogenesis.

Protocols

There are mainly two different protocols, the principles of which are based on the two successive actions of GnRH agonists: the immediate stimulatory action is used in the 'short' protocol, and the secondary inhibitory action in both the 'long' and 'short' protocols. Besides these two protocols, an 'ultra-short' protocol has been described in which the agonist is used only during the first 3 days of ovarian stimulation (MacNamee, 1989).

In the long protocol, the basic principle is to conduct the complete period of folliculogenesis with the lowest possible LH (Figure 1). The GnRH agonist is given first at the beginning of the cycle (Belaisch-Allart, 1988b) or at the end of the preceding cycle (Porter et al, 1984; Fleming and Coutts,

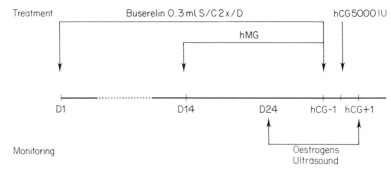

Figure 1. The gonadotrophin-releasing hormone (GnRH) agonist–human menopausal gonadotrophin (hMG) 'long protocol'. hCg, human chorionic gonadotrophin; D, day. From Hedon (1988b) with permission.

1986). After 2 or 3 weeks of administration, when hypophyseal desensitization is complete, follicular growth and maturation are induced by exogenous gonadotrophins, while administration of GnRH agonist is continued to prevent any premature LH rise. The administration of GnRH agonist is discontinued at the same time as human menopausal gonadotrophin (hMG) administration is stopped, when criteria of follicular maturity appear and it is decided to trigger ovulation with hCG. Either hMG or pure FSH can be used as the ovarian stimulus. Standard forms of GnRH agonists can be used, given either subcutaneously (Charbonnel, 1987; Belaisch-Allart, 1988b) or intranasally (Check, 1988). Long-acting forms of GnRH agonists, microspheres or implants can also be used (Fenichel et al, 1987; Chetkowski, 1989), but there is some concern that they might persist and affect the luteal phase of the cycle.

In the short protocol the immediate stimulatory action of the GnRH agonist serves as initial stimulus for follicular recruitment. Administration of GnRH agonist is begun on the first or second day of the cycle, together with hMG (Barriere et al, 1987a). Adequate follicular maturation is reached in 12 days on average, which should allow enough time for hypophyseal desensitization to be sufficient to prevent any inadequate LH rise before the physician decides to give hCG (Lopes et al, 1986; Barriere et al, 1987a, 1987b). In this type of protocol, only standard forms of GnRH agonists are used.

In both long and short protocols, the ovarian response is monitored by daily oestrogen measurements and daily ovarian ultrasonography. There is no need for LH or preovulatory progesterone evaluation since the GnRH agonist prevents any premature LH rise or premature luteinization. Investigators who have experience with the short protocol advocate early monitoring in order to adapt the doses of gonadotrophins to the intensity of the ovarian response (Barriere et al, 1987b). Early monitoring does not seem to be useful when the long protocol is used (Hedon et al, 1988).

The luteal phase can be shortened by giving GnRH agonists (Smitz, 1988). Some kind of luteal support is necessary (Devroey, 1988). This support can be by repeated injections of hCG during the luteal phase (1500 IU on the day of follicular aspiration, 1500 IU on the day of ET and again 1500 IU 4 days later). Others prefer to give progesterone (Belaisch-Allart, 1988b). There is no difference between the therapies in final results (Hedon, 1988a).

Results

Prospective randomized studies

The first prospective randomized study to compare the results of GnRH agonist (long protocol) with those of more classic protocols (same gonadotrophin regimen without pituitary desensitization) was published in 1986 (Hedon et al, 1986a, 1986b) and 1987 (Neveu et al, 1987) based on the work of our group in Montpellier (France). In this study 20 patients, 28–38 years of age, were selected according to strict criteria in order to minimize the influence of parameters independent of ovarian stimulation: tubal infertility, normal ovulation, normal husband semen, ovaries free of adhesions, and easy access to the uterine cavity for ET. These 20 patients were randomly divided into two groups. In group A, ten patients were stimulated with pure FSH (Metrodin®, Serono), 225 IU per day from day 2 to day 5 of the cycle, and then 150 IU on days 6 and 7. From the 8th day of the cycle, the amount of FSH was modified according to the degree of ovarian response obtained, as measured by urinary oestrogens (Cristol et al, 1985). In group B, ten patients were stimulated with pure FSH after pituitary desensitization. The GnRH agonist (Buserelin®, Hoechst) was administered at a dose of 0.3 ml subcutaneously twice a day for 14 days, beginning on day 1 or 2 of the cycle. On day 14 of Buserelin administration, FSH stimulation was started according to the same protocol as in group A. Buserelin treatment was continued until hCG was administered. The results of this study are summarized in Table 1.

Table 1. Results of the first randomized study comparing ovarian stimulation protocols.

	Group A: without GnRH agonist	Group B: with GnRH agonist
Number of cycles	10	10
Stimulation failure	2	0
Dose of hMG (IU)	1552 ± 220	1890 ± 280
Number of oocytes/aspiration	4.78 ± 2.2	8.2 ± 2.8
Number of embryos/transfer	3.29 ± 1.8	4.5 ± 2.1
Clinical pregnancies	1*	6**

* Single ongoing pregnancy; ** three singles, two twins, one triplet, all ongoing pregnancies.
GnRH, gonadotrophin-releasing hormone; hMG, human menopausal gonadotrophin.

Comparison of the two groups showed a larger number of oocytes retrieved and a larger number of embryos obtained by IVF in group B. In group A, only one pregnancy was achieved (one of ten stimulations, one of eight follicular aspirations, one of eight ETs). In group B six pregnancies were obtained (six of ten stimulations, six of ten follicular aspirations, six of nine ETs). This preliminary study was confirmed by a similar study undertaken in collaboration with the Clamart group (Paris) and our group in Montpellier. In this series 60 patients were selected by the same careful criteria as before and randomly divided into two groups. Group A was stimulated with a combination of pure FSH (Fertinine®, Searle) and hMG (Inductor®, Searle): FSH 150 IU and hMG 150 IU on days 3 and 4 and then hMG 150 IU from day 5 to day 7, and then daily adaptation from day 8 until hCG administration. Group B was stimulated with the same gonadotrophin regimen but after previous pituitary desensitization with a GnRH agonist (Buserelin) according to the protocol described previously. Results confirmed the findings of the first study (Table 2): the pregnancy rate was 10% per stimulation cycle, 13% per follicular aspiration, and 14.3% per ET in the first group, and 23%, 27% and 33.3% in the group with pituitary inhibition.

As far as the short protocol is concerned, the results of Barriere et al (1987b) show the same kind of trend. Similar studies have been undertaken with the ultrashort protocol, again with similar results (Loumaye, 1988).

Table 2. Results of the second randomized study comparing ovarian stimulation protocols.

	n	A(%)	B(%)	C(%)
FSH + hMG				
A, stimulation cycles	30			
B, oocyte retrievals	23	77%		
C, transfers	21	70%	91%	
Clinical pregnancies	3	10%	13%	14.3%
GnRH agonist + FSH + hMG				
A, stimulation cycles	30			
B, oocyte retrievals	26	87%		
C, transfers	21	70%	81%	
Clinical pregnancies	7	23%	27%	33.3%

FSH, follicle-stimulating hormone; hMG, human menopausal gonadotrophin; GnRH, gonadotrophin-releasing hormone.

Routine experience

Routine experience has confirmed the results of the randomized studies. Our group has used GnRH agonists on a large scale since 1985. From 1985 to 1988, nearly 2000 cycles were stimulated with the agonist long regimen; 5% of these cycles had to be cancelled because of inadequate responses, 1701 follicular aspirations were performed, producing 11 968 oocytes, the fecundation and cleavage rate of these oocytes was 46%, and 1242 ETs of one to five embryos could be done (3.3 embryos/ET), producing 421 clinical pregnancies (24.8% of egg collections and 33.9% of ETs). The implantation rate per transferred embryo was 14%; 82% of pregnancies produced living babies. Overall comparison of these results with those of more classical protocols not using GnRH agonists (combination of clomiphene citrate and hMG) shows that GnRH agonist protocols produce more oocytes (7.04 versus 4.75 per cycle), a similar fecundation and cleavage rate (46%), more

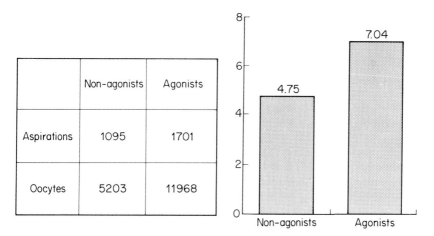

Figure 2. Montpellier-Languedoc-Roussillon in vitro fertilization. Results for period 1985–1988 (attempts 1–3): number of oocytes per aspiration.

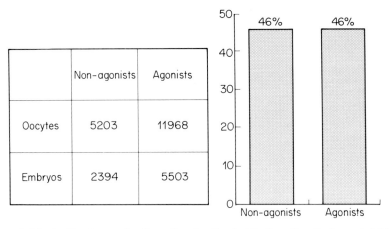

	Non-agonists	Agonists
Oocytes	5203	11968
Embryos	2394	5503

Figure 3. Montpellier-Languedoc-Roussillon in vitro fertilization. Results for period 1985–1988 (attempts 1–3): cleavage rates.

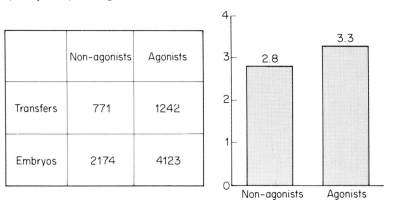

	Non-agonists	Agonists
Transfers	771	1242
Embryos	2174	4123

Figure 4. Montpellier-Languedoc-Roussillon in vitro fertilization. Results for period 1985–1988 (attempts 1–3): number of embryos per transfer.

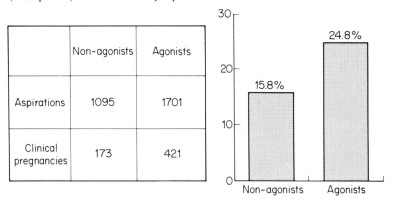

	Non-agonists	Agonists
Aspirations	1095	1701
Clinical pregnancies	173	421

Figure 5. Montpellier-Languedoc-Roussillon in vitro fertilization. Results for period 1985–1988 (attempts 1–3): pregnancy rate per aspiration.

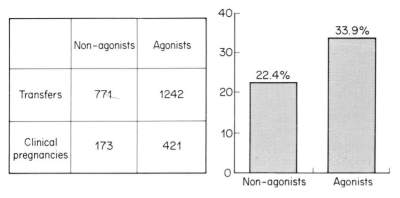

Figure 6. Montpellier-Languedoc-Roussillon in vitro fertilization. Results for period 1985–1988 (attempts 1–3): pregnancy rate per transfer.

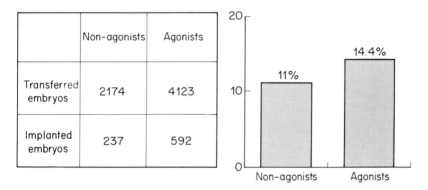

Figure 7. Montpellier-Languedoc-Roussillon in vitro fertilization. Results for period 1985–1988 (attempts 1–3): implantation rates.

embryos to be transferred (3.3 versus 2.8 per cycle) and a higher pregnancy rate (24.8 versus 15.8 per cycle) (Figures 2–7).

This experience of our group has been reproduced by many others, as shown by the FIVNAT annual results: in France in 1987 60.5% of ovarian stimulations for IVF used GnRH agonists, and in 1988 this proportion increased to 88%, with a majority of long protocols. Comparison of 'agonist protocols' with 'non-agonist protocols' shows an important reduction in the cycle cancellation rate (10.5% versus 18%), mainly by suppressing cancellations caused by inappropriate LH surge, and also an increase in the pregnancy rate per ET (29% versus 20%) (Mandelbaum, 1988).

Meta-analysis of all published series leads to the same conclusion, i.e., better results with agonist protocols (Zorn, 1987; Chetkowski, 1989; MacLachlan, 1989). All patients seem to profit from this therapy, although some profit more than others (Fenichel, 1988a).

Results in 'bad responder' patients

Use of a GnRH agonist in association with hMG has been reported to give good results in patients who had previously been classified as 'bad responders' (Antoine, 1988; Fenichel, 1988b; Loumaye, 1988; Smitz et al, 1988; Belaisch et al, 1989). The causes of cycle cancellations are (Hedon, 1988c):

1. Insufficient response. Follicular development does not take place (no increase in oestrogen secretion, no follicular development at ultrasonography) or is poor (only one follicle is recruited, oestrogen secretion remains low) and slow (no real oestrogen increase).
2. Excessive response. A large number of follicles are recruited. High oestrogen levels are obtained, usually before follicular maturation is complete. If hCG were injected, a hyperstimulation syndrome would develop.
3. Follicular atresia. The arrest of follicular growth is marked by a drop in oestrogen secretion. This phenomenon could appear at any stage of follicular maturation, especially if the ovarian response is weak or if there is a premature LH surge.
4. Spontaneous LH surge. If a spontaneous LH surge appears, it may be too early for the stage of follicular maturation; this maturation stops and the follicles undergo atresia. It can also be inconvenient for the organization of the medical team. For follicular aspirations to be performed after spontaneous LH surges complete availability of the medical staff is necessary, and precise monitoring of LH secretion would be compulsory in order to choose the precise timing for oocyte retrieval.

GnRH agonists suppress all cancellations related to a premature LH surge. However, cancellations related to an insufficient ovarian response or phenomena of atresia remain. The main usefulness of GnRH agonists is to make the situation clear, with no possible interference by endogenous phenomena on the type of ovarian response. Under GnRH agonist hypophyseal desensitization, the ovary is subjected only to the stimulatory influence of gonadotrophins, and if there is an inadequate response it is most often a result of inappropriate administration of drugs or ovarian deficiency. In this regard, the level of FSH at the beginning of a cycle, before any treatment is given, can be of good prognostic significance for the degree of ovarian activity. This level increases steadily during the years before menopause, long before the first modifications of the menstrual cycle appear. For this reason it can be a good indicator of the possibility of ovarian stimulation. When there is a higher level of FSH, one should give more hMG to obtain the desired ovarian response.

Comparison of long and short protocols

In several prospective randomized or retrospective studies, results obtained with the different types of protocols using GnRH agonists, mainly the so-called 'short' and 'long' protocols, have been compared. All of them demonstrate a higher pregnancy rate with the long protocol, despite the fact

Table 3. Comparison of short and long stimulation protocols.

	Short protocol (ongoing pregnancies/aspiration)	Long protocol (ongoing pregnancies/aspiration)
Hedon, 1988b	9%	32%
Foulot, 1988	14%	18%
Antoine, 1988	10%	22%
Belaisch-Allart, 1988a	16.5%	21.1%
Fivnat, 1988 (see Mandelbaum, 1988)	15.3%	22.5%

that the difference was not statistically significant for individual series (Table 3). However, with techniques such as IVF-ET, only large-scale studies can produce statistically significant results. Such studies are impossible for individual groups to undertake and necessitate multicentre trials which are very difficult to organize because of the great variety of techniques in use in different IVF centres (Daures et al, 1990).

GnRH AGONISTS AND INDUCTION OF OVULATION

Results of ovulation induction with hMG are better when the patient is totally anovulatory and when no pituitary function is retained. This observation is the main basis for the use of GnRH agonists to create a state of reversible hypophysectomy prior to ovulation induction (Lewinthal, 1988). The use of GnRH agonists can also have a variety of potentially beneficial effects: (1) reduction in the levels of endogenous LH and of androgens, hormones which can promote atresia when their level of secretion is above normal, as is the case in the polycystic ovary syndrome; and (2) suppression of premature LH surges and suppression of the risk of premature luteinization.

Using GnRH agonists together with hMG for ovulation induction is a unique occasion to suppress all extraovarian influences. If the factor responsible for the ovulatory defect is extraovarian, its suppression should leave an intact ovary to the influence of external gonadotrophins, and the same induction results should be obtained as if the cause of anovulation were hypothalamic deficiency.

Results

With a combination of GnRH agonists/hMG/hCG Fleming obtained 27 pregnancies during 80 cycles (34%) in 35 patients with hormonal anomalies of polycystic ovarian syndrome. Comparison of these results with the 19 pregnancies obtained among 120 non-randomized cycles (16%) in 45 women undergoing ovulation induction with hMG/hCG shows the superiority of the combined treatment. According to Fleming (1988) a possible explanation for the worse results of classical treatment is the frequency of premature luteinization. This phenomenon disappears totally when GnRH agonist is given. The same group also reports on the beneficial effects of the GnRH agonist combination for treatment of infertility with luteal insufficiency; 16 pregnancies were obtained among 26 women in 110 cycles of induction (15%) (Fleming, 1985).

Charbonnel (1987) draws somewhat different conclusions: despite five pregnancies obtained in eight women with polycystic ovarian syndrome, 33 cycles were necessary (15% pregnancy per induction cycle) and none of the habitual difficulties of ovulation induction in this type of disease was modified by the combination with the agonist. The frequency of multifollicular development, cyst formation and hyperstimulation syndrome remained unchanged. Our own results are similar (Gilbert, 1986; Hedon et al, 1989), as were the results of randomized studies (Hompes, 1986; Dodson, 1987). In fact, the majority of the studies reveal no differences when GnRH agonists plus hMG are used for ovulation induction (Alvarez, 1988). The only demonstrated effect is to prevent premature luteinization.

We can conclude the following from these results.

1. There is no reason to use GnRH agonists when there is a hypothalamic or a hypophyseal deficiency. When gonadotrophin deficiency is present, no ectopic LH surge can intervene. There is no use in further depressing gonadotrophin secretion.
2. When the defect is the ovary itself, suppression of endogenous gonadotrophins does not correct the default.
3. In polycystic ovarian syndrome the primary anomaly seems to be intraovarian. Suppression of higher influences does not modify the function of these ovaries, which respond to the stimulatory process with the same problems. Furthermore, with GnRH agonist the ovaries seem to respond even more intensely to gonadotrophin therapy, as is the case in stimulation procedures for IVF-ET. Multifollicular development and hyperstimulation syndromes might be even more frequent unless small quantities of gonadotrophins are used.

So, in the majority of cases of ovulation induction there is no real place for GnRH agonists, except when androgen or LH levels are very high or when there is repeated failure because of premature luteinization (Franks, 1987; Lanzone, 1987; Check, 1988; Weise, 1988).

GnRH agonists as a means of ovarian 'healing'

Filicori (1988) administered GnRH agonists for 3 months to a series of 21 patients having polycystic ovarian disease. Immediately after this treatment, ovulation induction was performed by pulsatile injection of GnRH. Results were much more favourable than when the same patients were treated without prior ovarian blockage (Filicori, 1988). After GnRH agonist therapy the LH/FSH ratio and testosterone levels were reduced, and there was a less explosive response on oestrogen secretion after the start of the induction treatment. The long ovarian blockage lets the ovaries heal from the atretic process. However, this process starts again very quickly once the blockage is removed, especially if the ovaries are stimulated (Shaw, 1987).

This observation does not extend to other kinds of ovarian disorders. In deficient ovaries with high gonadotrophin levels, as in premenopausal patients, no healing is observed even after prolonged suppression of gonadotrophins with GnRH agonists, and induction of ovulation remains just as difficult, usually with no ovarian response or very poor follicular recruitment and growth (Surrey, 1989).

CONCLUSIONS

The use of GnRH agonists plus hMG for ovarian stimulation is a new concept, allowing the ovaries to be stimulated with no possible interference from the hypothalamo–pituitary axis. Experience with this type of therapy has shown that it is particularly suited to the promotion of follicular growth and oocyte maturation when a stimulation effect is wanted. But the same is not true when induction of ovulation is wanted, because the suppression of influences from the hypothalamo–pituitary axis does not change the pathological condition responsible for the ovulatory disorder. In this regard, GnRH antagonists should have the same impact and the same place in the future as GnRH agonists have today.

REFERENCES

Alvarez S (1988) Y a-t-il intérêt à l'utilisation des analogues de la LHRH dans les dystrophies ovariennes polykystiques? *Journal of In Vitro Fertilization and Embryo Transfer* **26:** 285.

Antoine J (1988) Comparaison des profils hormonaux plasmatiques de fin de phase folliculaire au cours des inductions pour FIV en protocoles courts et longs utilisant des agonistes de la LHRH. *Contraception Fertilité Sexualité* **16:** 630.

Barriere P, Lopes P, Sagot P et al (1987a) Utilisation des analogues de la gonadoréline selon un protocole court pour la fécondation in vitro. *Contraception Fertilité Sexualité* **15:** 768–770.

Barriere P, Lopes P, Boiffard J et al (1987b) GnRH analogs in ovulation induction for in vitro fertilization: benefit of a short administration regimen. *Journal of In Vitro Fertilization and Embryo Transfer* **4:** 64–65.

Belaisch-Allart J (1988a) Intérêt de l'utilisation des agonistes du LHRH en protocole long, avec ou sans FSH, ou en protocole court dans un programme de FIV. *Contraception Fertilité Sexualité* **16:** 32.

Belaisch-Allart J (1988b) Effet de la supplémentation de la phase lutéale dans un programme de FIV après stimulation de l'ovulation par les agonistes du LHRH. Etude multicentrique. *Contraception Fertilité Sexualité* **16:** 654.

Belaisch-Allart J, Testart J & Frydman R (1989) Utilization of GnRH agonists for bad responders in an IVF program. *Human Reproduction* **4:** 33–34.

Charbonnel B (1987) Induction of ovulation in polycystic ovary syndrome with a combination of a LHRH analog and exogenous gonadotropins. *Fertility and Sterility* **47:** 920–924.

Check J (1988) The effect of leuprolide acetate in aiding induction of ovulation in hypergonadotropic hypogonadism: a case report. *Fertility and Sterility* **49:** 542.

Chetkowski RJ (1989) Improved pregnancy outcome with the addition of leuprolide acetate to gonadotropins for in vitro fertilization. *Fertility and Sterility* **52:** 250.

Cristol P, Hedon B, Chabab A et al (1985) Dosages enzymatiques es estrogènes urinaires. *Annales de Biologie Clinique* **43:** 841.

Daures JP, Hedon B, Arnal F et al (1990) Early or late monitoring of stimulation of ovulation for in-vitro fertilization? A methodological discussion of a randomized study. *Human Reproduction* **5:** 138–142.

Devroey P (1988) La phase lutéale après traitement à la buséréline. *Contraception Fertilité Sexualité* **16:** 46.

Dodson W (1987) The effect of Leuprolide acetate on ovulation induction with HMG in PCO syndrome. *Journal of Clinical Endocrinology and Metabolism* **65**: 95.

Fenichel P (1988a) Réponses ovariennes à la stimulation pour FIV: du protocole 'prêt à porter' au protocole 'sur mesure'. *Contraception Fertilité Sexualité* **16**: 621.

Fenichel P (1988b) Réponses inadéquates à la stimulation de l'ovulation: bilan hormonal prédictif et effets des analogues de la LHRH. *Contraception Fertilité Sexualité* **16**: 49.

Fenichel P, Grimaldi M, Olivero J et al (1987) Blocage hypophysaire par un analogue de la gonadoréline, le DTRP6-LHRH à libération prolongée avant induction de l'ovulation. *Contraception Fertilité Sexualité* **15**: 1033–1037.

Filicori M (1988) GnRH analog suppression renders PCO disease patients more susceptible to ovulation induction with pulsatile GnRH. *Journal of Clinical Endocrinology and Metabolism* **66**: 327.

Fleming R (1985) Successful treatment of infertile women with oligomenorrhoea using a combination of an LHRH agonist and exogenous gonadotrophins. *British Journal of Obstetrics and Gynaecology* **92**: 369.

Fleming R (1988) Combined GnRH analog and exogenous gonadotropins for ovulation induction in infertile women: efficacy related to ovarian function assessment. *American Journal of Obstetrics and Gynecology* **159**: 376.

Fleming R & Coutts J (1986) Induction of multiple follicular growth in normally menstruating women with endogenous gonadotropin suppression. *Fertility and Sterility* **45**: 226–230.

Foulot H (1988) Etude randomisée entre protocole court et protocole long de buséréline concernant 100 cycles de FIV. *Contraception Fertilité Sexualité* **16**: 628.

Franks S (1987) Use of LHRH agonists in the treatment of anovulation in women with PCO. *Hormone Research* **28**: 164.

Fraser H & Sandow J (1985) Suppression of follicular maturation by infusion of a LHRH agonist starting during the luteal phase in the stuptailed macaque monkey. *Journal of Clinical Endocrinology and Metabolism* **60**: 579.

Gibert F (1986) Induction de l'ovulation par les gonadotrophines ménopausales (HMG) après suppression de l'activité gonadotrope par les agonistes de la LHRH. *Annals of Endocrinology* **4**: 259.

Hedon B (1988a) Taux hormonaux en début de phase lutéale en fonction de divers protocoles de stimulation de l'ovulation en vue de FIV avec et sans agoniste de la GnRH. Effet de la supplémentation en progestérone. *Contraception Fertilité Sexualité* **16**: 660.

Hedon B (1988b) Comparaison randomisée protocole long-protocole court dans les stimulations de l'ovaire en association avec un agoniste de la GnRH en vue de FIV. *Contraception Fertilité Sexualité* **16**: 624.

Hedon B (1988c) Recurrent abnormal follicular maturation and ovarian stimulation for IVF. *Human Reproduction* **3**: 567.

Hedon B, Neveu S, Bringer J et al (1986a) L'inhibition de LH au cours de la stimulation de l'ovulation pour fécondation in vitro. *Hormones and Reproductive Metabolism* **3**: 173–177.

Hedon B, Bringer J, Neveu S et al (1986b) Utilisation de la GnRH et de ses agonistes pour stimulatio de l'ovulation en vue de fécondation in vitro. *Contraception Fertilite Sexualité* **14**: 683–688.

Hedon B, Arnal F, Simondon E et al (1988) Stimulation de l'ovulation par HMG après désensibilisation hypophysaire préalable par agonistes de la GnRH en vue de fécondation in vitro: monitorage précoce ou tardif? *Contraception Fertilité Sexualité* **16**: 43.

Hedon B., Badoc E, Bringer J et al (1989) Stérilité par syndrôme des ovaires polykystiques et fécondation in vitro. In Société Française de Gynécologie (eds) *Dystrophies Ovariennes*, pp 147–156. Paris: Masson Editeurs.

Hompes P (1986) The additional use of buserelin in HMG–HCG ovulation induction in PCO: a double blind controlled study. In Rolland R, Chadha D & Willemsen W (eds) Gonadotrophin down-regulation in gynecological practice, p 391. New York: Alan Liss.

Howles C, MacNamee M, Edwards R, Goswamy R & Steptoe P (1986) Effect of high tonic levels of luteinising hormone on outcome of in vitro fertilization. *Lancet* **ii**: 521–522.

Kenigsberg D, Littman B, Williams R & Hodgen G (1984) Medical hypophysectomy II: Variability of ovarian response to gonadotrophin therapy. *Fertility and Sterility* **42**: 116–126.

Lanzone A (1987) Successful induction of ovulation and conception with combined GnRH agonist plus highly purified FSH in patients with PCO disease. *Journal of Clinical Endocrinology and Metabolism* **65**: 1253.

Lewinthal D (1988) Induction of ovulation with luprolide acetate and HMG. *Fertility and Sterility* **49**: 585.

Lopes P, Barriere P, Charbonnel B & Paillard B (1986) Intérêt de l'utilisation brève d'un analogue de la gonadoréline dans un programme de fécondation in vitro. *Presse Médicale* **15**: 2074.

Loumaye E (1988) Résultats obtenus en FIV par administration à court terme de buséréline et HMG chez des patientes ayant présenté un échec de stimulation par clomifene-HMG ou HMG. *Contraception Fertilité Sexualité* **16**: 40.

MacLachlan V (1989) A controlled study of LHRH agonist (Buserelin) for the induction of folliculogenesis before IVF. *New England Journal of Medicine* **32**: 1233–1237.

MacNamee MC (1989) Short-term luteinizing-hormone-releasing hormone agonist treatment—prospective trial of novel ovarian stimulation regimen for in vitro fertilization. *Fertility and Sterility* **52**: 264.

Mandelbaum J (1988) Etat de la stimulation ovarienne dans la FIV. *Contraception Fertilité Sexualité* **16**: 579.

Monroe S, Henzl M, Martin M et al (1985) Ablation of folliculogenesis in women by a single dose of GnRH agonist: significance of time in cycle *Fertility and Sterility* **43**: 361.

Neveu S, Hedon B, Bringer J et al (1987) Ovarian stimulation by a combination of a gonadotrophin releasing hormone agonist and gonadotropins for in vitro fertilization. *Fertility and Sterility* **47**: 639–643.

Porter R, Smith W, Craft I, Abdulwahid N & Jacobs H (1984) Induction of ovulation for in vitro fertilization using buserelin and gonadotropins. *Lancet* **ii**: 1284–1285.

Shaw R (1987) Endocrine changes following pituitary desensitization with LHRH agonist and administration of purified FSH to induce follicular maturation. *British Journal of Obstetrics and Gynaecology* **94**: 682.

Smitz J (1988) The luteal phase and early pregnancy after combined GnRH agonist/HMG treatment for superovulation in IVF or GIFT. *Human Reproduction* **3**: 585.

Smitz J, Devroey P, Khan J et al (1988) Addition of buserelin to HMG in patients with failed stimulations for IVF or GIFT. *Human Reproduction* **3**: 35–38.

Stanger J & Yovich J (1985) Reduced in vitro fertilization of human ovocytes from patients with raised basal luteinizing hormone levels during the follicular phase. *British Journal of Obstetrics and Gynaecology* **92**: 385–393.

Surrey ES (1989) The effect of gonadotropin suppression on the induction of ovulation in premature ovarian failure patients. *Fertility and Sterility* **52**: 36.

Weise H (1988) Buserelin suppression of endogenous gonadotropin secretion in infertile women with ovarian feedback disorders given HMG/HCG treatment. *Fertility and Sterility* **49**: 399.

Zorn J (1987) Les analogues de la LHRH et les nouvelles techniques d'induction de l'ovulation pour la fécondation in vitro et le transfert intratubaire des gamètes. *Contraception Fertilité Sexualité* **15**: 771–773.

11

Induction of ovulation with pulsatile GnRH

ZEEV SHOHAM
ROY HOMBURG
HOWARD S. JACOBS

Following the discovery that hypothalamic extracts triggered release of gonadotrophins (McCann et al, 1960), years of effort were required before the neurotransmitter gonadotrophin-releasing hormone (GnRH) was finally isolated in 1971. Its chemical structure was described independently by Schally et al (1971) and Burgus et al (1971). GnRH is a single-chain decapeptide in which the amino acid sequence is identical in all mammalian species studied to date (Ory, 1985).

GnRH releases both follicle-stimulating hormone (FSH) and luteinizing hormone (LH), and so hopes were immediately raised that synthetic GnRH could be used for treatment of infertility caused by gonadotrophin deficiency. Although Kastin et al (1971) reported the first conception after treatment with GnRH, high-dose injections of GnRH given at infrequent intervals proved an unreliable form of treatment for inducing ovulation in patients with hypogonadotrophic hypogonadism (Mortimer et al, 1975; Nillius, 1979). The high expectations for GnRH treatment were not realized initially because the non-pulsatile administration of GnRH caused pituitary desensitization (Rabin and McNeil, 1980). Renewed hope that GnRH might prove therapeutically useful was provided by Knobil (1980) in a series of experiments in rhesus monkeys with experimental lesions of the arcuate nucleus. Administration of GnRH in a pulsatile mode activated episodic gonadotrophin secretion in these monkeys and resulted in ovulation. A new wave of interest then developed to determine the optimum dosage and frequency for GnRH administration to humans, as well as to establish whether the subcutaneous or intravenous route was the more satisfactory method of administration.

Leyendecker et al (1980a) were the first to show the effectiveness of pulsatile treatment with GnRH in stimulating ovulation in women. In the same year this group also reported the results in five women who were treated with GnRH intravenously with 10–15 μg of GnRH per pulse at 90-min intervals for 17–20 days (Leyendecker et al, 1980b). Since that time pulsatile GnRH treatment has become very popular for the management of patients suffering from various disturbances of GnRH secretion.

In this chapter we review current knowledge on the use of pulsatile

GnRH, concentrating on selection of patients, route and dose of administration, adverse effects, and outcome of treatment and pregnancy.

MODE OF ACTION OF GnRH

GnRH is a decapeptide in which the second and third amino acids, histidine and tryptophan, are critical for activation of the adenylate cyclase system and subsequent gonadotrophin release (Coy and Schally, 1978; Stewart, 1981). Pyroglutamic acid at position 1 and glycine in positions 6 and 10 are critical for maintaining the configuration of the molecule and its particular binding characteristics.

Studies in monkeys with experimental GnRH deficiency have shown that administration of GnRH, in the pulsatile mode in which the hormone is normally secreted, is essential for sustained gonadotrophin secretion (Nakai et al, 1978). These studies also demonstrated normal negative and positive feedback regulation of gonadotrophin secretion by oestrogen during pulsatile administration of uniform doses of GnRH, indicating that, in monkeys at least, ovarian feedback regulation solely at the pituitary level is sufficient for normal ovarian cyclicity. Feedback regulation at the hypothalamic level is therefore of secondary importance in this species (Nakai et al, 1978; Knobil, 1980). Knobil's group also studied the effect of different pulse frequencies of GnRH administration on gonadotrophin secretion (Knobil, 1980). They found that the optimum effect was obtained with a pulse interval of 60 min, and that each pulse of GnRH not only induced release but also synthesis of gonadotrophins (Rommler, 1978). Thus, using double GnRH stimulation tests, the LH response to a second GnRH bolus was maximal when the second bolus followed the first with an interval of 60–180 min. These observations were further substantiated by ultrastructural studies of rat pituitary gonadotrophs: parallel to the GnRH-induced extrusion of LH secretory granules, new secretory granules appeared 1–2 h after administration of GnRH (Rommler et al, 1978). These findings, which suggest that administration of GnRH induces functional cycles of release, synthesis, storage and intracellular degradation of gonadotrophins (Rommler et al, 1978), probably underlie the 'self-priming effect' of GnRH, which occurs only when GnRH is administered in a pulsatile fashion. In contrast, chronic GnRH infusion leads to desensitization of the gonadotroph, with, *inter alia*, down-regulation of GnRH receptors and a decrease in LH secretion (Belchetz et al, 1978).

The requirement for pulsatile stimulation of the pituitary gonadotrophs also explains why application of long-acting GnRH analogues results ultimately in impairment rather than enhancement of gonadotrophin secretion (Dericks-Tan et al, 1977). Since the above-mentioned pioneering work, it has been shown that sustained gonadotrophin secretion can be achieved with pulsatile GnRH administration in men, women and children with GnRH deficiency (Jacobson et al, 1979; Crowley and McArthur, 1980).

ROUTE OF ADMINISTRATION

GnRH is usually administered by computerized minipump via a chronic indwelling intravenous or subcutaneous catheter. The infuser is designed to deliver the drug in a pulsatile manner, in an amplitude and interval according to the investigator's demands. The pumps are designed to be worn under clothing or on a belt. The cannula is inserted either into the subcutaneous tissue or into a vein in the arm.

Several pumps are available. The Auto Syringe, model AS6H (Auto Syringe Inc., Hooksett, New Hampshire, USA), can be programmed to deliver 12–87 µl at seven different intervals. The Zyklomat Var Franconia (Ferring GmbH, Kiel, FRG) delivers a single pulse volume of 50 µl at various time intervals. The Provider PA 3000 (Pancretec, San Diego, California, USA) delivers a pulse volume of 62.5 µl with a single pulse frequency of 90 min. The battery-driven pump we use, developed by Sutherland et al (1984), delivers a range of volumes from 20 to 320 µl per pulse at intervals of 8.5–128 min (Figure 1).

Debate continues over whether the intravenous or subcutaneous route is preferable for induction of ovulation. Intravenous injections produce higher and more sharply focused serum GnRH pulse profiles than subcutaneous injections (Handelsman et al, 1984; Menon et al, 1984; Handelsman and Swerdloff, 1986). Since less GnRH is needed, treatment via the intravenous route costs less. In a pharmacokinetic study it was found that plasma GnRH levels rose rapidly after both subcutaneous and intravenous administration, reaching peak levels after 5–10 min and 2 min, respectively. The mean peak

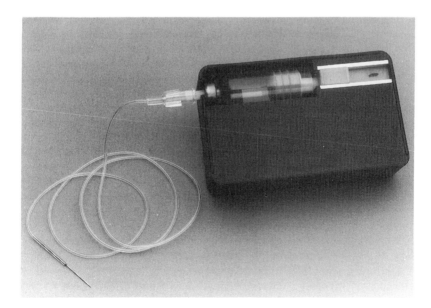

Figure 1. Mill Hill Pulsatile Infuser used for pulsatile administration of gonadotrophin-releasing hormone (GnRH).

GnRH levels were 80–170 pg/ml after subcutaneous doses of 5 and 10 μg, respectively, whereas the levels exceeded 1000 pg/ml 2–5 min after an intravenous injection of 10 μg of GnRH. With both routes of administration, GnRH levels fell rapidly after the peak. GnRH is well absorbed after subcutaneous administration, resulting in a pulsatile plasma profile with a duration only slightly longer than that after intravenous administration. Most importantly, subcutaneous and intravenous GnRH administration resulted in similar pulsatile profiles of LH (Hurley et al, 1984). In another study, subcutaneous injection of 20 μg of GnRH into the upper arm was compared with its injection into the lower abdominal wall. GnRH injected into the upper arm produced a pulse of greater peak height and shorter duration than after injecting it into the abdominal skin (Blunt et al, 1986). These results may in part explain the disappointing rates of ovulation reported by Menon et al (1984) who used the lower abdomen for the site of injection.

Investigators employing the subcutaneous route argue for its convenience and lack of invasiveness. Higher doses of GnRH are, however, often required (Hurley et al, 1984) and lower rates of ovulation have been reported (Leyendecker and Wildt, 1984). There may be prolonged absorption from the subcutaneous tissues (Reid et al, 1981; Handelsman et al, 1984). Intravenous administration yields a more predictable response with, it is claimed, a more physiological pattern of gonadotrophin secretion (Reid et al, 1981; Handelsman et al, 1984) and a higher rate of ovulatory cycles. In addition, GnRH dosage can be reduced, and the time to ovulation shortened (Handelsman et al, 1984; Leyendecker and Wildt, 1984; Crowley et al, 1985). In a study compiled from the literature by Lunenfeld (1984) a total of 293 patients who had been treated for 516 cycles by the intravenous route was reported: 405 ovulated (78.5%) and the pregnancy rate was 46.1% (135 patients). These results were compared with those in 97 patients who had been treated in 198 cycles by the subcutaneous route, of whom 129 ovulated (65.2%) with a pregnancy rate of 37.1% (36 patients). Several reasons may exist for the differences described. Most possible is that some investigators may have administered a dose too low for successful subcutaneous therapy. Another reason may be inappropriate patient selection (Mason et al, 1984a). Thus, Loucopoulos et al (1984) reported that their two patients with low serum gonadotrophin concentrations who did not ovulate on subcutaneous therapy did not respond to intravenous administration either.

In our own survey of the literature, we compared the results in 319 patients treated with subcutaneous GnRH for 934 cycles (Table 1) with those in 107 patients treated through the intravenous route for 304 cycles (Table 2). The rates of ovulation per cycle were 70.9 and 87.8% respectively (Fisher's exact test, two-tailed, $P < 0.0005$). This therapeutic gain of 17% (95% confidence limits 12.3–21.6%) was not, however, reflected in a difference in the pregnancy rate per cycle (23.6 and 27.6% respectively) or per ovulatory cycle (33.2 and 31.5%), and there was no significant difference in the pregnancy rate per patient (68.9 and 78.5% respectively, Fisher's exact (two-tailed) probability = 0.074). Based on these results, therefore,

Table 1. Pulsatile administration of gonadotrophin-releasing hormone (GnRH) via the subcutaneous route.

Authors	No. of patients	Total no. of cycles	Ovulatory cycles	No. of pregnancies	Pulse dose (µg)	Interval (min)	Luteal phase (P/hCG)	No. of multiple pregnancies	Miscarriages
Homburg et al (1989)	118	434	304	100	15	90	P	7	28
Reid et al (1981)	2	2	0		0.5–5	90–120			
Mason et al (1984b)	28	83	80	30	10–25	90	hCG	1	8
Hurley et al (1984)	14	36	30	13	5–15	90	hCG		2
Polsen et al (1986)	5	12	9		7.5–15	90	P		
Glasier et al (1987)	16	32	16	3		90	P		
Saffan and Seible (1986)	13	21	17	4	8.5–20	90–120	hCG		1
Eshel et al (1988)	48	141	73	23	15	90	P	1	10
Mason et al (1984a)	54	123	85	38	15	90	P		11
Skarin et al (1983)	14	38	36	8	1–20	90	P	1	3
Skarin et al (1982)	7	12	12	1	20	90	P		
Totals	319	934	662	220	0.5–25	90–120	P/hCG	10	63

P, pump; hCG, human chorionic gonadotrophin.

Table 2. Pulsatile administration of gonadotrophin-releasing hormone (GnRH) via the intravenous route.

Authors	No. of patients	Total no. of cycles	Ovulatory cycles	No. of pregnancies	Pulse dose (µg)	Interval (min)	Luteal phase (P/hCG)	No. of multiple pregnancies	Miscarriages
Gompel and Mauvais-Jarvis (1988)	37	117	110	41	5–20	90	P	1	11
Gindoff et al (1986)	1	3	2	1	5–20	90	P		
Miller et al (1983)	8	23	20	7	1–5	62–120	P/hCG		3
Leyendecker et al (1980b)	5	5	3		10–15	90	P		
Reid et al (1981)	2	2	2	2	0.5–55	90–120	hCG		
Jansen et al (1987)	36	113	102	28	2.5–5	60–120	P	4	4
Gerhard et al (1988)	18	41	28	5	5–40	90	P		2
Totals	107	304	267	84	0.5–55	60–120	P/hCG	5	20

P, pump; hCG, human chorionic gonadotrophin.

using intravenous GnRH provided no overall therapeutic gain. The dose of GnRH used in the subcutaneous route was 0.5–25 μg/pulse and in the intravenous route 1–5 μg/pulse. The pulse interval was almost the same in the two groups.

We advocate routine use of subcutaneous GnRH. We only employ intravenous treatment in patients who fail to respond to subcutaneous pulsatile GnRH therapy.

PULSE DOSE AND INTERVAL

Whereas there is clear evidence that the normal human ovulation cycle is characterized by phase-specific rates of gonadotrophin pulsatility—one LH pulse every 60–90 min in the follicular phase, one pulse every 3–4 h during the luteal phase (Crowley et al, 1985)—all the clinical results of pulsatile GnRH therapy reported to date have been obtained using a fixed pulse interval (usually of 90 min). There is thus a contrast between the subtle and variable pattern of endogenous gonadotrophin secretion and the remarkable clinical results achieved with administration of exogenous releasing hormone at fixed intervals (Figure 2). The paradox may be resolved in part by considering the doses of GnRH most clinicians use. For intravenous therapy a dose of 5 μg and for subcutaneous therapy a dose of 15 μg per pulse is usually administered. It is likely that if the doses were reduced to produce pituitary portal blood concentrations equivalent to those occurring

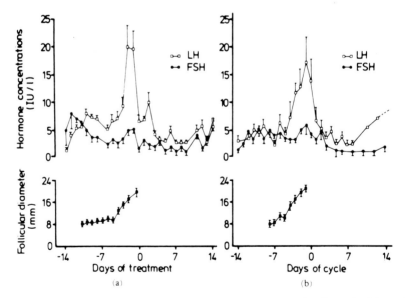

Figure 2. Gonadotrophin concentrations and follicular diameters (as determined by serial ultrasound scans) during gonadotrophin-releasing hormone (GnRH)-induced cycles: (a) ovulatory cycles, (b) ovulatory cycles in which conception occurred. LH, luteinizing hormone; FSH, follicle-stimulating hormone.

naturally, some adjustment of pulse interval might become necessary. In terms of the practicalities of clinical treatment, such considerations have generally been abandoned. In clinical terms, therefore, the remarkable flexibility of the pumps described earlier represents a degree of engineering redundancy similar to that exhibited by the body's own GnRH pulse generator. In our clinic we use a dose of 15 μg of GnRH per pulse, given every 90 min subcutaneously into the upper arm. When we have used the drug intravenously, we have changed neither the dose nor the interval.

PATIENT SELECTION AND PREGNANCY RATES

Optimal use of GnRH for ovulation induction requires its administration to women in whom all factors other than anovulation have been excluded. GnRH deficiency may be partial or complete, isolated or associated with other hormonal deficiencies. Impaired GnRH release may be found in weight-, stress- and exercise-related amenorrhoea. Acquired GnRH deficiency may be associated with organic disease of the hypothalamus and the pituitary stalk, as seen in tuberculous meningitis, post surgery, trauma and irradiation of the hypothalamic and pituitary areas. The clinical features of GnRH deficiency depend on several factors (Brook et al, 1987): age of onset (before, during or after puberty), severity of the GnRH deficiency and its association with other features, such as hyposmia in Kallman's syndrome (Crowley and McArthur, 1980) or with congenital adrenal hypoplasia (Burke et al, 1988). GnRH may also have a role in the treatment of patients with polycystic ovary syndrome and hyperprolactinaemia.

Hypogonadotrophic hypogonadism is a clinical syndrome whose abnormalities include a spectrum of defects of the amplitude and frequency of GnRH secretion (Backstrom et al, 1982). Women with weight-loss-related amenorrhoea may be classified under this heading and in some senses are considered ideal candidates for pulsatile GnRH therapy (Nillius and Wide, 1978; Nillius et al, 1985; Homburg et al, 1989). We found that patients who did not resume ovulation despite adequate weight gain achieved a cumulative rate of pregnancy of 95% after 6 months' treatment with pulsatile GnRH (Homburg et al, 1989). We do, however, advise deferring treatment until the patient's weight has increased sufficiently to give her a body mass index of 20 kg/m², the reason being the relatively poor obstetric outcome of underweight women undergoing induction of ovulation (van der Spuy et al, 1988).

In our survey of the current literature (Table 3) we found that the rate of ovulation among 464 cycles in 150 women with hypogonadotrophic hypogonadism (treated either via the subcutaneous or intravenous route) was 90.1% and the pregnancy rate per cycle was 28.6%. The pregnancy rate per ovulatory cycle was 32%. In our own experience of treating 39 patients with hypogonadotrophic hypogonadism, the cumulative conception rate after 6 months of treatment was 93% (Homburg et al, 1989).

Functional hypothalamic amenorrhoea is a common cause of infertility in which anovulation is associated with subnormal oestrogen levels and low or apparently normal serum gonadotrophin and prolactin concentrations,

Table 3. Pulsatile administration of gonadotrophin-releasing hormone (GnRH) in hypogonadotrophic hypogonadism (route of administration is either subcutaneous or intravenous).

Authors	No. of patients	Total no. of cycles	Ovulatory cycles	No. of pregnancies	Pulse dose (µg)	Interval (min)	Luteal phase (P/hCG)	No. of multiple pregnancies	Miscarriages
Homburg et al (1989)	33	129	112	38	15	90	P	4	6
Reid et al (1981)	2	2	0		0.5–5	90–120	hCG		
Reid et al (1981)	2	2	2	2	0.5–5	90–120	hCG		
Jansen et al (1987)	29	97	95	27	2.5–5	60–120	P	4	4
Gerhard et al (1988)	7	19	17	4	5–40	90	P		2
Glasier et al (1987)	8	21	11	2		90	P		
Saffan and Seible (1986)	10	16	15	4	12.5–20	90–120	hCG		1
Skarin et al (1983)	14	38	36	8	1–20	90	P	1	3
Miller et al (1983)	8	23	20	7	1–5	62–120	P/hCG		3
Gompel and Mauvais-Jarvis (1988)	37	117	110	41	5–20	90	P	1	11
Totals	150	464	418	133	0.5–40	60–120	P/hCG	10	30

P, pump; hCG, human chorionic gonadotrophin.

without evidence of a structural lesion of the pituitary or hypothalamus. A reduction in GnRH secretion may also be involved in the anovulation of hyperprolactinaemia. The pulse frequency of LH is reduced in most women with this condition (Klibanski et al, 1984; Sauder et al, 1984) and the endocrine findings in these patients are typified by low serum oestradiol and low–normal gonadotrophin concentrations with a normal pituitary response to exogenous GnRH (Jacobs et al, 1976). Suppression of hyperprolactinaemia by treatment with bromocriptine reduces elevated prolactin levels and restores menses in 80–90% of women (Vance et al, 1984). Ovulation can also be restored by pulsatile administration of GnRH (Gindoff et al, 1986). Such therapy, of great theoretical interest in that it helps to identify the mechanism of the impairment of fertility in women with hyperprolactinaemia, is, however, of little practical importance. The optimal method of treatment remains the suppression of excessive prolactin secretion with dopaminergic agonists such as bromocriptine (Franks and Jacobs, 1983) or the more recently introduced non-ergot dopamine agonist CV 205-502 (Homburg et al, 1990).

Organic disease in the hypothalamic–pituitary region may cause hypogonadotrophic amenorrhoea. In addition to prolactinoma and acromegaly, the causes include tuberculous meningitis, craniopharyngioma, non-functioning pituitary adenoma and Sheehan's syndrome. Morris et al (1987) treated 13 patients who had various organic lesions within the hypothalamic–pituitary area with pulsatile GnRH: eight ovulated and six conceived. The results of this study indicated that GnRH therapy may be applied successfully to carefully selected cases with structural hypothalamic–pituitary damage. In selecting such cases for treatment, it is important to remember that the amount of gonadotrophin released after a diagnostic test with GnRH offers no guide at all to the outcome of therapy (Abdulwahid et al, 1985). Homburg et al (1989) found that patients who had residual pituitary tissue after pituitary surgery benefited most from GnRH treatment. Those who had received irradiation or radical surgery benefited least.

Polycystic ovaries

Two patterns of ovarian appearance on ultrasound were described by Adams and her colleagues (1985). One, originally termed 'megalocystic ovaries' (Tucker et al, 1984) and more recently 'multicystic ovaries' is the appearance seen typically in girls going through puberty. The ovaries are enlarged by six to eight cysts of 6–8 mm diameter and, most crucially, there is no increase in the stromal echo. This appearance is seen only in the presence of demonstrable pulsatile gonadotrophin secretion, arising from spontaneous GnRH activity (Brook et al, 1987) or from pulsatile GnRH therapy. In adults this appearance is often seen in women emerging from the gonadotrophin deficiency of severe weight-related amenorrhoea, typically as the woman with anorexia nervosa approaches her target body mass index of 20 kg/m^2. As mentioned earlier, such patients respond very well to pulsatile GnRH therapy (Adams et al, 1985; Homburg et al, 1989).

Polycystic ovaries, as seen in patients with the Stein–Leventhal syndrome,

Table 4. Pulsatile administration of gonadotrophin-releasing hormone (GnRH) alone in polycystic ovary patients; route of administration is subcutaneous (104 patients) or intravenous (16 patients).

Authors	No. of patients	Total no. of cycles	Ovulatory cycles	No. of pregnancies	Pulse dose (μg)	Interval (min)	Luteal phase (P/hCG)	No. of multiple pregnancies	Miscarriages
Homburg et al (1989)	47	193	99	30	15	90	P	3	12
Jansen et al (1987)	5	14	7	1	2.5–5	60–120	P		
Gerhard et al (1988)	11	22	11	1	5–40	90	P		
Glasier et al (1987)	6	9	3	1		90	P		
Saffan and Seible (1986)	3	5	2		8.5–20	120	hCG	1	
Eshel et al (1988)	48	141	73	23	15	90	P		10
Totals	120	384	195	56	0.5–40	60–120	P/hCG	4	22

P, pump; hCG, human chorionic gonadotrophin.

present a different morphological picture on ultrasound. These ovaries are characteristically larger than normal (average volume of 12 ml versus 6 ml in normal women) and have a highly echodense central stroma surrounded by a necklace of cysts with an average diameter of 4–6 mm. The classical endocrine findings in these patients are raised serum concentrations of LH and testosterone with normal levels of FSH, prolactin and thyroxine. In our experience, only some 44% of these patients do in fact have hypersecretion of LH, but the complaint of infertility is significantly more common amongst these women compared with those with normal LH concentrations (Conway et al, 1989). Eshel et al (1988) found that the administration of pulsatile GnRH was only partially successful in inducing ovulation in patients with polycystic ovary syndrome. They identified obesity (body mass index over 30 kg/m^2), hyperandrogenaemia (serum total testosterone over 2.5 nmol/litre) and hypersecretion of LH as factors associated with an adverse outcome. Subsequently Homburg et al (1988a) found that the presence of a high pretreatment serum concentration of LH was associated with an impairment of the rate of conception and a striking increase in the rate of miscarriage.

The clinical implication of the above studies is that obese hyperandrogen-aemic women with polycystic ovary syndrome are unsuitable for treatment with pulsatile GnRH. Surveying the literature (Table 4) we found that, out of 120 patients with polycystic ovary treated for 384 cycles, the ovulation rate per treated cycle was 50.7%, the pregnancy rate per ovulatory cycle was 28.7% but the pregnancy rate per treated cycle was only 14.6%. A recent study by Filicori et al (1989) reported that pituitary–gonadal suppression with a superactive GnRH analogue improved the endocrine and clinical responses to subsequent treatment with pulsatile GnRH.

Miscellaneous

GnRH treatment may be associated with a prolonged follicular phase, regardless of the condition treated. In such cases administration of human menopausal gonadotrophin (hMG) together with GnRH has been success-ful in shortening the follicular phase and inducing ovulation and pregnancy (Eckstein et al, 1985).

Liu et al (1983) administered GnRH intravenously to normally ovulating women in an in vitro fertilization programme in a dose of 10 µg per pulse and achieved two to five preovulatory follicles in each patient, indicating that the drug is capable of overcoming the normal mechanisms responsible for unifollicular development.

MULTIPLE PREGNANCY

One of the main advantages of treatment with GnRH compared with other forms of inducing ovulation is the low rate of multiple pregnancies. In a retrospective international study (Braat et al, 1989) of results obtained in 22 centres, which included 223 pregnancies induced by GnRH (using both intravenous and subcutaneous routes), the rate of multiple pregnancy was 17.2% (30 out of 174) in patients with hypogonadotrophic amenorrhoea, but there were no multiples among the 21 pregnancies in the patients with polycystic ovaries. In our survey of the literature we found an overall rate of 5.0% for multiple pregnancies (15 multiple pregnancies among 304 pregnancies, Tables 1 and 2). In our own experience (Homburg et al, 1989) there were four multiple pregnancies in the group of patients with hypogonadotrophic hypogonadism who had conceived in the first cycle of treatment. This finding was consistent with that of Braat et al (1985) who collected national figures in The Netherlands for the outcome of treatment with GnRH. They too found a significant association of multiple pregnancies with the first cycle of treatment. The mechanism is uncertain but the association with the first cycle of treatment suggests that lack of a preceding luteal phase may result in either an exaggerated pituitary response to GnRH or an exaggerated ovarian response to normal gonadotrophic stimulation. A correlation has also been noted with the use of high doses of GnRH and luteal replacement of hCG (Braat et al, 1989). The low rate of multiple pregnancies among patients with polycystic ovary syndrome may be related to the poor pregnancy (Braat et al, 1985; Blankstein et al, 1986) and fertilization rates, as also found in an assisted fertility programme (Stanger and Yovitch, 1985).

We conclude that treatment with pulsatile GnRH is associated with a higher incidence of multiple pregnancies than normal but a lower rate than with gonadotrophin-induced pregnancies (25–38%; Oelsner et al, 1978; Blankstein et al, 1986). The small increase in the risk is particularly evident in the first cycle of treatment.

ABORTION RATE AND CONGENITAL MALFORMATIONS

Different rates of miscarriage have been reported by various authors. Reviewing the literature of pregnancies following GnRH treatment in patients with hypogonadotrophic hypogonadism, we found a rate of 22.2% (Table 3). In the multicentre study (Braat et al, 1989) the rate of abortion was 10% in patients with hypogonadotrophic hypogonadism and 8.7% in the group with polycystic ovaries. In our own literature survey, the rate of abortion among patients with polycystic ovaries was 39.2% (Table 4). There was no difference in the rate of abortion in the patients with hypogonadotrophic hypogonadism compared with normal (Wilcox et al, 1988). The miscarriage rate reported in patients with polycystic ovary syndrome varies between authors and different treatment groups and 20–50% (Garcia et al, 1977; Adams et al, 1985; Blankstein et al, 1986; Filicori et al, 1988). In our own results we found that the high rate of abortion among polycystic ovary patients was related to inappropriate secretion of LH during the follicular phase. Inappropriate LH secretion may also represent a subtle cause of infertility (Homburg et al, 1988a; Shoham et al, 1990).

Among 246 babies born after induction of ovulation with GnRH (Braat et al, 1989) four congenital malformations have been reported: congenita atresia of the oesophagus, double ureter, cleft lip and palate and undescended testicle. No congenital abnormalities were detected among 49 babies delivered in our unit (Homburg et al, 1989). We conclude that the risk of congenital malformations in pregnancies achieved after GnRH is no higher than in the general population.

MONITORING TREATMENT

The value of pelvic ultrasound for monitoring follicular activity in spontaneous and induced cycles is widely accepted. The rate of enlargement of the diameter of the dominant follicle in GnRH-induced cycles is not different from that observed in women undergoing spontaneous cycles (Adams et al, 1985). Increasing serum oestradiol secretion from the enlarging dominant follicle results in uterine growth and endometrial thickening. Thus changes in uterine size, endometrium and follicular diameter can be used as an in vivo bio-assay of GnRH action. Lack of uterine growth during GnRH therapy implies a failure of adequate ovarian stimulation (Adams et al, 1984, 1985). Measurements of LH, FSH, oestradiol and progesterone during treatment were found to be similar to those of normal subjects during a spontaneous cycle (Mason et al, 1984b).

LUTEAL PHASE

Almost all the investigators agree that the corpus luteum must be supported during GnRH treatment in GnRH-deficient patients. If treatment with GnRH is stopped at ovulation and luteal phase support is withheld a short luteal phase and menstruation ensue (Franks et al, 1985). This result has been confirmed in animal experiments (Hutchison and Zeleznik, 1985), in which it was shown that interrupting exogenous GnRH support in the GnRH-deficient rhesus monkey caused immediate failure of the corpus luteum. The question of whether to interrupt pulsatile administration of GnRH following ovulation and support the corpus luteum with hCG injections or to continue GnRH through the luteal phase is not infrequently raised. While such an approach can be successful—and restarting treatment with GnRH can rescue a corpus luteum that has begun to wane (Polsen et al, 1987)—the only possible clinical advantage of this technique is to reduce the patient's commitment to the pump, freeing it for another patient to use. In our experience, the advantages of this approach are illusory.

ADVERSE EFFECTS

Infection and haematoma

Apart from inflammation at the cannula site in a small number of the patients treated with subcutaneous pulsatile GnRH (Skarin et al, 1982,

1983; Hurley et al, 1984) there is a report by Jansen et al (1987) of eight episodes of fever among 113 cycles of treatment using GnRH. These patients were treated with antibiotics and none had a fever lasting more than 36 h. One of our patients developed septicaemia during treatment with intravenous GnRH and several have experienced minor infections at the subcutaneous injection site.

Antibody formation

Synthetic GnRH is a copy of the naturally occurring decapeptide and would not be expected to initiate an immune response. Despite this there are some reports in the literature of GnRH-specific immunoglobulin G (IgG) and E (IgE) antibodies to GnRH in men and women on long treatment with pulsatile GnRH therapy (Brown et al, 1977; Lindner et al, 1981; Claman et al, 1987). In one study of 163 patients (23 females, four men and 137 boys) treated with pulsatile GnRH for 3 weeks to 9 months, five (three males and two females) showed specific binding of GnRH to IgG antibodies (Meakin et al, 1985). It was proposed that the formation of antibodies to the small GnRH molecule was related to its mode of delivery. It was suggested that subclinical chronic inflammation at the tip of the needle led to complexing of GnRH to larger proteins, thus potentiating antigenicity of the decapeptide. It was therefore suggested that frequent needle changes may decrease the chance of antibody formation (Claman et al, 1987).

Hyperstimulation

Although hyperstimulation syndrome has been reported after GnRH therapy (Geisthovel et al, 1985) it occurs significantly less frequently than with gonadotrophin therapy (Bogchelman et al, 1982; Heineman et al, 1984; Jacobs et al, 1984). In the survey of the literature by Blankstein et al (1986) ten cases of hyperstimulation out of 917 treated cycles were reported (1.1%).

Desensitization

Desensitization may arise as a result of an inadequate dose or pulse frequency of GnRH or as a result of impaired absorption of the hormone. It is more likely to occur with excessive than with too little GnRH (Knobil, 1980; Wildt et al, 1981). Both pituitary and gonadal desensitization have been observed in monkeys (Knobil, 1980), rats (DeKoning et al, 1978) and in humans (Rabin and McNeil, 1980; Glasier et al, 1987) with GnRH given as a continuous infusion.

SUMMARY

The use of pulsatile GnRH to treat infertile women who do not ovulate has been shown to be safe, simple, and effective and the preferred method of inducing ovulation in appropriately selected patients who are resistant to treatment with clomiphene citrate. Treatment with GnRH is particularly effective for restoring ovulation in patients with idiopathic hypogonado-trophic hypogonadism and partially recovered weight-related amenorrhoea, but less successful in patients with polycystic ovary syndrome and organic hypothalamic pituitary disease. Based on personal experience, we advocate routine use of the subcutaneous route, using 15 μg per pulse every 90 min, and we monitor the patient's progress by serial ultrasound scanning and measurement of serum gonadotrophin and oestradiol concentrations. If the patient does not respond we recommend adding treatment with clomiphene citrate (Homburg et al, 1988b). Treatment with intravenous GnRH is reserved for women who do not respond to the above combination of drugs. We do not treat patients with GnRH until their body mass index is in the normal range (between 20–25) and we avoid GnRH treatment in patients with hyper-secretion of LH during the follicular phase. If LH concentrations are raised, an alternative method of treatment is recommended, such as ovarian diathermy (Armar et al, 1990).

Finally, the question of whether GnRH deficiency in patients with hypo-gonadotrophic hypogonadism is caused by a specific genetic lesion is not yet fully resolved. Yang-Feng et al (1986) used a cDNA clone encoding the human GnRH precursor molecule in order to assign the GnRH gene to a particular human chromosome. They found a single site for GnRH sequences in the human genome and that the gene coding for GnRH is located on the short arm of chromosome 8. Experiments in the congenitally hypogonadal mouse have shown that it is possible to restore gonadal development and gametogenesis by gene transfer (Mason et al, 1987). Clearly an abnormality at the level of the genome may be responsible for the secretory defect in patients with hypogonadotrophic hypogonadism, but it has yet to be defined (Weiss et al, 1989). Presumably elucidation awaits the development of more refined methods because both the genetics and the clinical associations of GnRH deficiency are most persuasive. Meanwhile replacement treatment with GnRH provides a simple and safe form of treatment for managing the clinical syndromes of GnRH deficiency.

REFERENCES

Abdulwahid NA, Armar NA, Morris DV, Adams J & Jacobs HS (1985) Diagnostic tests with luteinizing hormone releasing hormone should be abandoned. *British Medical Journal* **291:** 1471–1472.

Adams J, Mason WP, Tucker M, Morris DV & Jacobs HS (1984) Ultrasound assessment of changes in the ovary and the uterus during LHRH therapy. *Upsala Journal of Medical Science* **89:** 39–41.

Adams J, Polsen DW, Abdulwahid N et al (1985) Multifollicular ovaries: clinical and endocrine features and response to pulsatile gonadotropin releasing hormone. *Lancet* **ii:** 1375–1378.

Armar NA, McGarrigle HHG, Honour J, Holownia P, Jacobs HS & Lachelin GCL (1990) Laparoscopic ovarian diathermy in the management of anovulatory infertility in women with polycystic ovaries: endocrine changes and clinical outcome. *Fertility and Sterility* **53:** 42–49.

Backstrom CT, McNeilly AS, Leask RM & Baird DT (1982) Pulsatile secretion of LH, FSH, prolactin, oestradiol and progesterone during the human menstrual cycle. *Clinical Endocrinology* **17**: 29–42.

Belchetz PE, Plant TM, Nakai Y, Keogh EJ & Knobil E (1978) Hypophysial responses to continuous and intermittent delivery of hypothalamic gonadotropin-releasing hormone. *Science* **202**: 631–633.

Blankstein J, Mashiach S & Lunenfeld B (1986) Gonadotrophin-releasing hormone. In Blankstein J, Mashiach S & Lunenfeld B (eds) *Ovulation Induction and In Vitro Fertilization*, p 99–110. Chicago: Year Book Medical Publishers.

Blunt SM, Clayton RN & Butt WR (1986) Effect of injection site on the pharmacokinetics and pharmacodynamics of subcutaneous administration of luteinizing hormone releasing hormone. *Clinical Endocrinology* **25**: 589–596.

Bogchelman D, Lappohn RE & Janssens J (1982) Triple pregnancy after pulsatile administration of gonadotropin-releasing hormone. *Lancet* **ii**: 45–46.

Braat DDM, Boghelman D & Coelingh-Bennink HJT (1985) The outcome of pregnancies established in GnRH induced cycles with special reference to the multiple pregnancies in five Dutch centers. In Coelingh-Bennink HJT, Dogterom AA, Lappohn RE, Rolland R & Shoemaker J (eds) *Pulsatile GnRH*, pp 207–217. Haarlem: Ferring.

Braat DDM, Ayalon D, Blunt SM et al (1989) Pregnancy outcome in luteinizing hormone-releasing hormone induced cycles: a multicentric study. *Gynecological Endocrinology* **3**: 35–44.

Brook CGD, Jacobs HS, Stanhope R, Adams J & Hindmarsh P (1987) Pulsatility of reproductive hormones: applications to the understanding of puberty and to the treatment of infertility. *Baillière's Clinical Endocrinology and Metabolism* **1**: 23–41.

Brown GM, Van Loon GR, Hummel BCW, Grota LJ, Arimura A & Schally AV (1977) Characteristics of antibody produced during chronic treatment with LHRH. *Journal of Clinical Endocrinology and Metabolism* **44**: 784–790.

Burgus R, Butcher M, Ling N et al (1971) Structure moleculair du facteur hypothalamique (LRF) d'origine ovine controlant la secretion de l'hormone gonadotrope hypophysaire luteinisation (LH). *Comptes Rendues de l'Académie des Sciences* **273**: 1611–1613.

Burke BA, Wick MR, King R et al (1988) Congenital adrenal hypoplasia and selective absence of pituitary luteinizing hormone: a new autosomal recessive syndrome. *American Journal of Medical Genetics* **31**: 75–97.

Claman P, Elkind-Hirsch K, Oskowitz SP & Seible MM (1987) Urticaria associated with antigonadotropin-releasing hormone antibody in a female Kallman's syndrome patient being treated with long-term pulsatile gonadotropin-releasing hormone. *Obstetrics and Gynecology* **69**: 503–505.

Conway GS, Honour JW & Jacobs HS (1989) Heterogeneity of polycystic ovary syndrome: clinical, endocrine and ultrasound features in 556 cases. *Clinical Endocrinology* **30**: 459–470.

Coy DH & Schally AV (1978) Gonadotropin releasing hormone analogues. *Annals of Clinical Research* **10**: 139–144.

Crowley WF Jr & McArthur JW (1980) Stimulation of the normal menstrual cycle in Kallman's syndrome by pulsatile administration of luteinizing hormone-releasing hormone (LH-RH). *Journal of Clinical Endocrinology and Metabolism* **51**: 173–175.

Crowley WF, Filicori M, Spratt DI & Santoro NF (1985) The physiology of gonadotropin-releasing hormone (GnRH) secretion in man and women. *Recent Progress in Hormone Research* **41**: 473–477.

DeKoning J, van Dieten JAMJ & van Rees GP (1978) Refractoriness of the pituitary after continuous exposure to LHRH. *Journal of Endocrinology* **79**: 311–318.

Dericks-Tan JSE, Hammer E & Taubert H-D (1977) The effect of D-Ser (TBU)^6-LH-RH-EA^{10} upon gonadotropin release in normally cyclic women. *Journal of Clinical Endocrinology and Metabolism* **45**: 597–600.

Eckstein N, Vagman I, Eshel A, Naor Z & Ayalon D (1985) Induction of ovulation in amenorrheic patients with gonadotropin-releasing hormone and human menopausal gonadotropin. *Fertility and Sterility* **44**: 744–750.

Eshel A, Abdulwahid NA, Armar NA, Adams J & Jacobs HS (1988) Pulsatile luteinizing hormone-releasing hormone therapy in women with polycystic ovary syndrome. *Fertility and Sterility* **49**: 956–960.

Filicori M, Campaniello E, Michelacci L et al (1988) Gonadotropin-releasing hormone (GnRH) analog suppression renders polycystic ovarian disease patients more susceptible to ovulation induction with pulsatile GnRH. *Journal of Clinical Endocrinology and Metabolism* **66:** 327–333.

Filicori M, Flamigni C, Campaniello E et al (1989) The abnormal response of polycystic ovarian disease patients to exogenous pulsatile gonadotropin-releasing hormone: characterization and management. *Journal of Clinical Endocrinology and Metabolism* **69:** 825.

Franks S & Jacobs HS (1983) Hyperprolactinaemia. *Clinical Endocrinology* **12:** 641–668.

Franks S, van der Spuy ZM, Mason WP, Adams J & Jacobs HS (1985) Luteal function after ovulation induction by pulsatile luteinizing hormone releasing hormone. In Jeffcoate SL (ed.) *The Luteal Phase*, p 89–100. Chichester: John Wiley.

Garcia J, Jones GS & Wentz AC (1977) The use of clomiphene citrate. *Fertility and Sterility* **28:** 707–717.

Geisthovel F, Peters F & Breckwoldt M (1985) Ovarian hyperstimulation due to long-term pulsatile intravenous GnRH treatment. *Archives of Gynecology* **236:** 255–259.

Gerhard I, Hudea NH, Eggert-Kruse W & Runnebaum B (1988) Pulsatile gonadotrophin releasing hormone therapy in patients with hyperandrogenaemia or hypothalamic amenorrhoea. *Human Reproduction* **3:** 835–843.

Gindoff PR, Loucopoulos A & Jewelewicz R (1986) Treatment of hyperprolactinemic amenorrhea with pulsatile gonadotropin-releasing hormone therapy. *Fertility and Sterility* **46:** 1156–1158.

Glasier A, Baird DT & McNeilly AS (1987) Evidence for gonadal desensitization after pulsatile therapy in women with amenorrhoea? *Clinical Endocrinology* **26:** 441–451.

Gompel A & Mauvais-Jarvis P (1988) Induction of ovulation with pulsatile GnRH in hypothalamic amenorrhoea. *Human Reproduction* **3:** 473–477.

Handelsman DJ & Swerdloff RS (1986) Pharmacokinetics of gonadotropin-releasing hormone and its analogues. *Endocrine Reviews* **7:** 95–105.

Handelsman DJ, Jansen RPS, Boylan LM, Spaliviero JA & Turtle JR (1984) Pharmacokinetics of gonadotropin-releasing hormone: comparison of subcutaneous and intravenous routes. *Journal of Clinical Endocrinology and Metabolism* **59:** 739–746.

Heineman MJ, Bouckaert PXJM & Schellekens LA (1984) A quadruplet pregnancy following ovulation induction with pulsatile luteinizing hormone-releasing hormone. *Fertility and Sterility* **42:** 300–302.

Homburg R, Armar NA, Eshel A, Adams J & Jacobs HS (1988a) Influence of serum luteinizing hormone concentrations on ovulation, conception and early pregnancy loss in polycystic ovary syndrome. *British Medical Journal* **297:** 1024–1026.

Homburg R, Eshel A, Armar NA, Tucker M, Adams J & Jacobs HS (1988b) Synergism of pulsatile LHRH therapy with oral clomiphene treatment. *Gynecological Endocrinology* **2:** 59–66.

Homburg R, Eshel A, Armar NA et al (1989) One hundred pregnancies after treatment with pulsatile luteinizing hormone releasing hormone to induce ovulation. *British Medical Journal* **298:** 809–812.

Homburg R, West C, Brownell J & Jacobs HS (1990) A double-blind study comparing a new non-ergot, long-acting dopamin agonist, CV 205–502, with bromocriptine in women with hyperprolactinaemia. *Clinical Endocrinology* **32:** 565–571.

Hurley DM, Brian R, Outch K et al (1984) Induction of ovulation and fertility in amenorrheic women by pulsatile low dose gonadotropin-releasing hormone. *New England Journal of Medicine* **310:** 1069–1074.

Hutchison JS & Zeleznik AJ (1985) The corpus luteum of the primate menstrual cycle is capable of recovering from a transient withdrawal of pituitary gonadotropin support. *Endocrinology* **17:** 1043–1049.

Jacobs HS, Frank S, Murray MAF, Hull MGR, Steele SJ & Nabarro JDN (1976) Clinical and endocrine features of hyperprolactinemic amenorrhoea. *Clinical Endocrinology* **5:** 439–454.

Jacobs HS, Adams J, Franks S et al (1984) Induction of ovulation with LH-RH-problems, indications and contraindications. In Labrie F (ed.) *LH-RH and Its Analogs*, pp 464–478. Amsterdam: Excerpta Medica.

Jansen RPS, Handelsman DJ, Boylan LM, Conway A, Shearman RP & Fraser IS (1987) Pulsatile intravenous gonadotropin-releasing hormone for ovulation-induction in infertile women. I. Safety and effectiveness with outpatient therapy. *Fertility and Sterility* **48:** 33–38.

Jacobson RL, Seyler LE Jr, Tamborlane WV Jr, Gertner LM & Genel M (1979) Pulsatile subcutaneous nocturnal administration of GnRH by portable infusion pump in hypogonadotropic hypogonadism: initiation of gonadotropin responsiveness. *Journal of Clinical Endocrinology and Metabolism* **49:** 652–654.

Kastin AJ, Zarate A, Midgley AR, Canales ES & Schally AV (1971) Ovulation confirmed by pregnancy after infusion of porcine LH-RH. *Journal of Clinical Endocrinology and Metabolism* **33:** 980–982.

Klibanski A, Beitins IZ, Merriam GR, McArthur JW, Zervas NT & Ridgway EC (1984) Gonadotropin and prolactin pulsations in hyperprolactinemic women before and during bromocriptine therapy. *Journal of Clinical Endocrinology and Metabolism* **58:** 1141–1147.

Knobil E (1980) The neuroendocrine control of the menstrual cycle. *Recent Progress in Hormone Research* **36:** 53–88.

Leyendecker G & Wildt L (1984) Pulsatile administration of GnRH in hypothalamic amenorrhea. *Upsala Journal of Medical Science* **89:** 19.

Leyendecker G, Wildt L & Hansmann M (1980a) Pregnancy following chronic intermittent (pulsatile) administration of Gn-RH by means of a portable pump (ZYKLOMAT)—a new approach to the treatment of infertility in hypothalamic amenorrhea. *Journal of Clinical Endocrinology and Metabolism* **51:** 1214–1216.

Leyendecker G, Struve T & Plotz EJ (1980b) Induction of ovulation with chronic intermittent (pulsatile) administration of LH-RH in women with hypothalamic and hyperprolactinemic amenorrhea. *Archives of Gynecology* **229:** 177–190.

Lindner J, McNeil LW, Marney S et al (1981) Characterization of human anti-luteinizing hormone-releasing hormone (LRH) antibodies in the serum of a patient with isolated gonadotropin deficiency treated with synthetic LRH. *Journal of Clinical Endocrinology and Metabolism* **52:** 267–270.

Liu JH, Durfee R, Muse K & Yen SSC (1983) Induction of multiple ovulation by pulsatile administration of gonadotropin releasing hormone. *Fertility and Sterility* **40:** 18–22.

Loucopoulos A, Ferin M, Vande Wiele RL et al (1984) Pulsatile administration of gonadotropin-releasing hormone for induction of ovulation. *American Journal of Obstetrics and Gynecology* **148:** 895–900.

Lunenfeld B (1984) Ovulation induction evaluation of drug efficacy. *Proceedings of the ESCO Meeting*, Monte Carlo.

Mason WP, Adams J, Tucker M & Jacobs HS (1984a) The role of subcutaneous luteinizing hormone releasing hormone in the induction of ovulation. *Uppsala Journal of Medical Science* **89:** 33–37.

Mason P, Adams J, Morris DV et al (1984b) Induction of ovulation with pulsatile luteinizing hormone releasing hormone. *British Medical Journal* **288:** 181–185.

Mason AJ, Pitts SL, Nikolics K et al (1987) Gonadal development and gametogenesis in the hypogonadal mouse are restored by gene transfer. *Annals of the New York Academy of Science* **513:** 16–26.

McCann SM, Talersnik S & Friedman HM (1960) LH releasing activity in hypothalamic extracts. *Proceedings of the Society for Experimental Biology and Medicine* **104:** 432–437.

Meakin JL, Keogh EJ & Martin CE (1985) Human anti-luteinizing hormone-releasing hormone antibodies in patients treated with synthetic luteinizing hormone-releasing hormone. *Fertility and Sterility* **43:** 811–813.

Menon V, Butt WR, Clayton RN, Edwards RL & Lynch SS (1984) Pulsatile administration of GnRH for the treatment of hypogonadotrophic hypogonadism. *Clinical Endocrinology* **21:** 223–232.

Miller DS, Reid RR, Cetel NS, Rebar RW & Yen SSC (1983) Pulsatile administration of low-dose gonadotropin-releasing hormone. *Journal of the American Medical Association* **250:** 2937–2941.

Morris DV, Abdulwahid NA, Armar A & Jacobs HS (1987) The response of patients with organic hypothalamic–pituitary disease to pulsatile gonadotropin-releasing hormone therapy. *Fertility and Sterility* **47:** 54–59.

Mortimer CH, Besser GM & McNeilly AS (1975) Uses. In Motta M, Crosignani PG & Martini L (eds) *Hypothalamic Hormones: Chemistry, Physiology, Pharmacology and Clinical Uses*, pp 325–335. New York: Academic Press.

Nakai Y, Plant TM, Hess DL, Keogh EJ & Knobil E (1978) On the sites of negative and positive feedback actions of estradiol in the control of gonadotropin secretion in the rhesus monkey. *Endocrinology* **102:** 1008–1014.

Nillius SJ (1979) Gonadotropin releasing hormone for induction of ovulation in women. In Hafez ESE (ed.) *Human Ovulation*, pp 385–404. Amsterdam: Elsevier North-Holland Biochemical Press.

Nillius SJ & Wide L (1978) Effects of prolonged luteinizing hormone-releasing hormone therapy on follicular maturation, ovulation and corpus luteum function in amenorrhaeic women with anorexia nervosa. *Upsala Journal of Medical Science* **84:** 21–35.

Nillius SJ, Fries H & Wide L (1975) Successful induction of follicular maturation and ovulation by prolonged treatment with LH-releasing hormone in women with anorexia nervosa. *American Journal of Obstetrics and Gynecology* **122:** 921–928.

Oelsner G, Serr DM, Mashiach S, Blankstein J, Snyder M & Lunenfeld B (1978) The study of induction of ovulation with menotropins: analysis of results of 1897 treatment cycles. *Fertility and Sterility* **30:** 538–544.

Ory SJ (1985) Clinical uses of luteinizing hormone-releasing hormone. In Wallach E & Kempers R (eds) *Modern Trends in Infertility and Conception Control*, Volume 3, pp 191–205. Birmingham, Alabama: American Fertility Society.

Polson DW, Sagle M, Mason HD, Adams J, Jacobs HS & Franks S (1986) Ovulation and normal luteal function during LHRH treatment of women with hyperprolactinaemic amenorrhoea. *Clinical Endocrinology* **24:** 531–537.

Polson DW, Sagle M, Mason HD, Kiddy D & Franks S (1987) Recovery of luteal function after interruption of gonadotrophin secretion in the mid-luteal phase of the menstrual cycle. *Clinical Endocrinology* **26:** 597–600.

Rabin D & McNeil LW (1980) Pituitary and gonadal desensitisation after continuous luteinizing hormone-releasing hormone infusion in normal females. *Journal of Clinical Endocrinology and Metabolism* **51:** 873–876.

Reid RL, Leopold GR & Yen SSC (1981) Induction of ovulation and pregnancy with pulsatile luteinizing hormone releasing factor: dosage and mode of delivery. *Fertility and Sterility* **36:** 553–559.

Rommler A (1978) Short-term regulation of LH and FSH secretion in cyclic women. I. Altered pituitary response to a record of two LH-RH injections at short intervals. *Acta Endocrinologica* **87:** 248–258.

Rommler A, Seinsch W, Hasan AS & Haase F (1978) Ultrastructure of rat pituitary gonadotrophs in relation to serum and pituitary LH levels following repeated LH-RH stimulation. *Cell and Tissue Research* **190:** 135–149.

Saffan D & Seible MM (1986) Ovulation induction with subcutaneous pulsatile gonadotropin-releasing hormone in various ovulatory disorders. *Fertility and Sterility* **45:** 475–482.

Sauder SE, Frager M, Case GD, Kelch RP & Marshall JC (1984) Abnormal patterns of pulsatile luteinizing hormone secretion in women with hyperprolactinemia and amenorrhea: responses to bromocriptine. *Journal of Clinical Endocrinology and Metabolism* **59:** 941–948.

Schally AV, Arimura A, Kastin AJ et al (1971) Gonadotropin-releasing hormone: one polypeptide regulates secretion of luteinizing and follicle stimulating hormones. *Science* **173:** 1036–1037.

Shoham Z, Borenstein R, Lunenfeld B & Pariente C (1990) Hormonal profiles following clomiphene citrate therapy in conception and nonconception cycles. *Clinical Endocrinology* (in press).

Skarin G, Nillius SJ & Wide L (1982) Pulsatile low dose luteinizing hormone releasing hormone treatment for induction of follicular maturation and ovulation in women with amenorrhoea. *Acta Endocrinologica* **101:** 78–86.

Skarin G, Nillius SJ & Wide L (1983) Pulsatile subcutaneous low-dose gonadotropin-releasing hormone treatment of anovulatory infertility. *Fertility and Sterility* **40:** 454–460.

Stanger JD & Yovitch JL (1985) Reduced in vitro fertilization of human oocytes from patients with raised basal luteinizing hormone levels during the follicular phase. *British Journal of Obstetrics and Gynecology* **92:** 385–393.

Stewart JM (1981) Pharmacology of LH-RH and analogs. In Zatuchni GI, Shelton JD & Sciarra JJ (eds) *LHRH Peptides as Female and Male Contraceptives*, pp 3–15. Philadelphia: Harper and Row.

Sutherland IA, White S, Chambers GR et al (1984) A miniature infuser for the pulsatile administration of LHRH. *Journal of Biomedical Engineering* **6:** 129–133.

Tucker M, Adams J, Mason WP & Jacobs HS (1984) Infertility, megalocystic and polycystic ovaries: differential response to LH-RH therapy. *Upsala Journal of Medical Science* **89:** 43–46.

Vance M, Evans W & Thorner M (1984) Bromocriptine. *Annals of Internal Medicine* **100:** 78–91.

van der Spuy ZM, Steer PJ, McCusker M, Steele SJ & Jacobs HS (1988) Pregnancy outcome in underweight women following spontaneous and induced ovulation. *British Medical Journal* **296:** 962–965.

Weiss J, Crowley WF Jr & Jameson JL (1989) Normal structure of the gonadotropin-releasing hormone (GnRH) gene in patients with GnRH deficiency and idiopathic hypogonadotropic hypogonadism. *Journal of Clinical Endocrinology and Metabolism* **69:** 299–303.

Wilcox AJ, Weinberg CR, O'Connor JF et al (1988) Incidence of early loss of pregnancy. *New England Journal of Medicine* **319:** 189–194.

Wildt L, Hausler A, Marshall G et al (1981) Frequency and amplitude of gonadotropin-releasing hormone stimulation and gonadotropin secretion in the rhesus monkey. *Endocrinology* **109:** 376–385.

Yang Feng TL, Seeburg PH & Francke U (1986) Human luteinization hormone-releasing hormone gene (LHRH) is located on short arm of chromosome 8 (region 8p11.2----p21). *Somatic Cell Molecular Genetics* **12:** 95–100.

12

Common problems in induction of ovulation

DIANA HAMILTON-FAIRLEY
STEPHEN FRANKS

This chapter is concerned with common problems encountered during the treatment of women with anovulatory infertility. Anovulation is the principal cause of infertility in about one third of couples (Hull, 1981). Successful treatment depends primarily on the correct identification of the underlying abnormality causing anovulation. Nevertheless, even when the appropriate treatment has been selected there remain some women who respond very poorly or in an atypical fashion to conventional induction of ovulation. The possible mechanisms of the failure to respond and the means by which treatment can be modulated to obtain optimum rates of ovulation will be examined. The particular diagnostic categories to be considered in this chapter are hypogonadotrophic hypogonadism (HH), polycystic ovary syndrome (PCOS) and primary ovarian failure (hypergonadotrophic hypogonadism).

HYPOGONADOTROPHIC HYPOGONADISM

This disorder is defined as anovulation associated with low or normal basal gonadotrophin levels and oestrogen deficiency. The commonest cause of this condition is reduced body weight (weight-related amenorrhoea (WRA), see Chapter 1 by Frisch, this issue). Marked weight loss leading to a body mass index (BMI) of < 16 kg/m^2 is associated with profound gonadotrophin deficiency (Nillius and Wide, 1977) in which gonadotrophin-releasing hormone (GnRH) secretion, as defined by analysis of pulses of luteinizing hormone (LH) and follicle stimulating hormone (FSH), is severely inhibited and displays a prepubertal pattern (Boyar et al, 1974; Mason et al, 1988). Hypothalamic amenorrhoea may also arise in women with a lesser degree of, or partially recovered, weight loss. The endocrine picture is characterized by a slightly impaired LH response to exogenous GnRH (Nillius and Wide, 1977) and reduced frequency of LH pulses (Mason et al, 1988).

The single most important and effective treatment for this group is weight gain, although this may be a rather protracted process (Hull, 1981) and meet with initial hostility from the patient (see Chapter 1). It may be tempting to induce ovulation in these patients using pulsatile GnRH since this treatment is highly successful (Adams et al, 1985; Homburg et al, 1989). However, there are at least two very good reasons why this temptation should be resisted. Firstly, women with a history of an eating disorder and who are still underweight have been shown to have considerable difficulties caring adequately for their offspring (Stein and Fairburn, 1989) and may still need the support of psychotherapy to recover fully. Secondly, a woman who conceives while still underweight has a significantly higher risk of having an underweight baby than a woman of normal weight (van der Spuy et al, 1988). However, there are some women who regain their premorbid weight and do not regain ovulatory cycles, and it is this group which deserves consideration for treatment. This should ideally be pulsatile GnRH because of its high success rate and low incidence of multifollicular development and subsequent hyperstimulation (Homburg et al, 1989).

Other causes of hypogonadotrophic hypogonadism include idiopathic hypogonadotrophic hypogonadism (IHH) and Kallmann's syndrome and its variants. The latter is rare and is characterized by a lack of GnRH usually associated with anosmia and other congenital abnormalities (Kallmann et al, 1944; Rogol et al, 1982). This condition, together with the more common IHH, are best treated by pulsatile administration of GnRH but will, of course, also respond to exogenous gonadotrophins such as human menopausal gonadotrophins (hMG) or FSH.

Poor responders to GnRH or hMG

Low basal gonadotrophin levels may also be a consequence of organic pituitary disease, e.g. following surgery or radiotherapy to the pituitary. In these circumstances the pituitary reserve of gonadotrophins may be insufficient to respond adequately to pulsatile GnRH. However, it should be noted that about 50% of hypogonadotrophic patients with organic pituitary disease will ovulate in response to GnRH (Homburg et al, 1989). Pulsatile GnRH may therefore be administered in such cases, but if the response is poor exogenous gonadotrophin therapy should be given.

In other cases of HH results of treatment using pulsatile GnRH are extremely good and normal fertility is effectively restored to these women regardless of the diagnosis (Leyendecker et al, 1980a; Bergh et al, 1984; Mason et al, 1984; Homburg et al, 1989). Exogenous gonadotrophins have a similar success rate (Lunenfeld et al, 1982) but the incidence of multiple pregnancy and hyperstimulation syndrome is significantly higher on this treatment. Multiple pregnancy is not avoided altogether using pulsatile GnRH (Coelingh-Bennink, 1983; Homburg et al, 1989) but the main risk seems to be in the first cycle of treatment when multiple follicular development is more common (Coelingh-Bennink, 1983; Armar and Eshel, 1988).

There are a few patients who, for no obvious reason, do not respond to treatment with GnRH. Most patients with HH will ovulate after subcutaneous administration of pulsed GnRH, which is clearly more convenient than intravenous therapy and should be considered in the first instance. Intravenous therapy should still be considered in women who fail to respond to subcutaneous pulsatile GnRH (Homburg et al, 1989).

Clomiphene has been used to supplement subcutaneous pulsatile GnRH treatment in women who do not ovulate on GnRH alone. Despite the reported success of this approach most centres opt for intravenous therapy with GnRH if subcutaneous administration is unsuccessful (Homburg et al, 1988a, 1989).

Should intravenous GnRH therapy prove impractical or unsuccessful, exogenous gonadotrophins may be administered, but there is still a small group of subjects who prove resistant to treatment with conventional doses of hMG (Pellicer et al, 1987). The reasons for this lack of response to gonadotrophins remains obscure, but recent studies have drawn attention to the potential importance of paracrine growth factors, particularly insulin-like growth factor (IGF-I) in modulating gonadotrophin action on the ovary (Adashi et al, 1985). Stimulation of oestradiol production from rat granulosa cells by FSH can be augmented by coincubation with IGF-I. In addition, treatment of rats with growth hormone (GH) enhances granulosa cell production of IGF-I (Davoren and Hsueh, 1986). Thus GH seems to be able to stimulate production of IGF-I by the ovary as well as by the liver. With this in mind, Homburg et al (1988b) devised a treatment protocol for these 'gonadotrophin-resistant' women with hypogonadotrophic hypogonadism. Seven patients were treated, four attempting in vivo fertilization and three

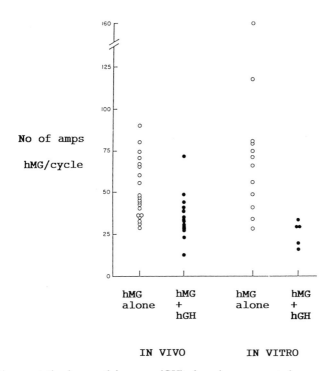

Figure 1. Augmentation by growth hormone (GH) of ovarian response to human menopausal gonadotrophin (hMG). In both in vivo and in vitro fertilization GH reduces the gonadotrophin requirement. From Homburg et al (1988b) with permission.

in vitro fertilization. A conventional regimen for ovulation induction was used together with 20 IU GH on alternate days for 2 weeks. In the groups treated for both in vivo and in vitro fertilization the gonadotrophin requirement fell significantly with added GH (Figure 1). In the in vitro group the number of oocytes collected rose from a mean of 3 to 7.4 per cycle with an apparent improvement in fertilization rates. Homburg et al (1988b) concluded from this that treatment with GH can augment the ovarian response to exogenous gonadotrophins. These findings have been confirmed in a larger, controlled study carried out by the same group (Homburg et al, 1990) and in a case report from Blumenfeld and Lunenfeld (1989). A multicentre randomized controlled trial is being conducted at present to determine the optimum dose of GH required to achieve this effect.

However, the place of GH therapy has not yet been fully validated and, in any case, is not readily available to all clinics. An alternative approach is to 'prime' the ovary with prolonged low-dose gonadotrophin treatment. We have attempted this in two women who were resistant to conventional doses

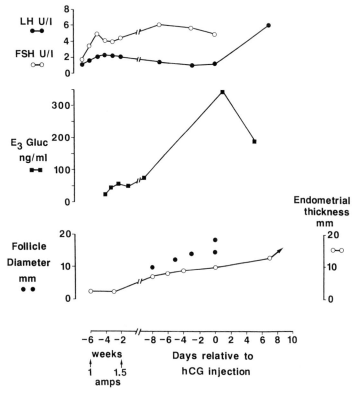

Figure 2. Profile of a patient with hypogonadotrophic hypogonadism on low-dose gonadotrophin therapy with an initial 'priming dose' of one ampoule for 4 weeks. Serum luteinizing hormone (LH) and follicle-stimulating hormone (FSH) levels and urinary oestrone glucuronide (E_3 Gluc) are shown relative to day of human chorionic gonadotrophin (hCG) (day 0). Only one follicle of > 16 mm was present on day of hCG.

of hMG. One woman failed to respond to a daily dose of 6 ampoules per day and the other to a dose of 12 ampoules per day. Our regimen was based on the assumption that pretreatment gonadotrophin levels in these women were low enough to prohibit the development of antral follicles, a process which may take up to 10 weeks (Gujeon, 1982). Both women were subsequently started on a daily dose of one ampoule per day (75 IU) and this was maintained for 4 weeks before increasing the dose by 0.5 ampoules every 7 days until an ovarian response was seen on ultrasound (Polson et al, 1987a). That dose was then continued until a follicular diameter of 20 mm was achieved (threshold dose) when human chorionic gonadotrophin (hCG) 5000 U was given. Further doses of hCG 2000 U were given on days 3 and 6 post-hCG as luteal support (Polson et al, 1987b). The first patient responded to a threshold dose of 1.5 ampoules (112.5 IU) per day, although a total dose of 50 ampoules was required. She developed a single dominant follicle and conceived in that cycle. The details of this cycle are illustrated in Figure 2. The second patient had a threshold dose of three ampoules a day (total dose 82 ampoules) with development of a single follicle and a progesterone of 46 nmol/litre on day 7 post-hCG, but she did not conceive. While the length of treatment is very long (6 weeks and 8 weeks, respectively) the patients both tolerated it well and were rewarded with ovulatory cycles and, in the first case, pregnancy. The dosage requirement is still high, but this regimen does offer some hope to the gonadotrophin-resistant hypogonadotrophic patient until the role of GH treatment has been more clearly established and the hormone is more readily available.

POLYCYSTIC OVARY SYNDROME

PCOS is the most common cause of anovulation (Adams et al, 1986; Hull, 1987). It is associated with oligomenorrhoea or secondary amenorrhoea. The diagnosis of PCO remains controversial, but our group has used ultrasound imaging of the ovaries as the primary criterion (Adams et al, 1986; Franks, 1987). If appropriate ultrasound imaging is not available then the biochemical finding of a raised LH (with a normal FSH) and a raised serum testosterone level help to confirm the diagnosis, but a small minority of patients with typical clinical and ultrasound features of PCO may have normal LH and testosterone on random sampling (Franks, 1989).

Women with PCOS are neither hypogonadotrophic nor oestrogen-deficient, and most will ovulate in response to anti-oestrogens such as clomiphene. However, more than 20% of women with PCO do not ovulate after clomiphene and should be considered for gonadotrophin therapy. These women can readily develop multiple follicles in response to gonadotrophin therapy and consequently they have a higher rate of complications. The complications include particularly an increased risk of multiple pregnancy (10–50% in published series: see Table 1) and the development of hyperstimulation syndrome. The majority of cases of the latter are mild (8–23%) or moderate (6–7%), but about 2% of cycles are associated with severe hyperstimulation requiring hospitalization.

Table 1. Summary of published results obtained with gonadotrophin therapy, 1966–1984.

Year	Authors	Patients conceiving (%)	Spontaneous miscarriage (%)	Multiple pregnancies (%)	Hyperstimulated cycles (%)
1966	Gemzell and Ross	50		50	
1967	Rabau et al	35	26	36	
1968	Tyler	16	28	21.7	
1969	Brown et al	78	14	26	3
1969	Gemzell	44.3	29.7	33.8	
1970	Thompson and Hanson	25	30	31	1.3
1974	Spadoni et al	35.4	11.5	34.7	
1975	Ellis and Williamson	48	12	39	5.6
1978	Oelsner et al	36	28	32.5	5
1980	Schwartz et al	58.6		31	
1980	Wang and Gemzell	65.9	24.1	36.3	3
1981	Schwartz and Jewelewicz	27.9	25.4	31	
1983	Bergquist et al	57	30	30	
1984	West and Baird	72	21	36	9.4

Note: these figures include women with hypogonadotrophic hypogonadism and it is difficult to isolate the figures for those women with polycystic ovary syndrome. The hyperstimulation data are for severe hyperstimulation only.

Brown et al (1969) felt that 'these complications result from failure to reproduce the precise dosage requirements which are normally maintained by feedback regulation'. Despite his attempts to achieve these 'precise dosage requirements' the multiple pregnancy rate was 26% and there was a 3.2% rate of hyperstimulation in his series. The majority of units offering in vivo ovulation induction commence treatment at a dose of 2 ampoules per day (150 IU), increasing the dose at 5-day intervals by one ampoule until the serum (or urinary) oestrogen levels start to increase. This dose is then maintained until follicular rupture (threshold dose).

Low-dose gonadotrophin therapy for induction of ovulation in PCO

In view of the high rate of complications found in this group of women we developed a low-dose protocol for the administration of hMG or FSH starting at one ampoule per day (Polson et al, 1987a, 1989). The ovulation rate using this protocol was high, with the majority of cycles (60%) being uniovulatory. The pregnancy rate in the initial studies was 41.5% (12 of 29 patients) with only two sets of twins and no higher-order pregnancies. There were no cases of severe or moderate hyperstimulation and only three cycles were associated with mild hyperstimulation. Following these results the protocol was adopted for all patients requiring ovulation induction using gonadotrophins.

Since then a total of 69 anovulatory women with clomiphene-resistant PCO have been treated with low-dose gonadotrophins given by daily intramuscular injection. This route of administration was chosen following a randomized trial we conducted comparing subcutaneous pulsatile administration with daily intramuscular injections (Polson et al, 1989). No difference in the rate of ovulation, single follicular development and preg-

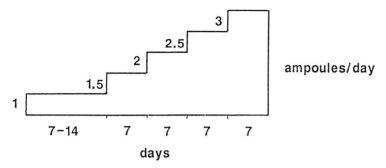

Figure 3. Diagram representing the regimen for administration of low-dose gonadotrophin. The initial dose of one ampoule is continued for 14 days in the first cycle to minimize the risk of multiple follicular development. In subsequent cycles this dose is only maintained for 7 days before increasing in a step-wise fashion as shown.

nancy was found between the two groups. Patients preferred the intramuscular route as it was less intrusive on their life-style. The protocol used is shown diagrammatically in Figure 3. All cycles were started at a dose of 1 ampoule per day (75 IU) regardless of the maximum dose used in previous cycles. This dose was maintained for 7 days, except in the first cycle when it was continued for 14 days. If there was no sign of ovarian response on ultrasound, i.e. no follicle >11 mm in diameter, the dose was increased to 1.5 ampoules per day (112.5 IU). This dose was again maintained for 7 days before increasing by 0.5 ampoules. This stepwise increase was continued as appropriate to a maximum dose of 3 ampoules. If the patient failed to respond at this dose then she was considered unresponsive and the treatment stopped. Once ovarian activity was seen on ultrasound, the dose ('threshold' dose) was maintained until follicular maturation was complete. hCG 5000 U was given to induce ovulation. No luteal support was given. A serum sample for progesterone analysis was taken 5–8 days after hCG and was considered ovulatory at a level >30 nmol/litre in the presence of a single follicle and >40 nmol/litre when two or three follicles were released. hCG was withheld in the presence of more than three follicles of 18 mm in diameter.

Treatment was monitored primarily by serial ultrasound scanning. On each occasion the uterine cross-sectional area, endometrial thickness and the diameter of any follicle present was measured in three dimensions. The

Table 2. Results of low-dose gonadotrophin therapy in 69 women with anovulatory polycystic ovary syndrome.

No. of cycles	280
Ovulatory cycles	184 (65.7%)
Uniovulatory cycles	140 (76%)
Mean maximum daily dose, IU/day (range)	93.5 (52.5–225 IU)
Mean total dose (range)	17.2 (5–82 ampoules)
Pregnancies	24
Multiple pregnancy	3 (twins)
Early pregnancy loss	9 (37.5%)

results of treatment are shown in Table 2. Of the 280 cycles induced in 69 patients using hMG, 70% were ovulatory and 71% of these were uni-ovulatory. The mean threshold dose was <1.5 ampoules per day. Three patients were found to produce multiple follicles within the first week on a dose of 1 ampoule, and so subsequent cycles were started at 0.7 ampoules. There was minimal variation in the threshold dose for each patient in sequential cycles.

The mean total dose for each cycle was 17 ampoules, and this compares very favourably with published data. Only two women required 3 ampoules per day, and they represent the upper value for both the threshold dose and the total dose. The vast majority (96%) of the patients responded to <2 ampoules with a mean follicular phase duration of 14.8 days (range 5–34 days).

During treatment three women were found to have an intermittently raised FSH and treatment was stopped. Nine women did not respond, and five women were found to have persistently negative post-coital tests despite normal semen analyses prior to the commencement of treatment.

In this series of patients only two women had a premature LH surge (an LH level >11 IU/litre in the presence of a follicle of <16 mm in diameter). The mean LH level 5 days and 2 days prior to hCG were within the normal range at 6.5 ± 3.3 and 5.2 ± 2.7 respectively ($\pm$SD). An appropriate LH surge was seen in 19 of 94 cycles analysed (20%).

The cumulative conception rate at 8 months by life table analysis was 38.7% for all patients and 49.6% excluding the anovulatory patients and those with a male factor. The early pregnancy loss rate was high at 37%, which is similar to that found in other series for women with PCO (Tyler, 1968; Gemzell, 1969; Thompson and Hanson, 1970; Oelsner et al, 1978; Dor et al, 1980; Schwartz et al, 1980; Wang and Gemzell, 1980). The precise reason for this high rate of pregnancy loss remains to be elucidated, but high follicular-phase LH levels have been implicated (Homburg et al, 1988c).

There were three multiple pregnancies (all twin pregnancies) in this series, and only two cycles (0.007%) were complicated by moderate hyper-stimulation and eight by mild hyperstimulation (0.03%). There were no cases of severe hyperstimulation and only one patient with moderate hyper-stimulation required hospitalization overnight for severe discomfort. This settled spontaneously within 48 h of initial onset and was not associated with any disturbance of electrolytes.

It would therefore seem that this low-dose protocol can successfully overcome the high rates of multiple pregnancy and hyperstimulation found in other series. The total number of ampoules used can be considerably less than on conventional therapy, and the length of treatment per cycle is similar. The pregnancy rate is comparable but the high rate of miscarriage remains an unsolved problem.

In women with PCO, who often have a raised basal LH level, it was thought that purified FSH alone might have a favourable advantage over hMG in terms of pregnancy rates and reduced pregnancy losses. Several studies have been conducted comparing the two, but none of these was randomized or controlled. It has been claimed that there is a reduced multiple pregnancy rate with FSH (Garcea et al, 1985; Seibel et al, 1985) but Seibel used a much lower starting dose of FSH (40–50 IU) compared with hMG (150–225 IU) which, from our data, would make this an expected finding. Hyperstimulation was not prevented, with an incidence of mild hyperstimulation in 23% of cycles.

Blunt et al (1987) treated nine patients with alternating hMG and FSH. The ovulation rates—86% FSH and 71% hMG—were similar. There was no difference in the pregnancy rate nor the incidence of premature luteinization. Our own data from a randomized prospective study of hMG and FSH in 30 women (Sagle et al, 1988) support the conclusion of Blunt et al (1987). There is therefore no firm evidence for an advantage of FSH over hMG.

Combined treatment with LH-releasing hormone (LHRH) analogues and gonadotrophins

In 1985 Fleming et al treated eight women who had PCOS with raised basal levels of LH and normal FSH with an LHRH analogue prior to commencing gonadotrophin therapy. Once endogenous gonadotrophin levels had been suppressed the women were treated with hMG. They found that seven of eight patients conceived rapidly without premature luteinization and without excessive ovarian enlargement. A similar pregnancy rate was found by Charbonnel et al (1987), but these workers reported a significant risk of hyperstimulation. Fleming and Coutts (1988) subsequently reported the results of treatment of 40 women with the combined treatment. They found a pregnancy rate of 82% of patients in six cycles, approximately double the rates published for hMG alone in PCOS (Dor et al, 1980; Diamond and Wentz, 1986). No significant difference was found in the rate of multiple follicular development (Coutts, 1989) or in the number of early pregnancy losses on combined treatment compared to hMG alone. Premature luteinization of the follicle was not observed in the combined group but was found in 33% of cycles induced with hMG alone (Fleming and Coutts, 1988). The remarkably high pregnancy rate has not been obtained by other groups (Buckler et al, 1989). Our own data show a pregnancy rate of 37.5% of patients on combined treatment, similar to that seen on hMG alone. In our series, however, the low-dose gonadotrophin protocol was used and the rate of multiple follicular development was lower than that reported by Fleming and Charbonnel (Franks et al, 1985). This combined treatment appears promising, but as yet there are insufficient data to justify its routine use as primary therapy in patients with PCOS, particularly as such treatment is considerably more expensive than hMG alone. Our practice is to use the combined treatment for women with PCOS who have been found to have persistently raised follicular phase LH levels, proven premature LH surges on hMG treatment alone, an inadequate luteal phase (Heasley et al, 1987), or those who have had two or more early pregnancy losses on clomiphene or hMG.

A combination of an LHRH analogue and hMG may overcome the problems of premature luteinization and inadequate luteal phases, but its true advantages over hMG alone, in ovulation induction (in vivo), have yet to be fully established.

Ovarian wedge resection and its variants

Wedge resection of the ovaries has been used for many years as a way of inducing ovulation in women with PCO. The reported ovulation rate is 30–90% but many of the studies are difficult to assess because the criteria for selection of patients are not always clear. To the authors' knowledge there has been no study comparing the effects of wedge resection with gonadotrophin therapy. Since wedge resection involves major surgery, and the risk of tubal damage secondary to adhesion formation is high, it seems sensible to confine this treatment to the small subgroup of women with PCO who fail to ovulate with gonadotrophin therapy.

A number of more recent and less traumatic modifications of wedge resection have been reported, again with encouragingly high rates of ovulation (Buttram and Vaquero, 1975; Adashi et al, 1981; Lunde 1982; Tanaka et al, 1988). Briefly, these techniques range from laparoscopic biopsy to placing lesions in the surface of the ovary by electrocautery or laser under laparoscopic guidance. It is too early to assess the long-term results of such therapies, but they carry the obvious advantage of less radical surgery than that associated with classic wedge resection.

At present there is no evidence that the success of these treatments is any greater than that resulting from induction of ovulation with gonadotrophins. It seems sensible, therefore, to reserve ovarian surgery for those women who have failed to conceive after six cycles of gonadotrophin therapy.

In vitro fertilization for women with PCOS

In vitro fertilization (IVF) has no established place in the treatment of patients with PCO who have not conceived on gonadotrophin therapy. However, it should be remembered that women with PCO may also have tubal problems or other factors causing their infertility with or without anovulation. Women with PCO tend to develop more follicles, have higher follicular-phase LH levels and a greater incidence of premature luteinization than women with normal ovaries. The latter two conditions may be improved by combined treatment with an LHRH analogue and gonadotrophins, but hyperstimulation remains a constant threat. This may be overcome by egg collection, fertilization and subsequent freezing of embryos for replacement at a later time when the danger of hyperstimulation has passed.

PRIMARY OVARIAN FAILURE (HYPERGONADOTROPHIC HYPOGONADISM)

Primary ovarian failure is defined as the cessation of ovarian function prior to the age of 40 by means other than surgical intervention. It is characterized by primary or secondary amenorrhoea with elevated serum gonadotrophin levels.

Ovarian failure is, fortunately, a rare entity. A population study carried out in the USA calculated a cumulative risk, based on age-specific incidence rates, of 1% before the age of 40. The incidence rates were 10 per 100 000 person years aged 15–29 and 76 per 100 000 in ages 30–39. Over the age of 40 the rate increased tenfold (Coulam et al, 1986). This, however, only applies to the incidence of idiopathic ovarian failure and does not include the medical, surgical and chromosomal causes of ovarian failure. Millot and Daux (1959) quoted an overall incidence of 3.9% before the age of 30.

Many causes of ovarian failure are known, but in most cases the exact aetiology remains obscure. Women with ovarian dysgenesis have a decreased complement of ova from birth. Follicular atresia may be induced by exposure to external irradiation or cytotoxic chemotherapy. Ovarian function may be destroyed by viral infection or surgery. During the last decade increasing interest has been focused on an autoimmune process underlying ovarian destruction. An association between ovarian failure and autoimmune disease has been reported many times (Duff and Bernstein, 1933; Ruehsen and Jones, 1967; Irvine et al, 1968; Vasquez and Kenny, 1973; Vaidya et al, 1977; McNatty et al 1978; Wolfsdorf et al, 1978; Austin et al, 1979; Collen et al, 1979; Taylor et al, 1989). In 1979 Coulam and Ryan reported circulating antibodies to ovarian tissue in 15 women with ovarian failure. In 1985 Alper and Garner showed that these patients also produce autoantibodies to tissues other than ovary and steroid-producing cells. The exact mechanism and importance of the autoimmune process remains unknown, but it has been suggested that those women with 'autoimmune' ovarian failure may have a greater chance of a spontaneous resumption of ovulation than the other groups (Johnson and Peterson, 1979; Zourlas and Mantzavinos, 1980). The diagnosis is made on the basis of an elevated serum concentration of FSH. This finding should be confirmed on one or more subsequent measurements.

Ovarian biopsy, whether obtained by laparoscopy or laparotomy, has been used in the past to differentiate premature menopause from the 'resistant ovary syndrome'. Originally it was felt that if primordial follicles were found in the biopsy specimen then high-dose gonadotrophin therapy might successfully induce ovulation (Johnson and Peterson, 1979; Zourlas and Mantzavinos, 1980). However, no controlled trial has ever been conducted to show that any one treatment is better than another, or better than no treatment at all (O'Herlihy et al, 1980). The risks of surgery far outweigh any benefit to the patient, particularly as a biopsy specimen may not be representative of the whole ovary (Aiman and Smentek, 1985). The risk of peritubular adhesions affecting future fertility, if ovarian function returns spontaneously, should also be considered. Since the histological findings have little influence on management of the patient it would seem difficult to justify performing an ovarian biopsy. The presence of antral follicles within the ovaries, which is thought to indicate a better prognosis for resumption of ovulatory cycles, can, in any case, often be detected by ovarian ultrasound scanning.

Treatment

There have been many reports in the literature of women with primary ovarian failure who resume menses or occasionally become pregnant (Wright and Jacobs, 1979; Menon et al, 1984). It is important to remember that menstruation can occur without ovulation and with slightly (or greatly) raised levels of FSH. Attempts at ovulation induction are usually unsuccessful in this situation. In a review of 93 women with primary ovarian failure Hague et al (1987) found that none of the cases of primary amenorrhoea resumed ovarian activity but 20 out of 73 cases (17.1%) with secondary amenorrhoea had some evidence of spontaneous recovery of ovarian function. They resumed menses and/or showed follicular and uterine growth with increasing endometrial thickness on scan. These findings were associated with a fall in gonadotrophin levels.

Other case studies have reported a resumption of ovarian function following the use of oestrogens (Shangold et al, 1977; Starup et al, 1978; Evers and Rolland, 1981; Alper et al, 1986; Navot et al, 1986). It has been suggested that ovulation results from the 'rebound' rise in gonadotrophin concentration which occurs after withdrawal of these steroids, but no controlled studies have been performed and such resumption of ovarian activity may well be coincidental. Following reports of the success of ovulation induction in anovulatory women following treatment with a GnRH analogue, Menon et al (1983) treated four women who had primary ovarian failure with Buserelin for 28 days. FSH and LH levels were suppressed in all cases. One woman ovulated on day 8 following cessation of treatment, while the other three had rapidly rising gonadotrophin levels with no signs of ovarian activity. More recently Surrey and Cedars (1989) have treated 14 women with high-dose hMG following gonadotrophin suppression with steroids or Buserelin. Only one woman ovulated without conception. There is, therefore, no evidence for a successful method for ovulation induction in these women. Oestrogen replacement is very important for these women if they are going to escape the long-term consequences of oestrogen deficiency.

The outlook for these women in terms of fertility is poor and no therapy offers them any improvement in this prognosis. It is therefore important to consider the impact of a prolonged menopausal state on the metabolism of these women. It is well recognized that menopausal women develop osteoporosis and have an increased risk of cardiovascular disease compared to premenopausal women. This is almost certainly secondary to lower oestrogen levels. These women should therefore be advised to take hormone replacement therapy with a combined low-dose oestrogen and progestagen preparation and, if necessary, given counselling to help them come to terms with their infertility.

Ovum donation

The recent development of ovum and embryo donation (Lutjen et al, 1984; Chan et al, 1987) has offered these women a chance of fertility. The difficulties in finding donors are much greater than for semen donors, and despite the initial hopes of being able to start ovum banks (Chen, 1986) cryopreservation of ova remains very difficult and unpredictable. The waiting lists for donation are long and the procedure is expensive. Successes have been reported (Chan et al, 1987) but increasing parliamentary and media concern over the legal and ethical issues may add an extra difficulty for an already oversubscribed service.

SUMMARY

There are many groups of women with anovulatory infertility who respond abnormally to conventional treatment. It is important to diagnose the underlying disorder correctly before commencing treatment. In this chapter we have discussed the various treatment modalities available and how they may be adapted to fit the particular clinical needs.

In women who are profoundly hypo-oestrogenic, the 'priming' of the ovary using prolonged low-dose gonadotrophins offers a possible solution if both subcutaneous and intravenous pulsatile GnRH therapy has failed. It may also reduce the incidence of multiple pregnancies in these women. Growth hormone seems to augment the response to gonadotrophin in these women and may prove a useful adjunct to therapy once further experience of its use has been reported.

Women with PCO have been a difficult group to treat because of their tendency to hyperstimulate. The low-dose gonadotrophin regimen outlined in this chapter overcomes the majority of these problems without reducing the rate of conception. This group continue to have an increased incidence of miscarriage. The introduction of combined therapy of hMG with a GnRH analogue may improve this situation, but the data from randomized controlled studies are still awaited.

Ovarian failure remains an untreatable cause of infertility. A few women may become pregnant spontaneously, but these are the exception rather than the rule. Hormone replacement therapy should be offered to all these women because of the long-term problems of osteoporosis and cardiovascular disease. Products containing a low dose of oestrogen (e.g. Premarin 0.625 mg) will not interfere with ovulation if there should be a spontaneous resumption of ovarian activity.

REFERENCES

Adams J, Franks S, Polson DW et al (1985) Multifollicular ovaries: clinical and endocrine features and responses to pulsatile gonadotrophin releasing hormone. *Lancet* **ii:** 1375–1378.

Adams J, Polson DW & Franks S (1986) Prevalence of polycystic ovaries in women with anovulation and idiopathic hirsutism. *British Medical Journal* **293:** 355–359.

Adashi EY, Rock JA, Guzick D et al (1981) Fertility following bi-lateral ovarian wedge resection: a critical analysis of 90 consecutive cases of the polycystic ovary syndrome. *Fertility and Sterility* **36:** 320–325.

Adashi EY, Resnick EE, D'Ercole AJ et al (1985) Insulin-like growth factors as intra-ovarian regulators of granulosa cell growth and function. *Endocrine Reviews* **6(3):** 400–420.

Aiman J & Smentek C (1985) Premature ovarian failure. *Obstetrics and Gynecology* **66:** 9–14.

Alper MM & Garner PR (1985) Premature ovarian failure: its relationship to autoimmune disease. *Obstetrics and Gynaecology* **66:** 27–30.

Alper MM, Jolly EE & Garner PR (1986) Pregnancies after premature ovarian failure. *Obstetrics and Gynecology* **67 (supplement):** 59S.

Armar NA & Eshel A (1988) Induction of fertility with pulsatile LHRH. In Cheng WC & Tan SL (eds) *Advances in Reproductive and Perinatal Medicine*, pp 61–76. Singapore: PG Publishing.

Austin GE, Coulam CB & Ryan RJ (1979) A search for antibodies to luteinizing hormone receptors in premature ovarian failure. *Mayo Clinic Proceedings* **54:** 394–396.

Bergh T, Skarin G, Nillius SJ et al (1984) Pulsatile LRH administration to women with bromocriptine-resistant hyperprolactinaemia. In Lamberts SW, Tilders FHJ, van der Veen EA & Assies J (eds) *Trends in Diagnosis and Treatment of Pituitary Adenomas*, pp 195–198. Amsterdam: Free University Press.

Bergquist C, Nillius SJ & Wide L (1983) Human gonadotrophin therapy. *Fertility and Sterility* **39:** 761–766.

Blumenfeld Z & Lunenfeld B (1989) The potentiating effect of growth hormone on follicle stimulation with human menopausal gonadotrophin in a panhypopituitary patient. *Fertility and Sterility* **52:** 328–331.

Blunt SM, Rudd BT, Habowbi N & Butt WR (1987) Comparison between human menopausal gonadotrophin and purified FSH in the treatment of women with polycystic ovarian disease. *Journal of Endocrinology* **112:** 5226.

Boyar RM, Katz J, Finkelstein JW et al (1974) Immaturity of the 24 hour luteinizing hormone secretory pattern in anorexia nervosa. *New England Journal of Medicine* **291:** 861–865.

Brown JB, Evans JH, Adey FD et al (1969) Factors involved in the induction of fertile ovulation with human gonadotrophins. *Journal of Obstetrics and Gynaecology of the British Commonwealth* **76:** 289–306.

Buckler HM, Phillips SE, Kovacs GT et al (1989) GnRH agonist administration in polycystic ovary syndrome. *Clinical Endocrinology* **31:** 151–163.

Buttram VC Jr & Vaquero C (1975) Post ovarian wedge resection adhesive disease. *Fertility and Sterility* **26:** 874–879.

Chan CLK, Cameron IT, Findlay JK et al (1987) Oocyte donation and in vitro fertilization for hypergonadotrophic hypogonadism. *Obstetrics and Gynecology* **42:** 350–362.

Charbonnel B, Krempf M, Blanchard P et al (1987) Induction of ovulation in polycystic ovary syndrome with a combination of a luteinising hormone releasing analog and exogenous gonadotrophins. *Fertility and Sterility* **47:** 920–924.

Chen C (1986) Pregnancy after oocyte cryopreservation. *Lancet* **i:** 224.

Coelingh-Bennink HJT (1983) Induction of ovulation by pulsatile intravenous administration of LHRH in polycystic ovarian disease. *65th Annual Meeting Endocrinology Society*, San Antonio, USA (abstract 81).

Collen RJ, Lippe BM & Kaplan SA (1979) Primary ovarian failure. Juvenile rheumatoid arthritis and vitiligo. *American Journal of Diseases of Childhood* **13:** 598–601.

Coulam CB & Ryan RJ (1979) Premature menopause 1, etiology. *American Journal of Obstetrics and Gynecology* **133:** 639–643.

Coulam CB, Adamson SC & Anneges JF (1986) Incidence of premature ovarian failure. *Obstetrics and Gynaecology* **67:** 604–606.

Coutts JRT (1989) The use of LHRH analogues in ovulation induction and induction of multiple follicular growth for in vitro fertilisation. In Shaw RW & Marshal JG (eds) *LHRH and its Analogues*, pp 198–213. London: Wright.

Davoren B & Hsueh AJW (1986) Growth hormone increases ovarian levels of immunoreactive somatomedin c/insulin-like growth factor-I in vitro. *Endocrinology* **118:** 888–890.

Diamond MP & Wentz AC (1986) Ovulation induction with human menopausal gonado-trophins. *Obstetrical and Gynaecological Survey* **41:** 480–490.

Dor J, Itzkowic DJ, Mashiach S et al (1980) Cumulative conception rates following gonado-trophin therapy. *American Journal of Obstetrics and Gynecology* **136:** 102–105.

Duff GL & Bernstein C (1933) Five cases of Addison's disease with so called atrophy of adrenal cartels. *Johns Hopkins Medical Journal* **52:** 67–69.

Ellis JD & Williamson JG (1975) Factors influencing the pregnancy and complication rates with human menopausal gonadotrophin therapy. *British Journal of Obstetrics and Gynaecology* **82:** 52–57.

Evers JLH & Rolland R (1981) The gonadotrophin resistant ovary syndrome: a curable disease. *Clinical Endocrinology* **14:** 99–103.

Fleming R & Coutts JT (1988) LHRH analogues for ovulation induction with particular reference to Polycystic Ovary Syndrome. *Baillière's Clinical Obstetrics and Gynaecology* **2:** 677–687.

Fleming R, Haxton MJ, Hamilton MPR et al (1985) Successful treatment of infertile women with oligomenorhoea using a combination of an LHRH agonist and exogenous gonadotrophins. *British Journal of Obstetrics and Gynaecology* **92:** 369–379.

Franks S (1987) Primary and secondary amenorrhoea. *British Medical Journal* **294:** 815–819.

Franks S (1989) Polycystic ovary syndrome: a changing perspective. *Clinical Endocrinology* **31:** 87–120.

Franks S, Adams J, Mason HD et al (1985) Ovulatory disorders in women with polycystic ovary syndrome. *Clinics in Obstetrics and Gynaecology* **12(3):** 605–632.

Franks S, Sagle M, Mason HD et al (1987) Use of LHRH agonists in the treatment of anovulation in women with polycystic ovary syndrome. *Hormone Research* **28:** 164–168.

Garcea N, Campo S, Paretta V et al (1985) Induction of ovulation with purified urinary follicle-stimulating hormone in patients with polycystic ovarian syndrome. *American Journal of Obstetrics and Gynecology* **151:** 635–640.

Gemzell C (1969) Treatment of female and male sterility with human gonadotrophins. *Acta Obstetrica et Gynaecologica Scandinavica* **68 (supplement 1):** 1.

Gemzell C & Ross P (1966) Pregnancies following treatment with human gonadotrophins with special reference to the problem of multiple birth. *American Journal of Obstetrics and Gynecology* **94:** 86–90.

Gujeon AL (1982) Rate of follicular growth in the human ovary. In Rolland R, van Hall EV, Hillier SG et al (eds) *Follicular Maturation and Ovulation*, pp 155–163. Amsterdam: Excerpta Medica.

Hague WM, Tan SL, Adams J et al (1987) Hypergonadotrophin amenorrhoea: aetiology and outcome in 93 young women. *International Journal of Obstetrics and Gynaecology* **25:** 121–125.

Heasley RN, Boyle DD & Thompson W (1987) LHRH analogue therapy in infertile women with luteal phase defects. *Clinical Reproduction and Fertility* **5:** 133–137.

Homburg R, Eshel A, Armar NA et al (1988a) Synergism of pulsatile LHRH therapy with oral Clomiphene treatment. *Gynecological Endocrinology* **2:** 59–64.

Homburg R, Eshel A, Abdalla HI et al (1988b) Growth hormone facilitates ovulation induction by gonadotrophins. *Clinical Endocrinology* **29:** 113–117.

Homburg R, Armar NA, Eshel A, Adams J & Jacobs HS (1988c) The influence of serum luteinising hormone concentrations on ovulation, conception and early pregnancy loss in patients with polycystic ovary syndrome. *British Medical Journal* **297:** 1024–1026.

Homburg R, Eshel A, Armar NA et al (1989) One hundred pregnancies after treatment with pulsatile luteinising hormone releasing hormone to induce ovulation. *British Medical Journal* **298:** 809–812.

Homburg R, West C, Torreson T et al (1990) Cotreatment with human growth hormone and gonadotrophins for induction of ovulation: a controlled clinical trial. *Fertility and Sterility* **53:** 254–260.

Hull MGR (1981) Ovulation failure and induction. *Clinics in Obstetrics and Gynaecology* **8(3):** 753–786.

Hull MGR (1987) Epidemiology of infertility and polycystic ovarian disease: endocrinological and demographic studies. *Gynecological Endocrinology* **1:** 235–245.

Irvine WJ, Chan MM, Scarth L et al (1968) Immunological aspects of premature ovarian failure associated with idiopathic Addison's disease. *Lancet* **ii:** 883–885.

Johnson TR & Peterson EP (1979) Gonadotrophin induced pregnancy following 'premature ovarian failure'. *Fertility and Sterility* **31:** 351.

Kallman FJ, Schoenfeld WA & Barrera SE (1944) The genetic aspects of primary eunuchoidism. *American Journal of Mental Deficiency* **48:** 203–236.

Leyendecker G, Struve T & Plotz EJ (1980a) Induction of ovulation with chronic intermittent (pulsatile) administration of LHRH in women with hypothalamic and hyperprolactinaemic amenorrhoea. *Archives of Gynaecology* **229:** 172–190.

Leyendecker G, Wildt L & Hausmann M (1980b) Pregnancies following chronic intermittent (pulsatile) administration of GnRH by means of a portable pump (Zyclomat)—a new approach to the treatment of infertility in hypothalamic amenorrhoea. *Journal of Clinical Endocrinology and Metabolism* **51:** 1214–1216.

Lunde O (1982) Polycystic ovarian syndrome: a retrospective study of the therapeutic effect of ovarian wedge resection after unsuccessful treatment with clomiphene citrate. *Gynecology* **38:** 483–487.

Lunenfeld B, Eshkol A, Tikotzky D et al (1982) Induction of ovulation: human gonadotrophins. In Flamigni C & Givens JR (eds) *The Gonadotrophins: Basic Science and Clinical Aspects in Females*, pp 395–403. London: Academic Press.

Lutjen P, Trowdon A, Leeton J et al (1984) The establishment and maintenance of pregnancy using in vitro fertilisation and embryo donation in a patient with primary ovarian failure. *Nature* **307:** 174–177.

Mason P, Adams J, Morris DV et al (1984) Induction of ovulation with pulsatile luteinizing hormone-releasing hormone. *British Medical Journal* **288:** 181–185.

Mason HD, Sagle M, Polson DW et al (1988) Reduced frequency of luteinizing hormone pulses in women with weight loss-related amenorrhoea and multifollicular ovaries. *Clinical Endocrinology* **28:** 611–618.

McNatty KP, Short RV, Barnest W et al (1978) The cytotoxic effect of serum from patients with Addison's disease and autoimmune ovarian failure on human granulosa cell culture. *Clinical and Experimental Immunology* **22:** 378–380.

Menon V, Edwards RL, Lynch SS et al (1983) Luteinizing hormone releasing hormone analogue in treatment of hypergonadotrophic amenorrhoea. *British Journal of Obstetrics and Gynaecology* **90:** 539–542.

Menon V, Edwards RL, Butt WR et al (1984) Review of 59 patients with hypergonadotrophic hypogonadism. *British Journal of Obstetrics and Gynaecology* **91:** 63.

Millot J & Daux JL (1959) Influence de la ménopause précose, naturelle on chirurgicale sur le déclenchement des coronantes. *Archives des Maladies du Coeur* **52:** 297–300.

Navot D, Laufer N, Koplovic J et al (1986) Artificially induced endometrial cycles and establishment of pregnancies in the absence of ovaries. *New England Journal of Medicine* **314:** 806–808.

Nillius SJ & Wide L (1977) The pituitary responsiveness to acute and chronic administration of gonadotrophin releasing hormone in acute and recovery stages of anorexia nervosa. In Vigersky RA (ed.) *Anorexia Nervosa*, pp 225–241. New York: Raven Press.

Oelsner G, Serr DM, Mashiach S et al (1978) The study of induction of ovulation with menotropins: analysis of results of 1897 treatment cycles. *Fertility and Sterility* **30:** 538–541.

O'Herlihy C, Pepperell RJ, Evans JH (1980) The significance of FSH elevation in young women with disorders of ovulation. *British Medical Journal* **281:** 1447–1450.

Pellicer A, Lightman A, Diamond MP et al (1987) Outcome of in vitro fertilisation in women with low response to ovarian stimulation. *Fertility and Sterility* **47:** 812–815.

Polson DW, Mason HD, Saldahna MBY & Franks S (1987a) Ovulation of a single dominant follicle stimulating hormone in women with polycystic ovary syndrome. *Clinical Endocrinology* **26:** 205–212.

Polson DW, Sagle M, Mason HD et al (1987b) Recovery of luteal function after interruption of gonadotrophin secretion in the mid-luteal phase of the menstrual cycle. *Clinical Endocrinology* **26:** 597–600.

Polson DW, Mason HD & Kiddy DS (1989) Low-dose follicle-stimulating hormone in the treatment of polycystic ovary syndrome: a comparison of pulsatile subcutaneous with daily intramuscular therapy. *British Journal of Obstetrics and Gynaecology* **96(6):** 746–748.

Rabau E, David A, Serr DM et al (1967) Human menopausal gonadotrophins for anovulation and sterility. *American Journal of Obstetrics and Gynecology* **94:** 490–495.

Rogol AD, White BJ, Lieblich JM et al (1982) The Kallman syndrome: a clinical genetic and endocrine view of nine affected women. In Flamigni C & Givens JR (eds) *The Gonadotrophins: Basic Science and Clinical Aspects in Females*, pp 233–244. London: Academic Press.

Ruehsen MDM & Jones GES (1967) Premature ovarian failure. *Fertility and Sterility* **18:** 440–446.

Sagle M, Kiddy DS & Franks S (1988) A prospective randomized comparative study of low dose HMG and FSH in polycystic ovary syndrome (PCOS). *Journal of Endocrinology* **121 (supplement):** abstract 307.

Schwartz M & Jewelewicz R (1981) The use of gonadotrophins for induction of ovulation. *Fertility and Sterility* **35:** 3–12.

Schwartz M, Jewelewicz R, Dyrenfirth I et al (1980) The use of human menopausal and chorionic gonadotrophin for induction of ovulation. *Journal of Obstetrics and Gynaecology* **138:** 801–807.

Shangold M, Turksoy RN, Bashford RA et al (1977) Pregnancy following the insensitive ovary syndrome. *Fertility and Sterility* **28:** 1179–1181.

Seibel MM, McArdle C & Smith D (1985) Ovulation induction in polycystic ovary syndrome with urinary follicle stimulating hormone or human menopausal gonadotrophin. *Fertility and Sterility* **45:** 703–708.

Spadoni LR, Cox DW & Smith DC (1974) Use of human menopausal gonadotrophins for the induction of ovulation. *Journal of Obstetrics and Gynaecology* **120:** 988–993.

Starup J, Philip J & Sele V (1978) Oestrogen treatment and subsequent pregnancy in two patients with severe hypergonadotrophic ovarian failure. *Acta Endocrinologica* **89:** 149–157.

Stein A & Fairburn CG (1989) Children of mothers with bulimia nervosa. *British Medical Journal* **299:** 777–778.

Surrey ES & Cedars MI (1989) The effect of gonadotrophin suppression on the induction of ovulation in premature ovarian failure patients. *Fertility and Sterility* **52:** 36–40.

Tanaka T, Oikawa M, Sakuraji N et al (1988) May wedge resection still be useful in patients with polycystic ovarian disease refractory to clomiphene citrate? *XII World Congress of Gynecology and Obstetrics*, Rio de Janeiro.

Taylor R, Smith NM, Angus B et al (1989) Return of fertility after 12 years of autoimmune ovarian failure. *Clinical Endocrinology* **31:** 305–308.

Thompson CR & Hanson LM (1970) Pergonal (menotropins): a summary of clinical experience in the induction of ovulation and pregnancy. *Fertility and Sterility* **21:** 844–847.

Tyler E (1968) Treatment of anovulation with menotrophins. *Journal of the American Medical Association* **205:** 86–93.

Vaidya RA, Aloorka SD, Rege NR et al (1977) Premature ovarian failure. *Reproductive Medicine* **19:** 348–355.

van der Spuy Z, Steer PJ, McCusker M et al (1988) Pregnancy outcome in underweight women following spontaneous and induced ovulation. *British Medical Journal* **296:** 962–965.

Vasquez AM & Kenny FM (1973) Ovarian failure and anti-ovarian antibodies in association with hypoparathyroidism, moniliasis and Addison's and Hashimoto's disease. *Obstetrics and Gynecology* **41:** 414–418.

Wang CF & Gemzell C (1980) The use of human gonadotrophins for the induction of ovulation in women with polycystic ovarian disease. *Fertility and Sterility* **33:** 479–486.

West CP & Baird DT (1984) Induction of ovulation with gonadotrophins a 10 year review. *Scottish Medical Journal* **29:** 212–220.

Wolfsdorf JI, Rosenfeld RL, Fang VS et al (1978) Partial gonadotrophin resistance in pseudohypoparathyroidism. *Acta Endocrinology* **88:** 321–325.

Wright CS & Jacobs HS (1979) Spontaneous pregnancy in a patient with hypergonadotrophic amenorrhoea. *British Journal of Obstetrics and Gynaecology* **86:** 389–390.

Zourlas PA & Mantzavinos T (1980) Pregnancies in primary amenorrhoea with normally developed secondary sexual characteristics. *Fertility and Sterility* **34:** 112–115.

13

Accidental hyperstimulation during ovulation induction

J. SALAT-BAROUX
J. M. ANTOINE

FREQUENCY

After simple stimulation of ovulation, Navot et al (1988) reported a 3% hyperstimulation rate in 1822 cycles induced by human menopausal gonadotrophin (hMG). However, the severe form occurs in only 0.84% (Lunenfeld, 1986).

After in vitro fertilization, the first case of severe hyperstimulation was reported by Friedman et al (1984) in a 36-year-old patient with abnormal cycles treated by hMG in gradually increasing doses. Ovulation was induced with a plasma oestradiol level of 3010 pg/ml. We made a similar observation in a patient with polycystic ovarian syndrome (PCO) treated by pure follicle-stimulating hormone (FSH; a total of 14 ampoules), with a polycystic response by ultrasound and plasma oestradiol of 2600 pg/ml on the day of ovulation induction (Salat-Baroux et al, 1987). In both cases, embryo transfer was followed by pregnancy.

Paradoxically, despite the use of high-dose ovarian stimulation during in vitro fertilization to achieve biological hyperstimulation, severe ovarian hyperstimulation syndrome is a rare occurrence. The usual explanation for this is that aspiration of all the follicles prevents initiation of the hyper-stimulation phenomenon. However, it is not possible to exclude a bias of recruitment, because classical ovulation stimulation is indicated for dis-ovulation or anovulation whereas in vitro fertilization is essentially pro-posed for cases of fertility with normal ovulation, that is, for tubal, idiopathic or male factor infertility.

PREDISPOSING FACTORS

Underlying conditions

It seems as if PCO constitutes the most important risk factor. The physiopathology of this is still imperfectly understood. Many factors are involved, including high endogenous luteinizing hormone (LH), a defective aromatization pathway giving a tendency to follicular atresia, high intra-follicular inhibin levels, hyperandrogenaemia (sometimes with an adrenal component), increased peripheral conversion to oestrogens, and an increased resistance to insulin related to obesity. Recently modifications of intrafollicular growth factors have been demonstrated: high epidermal growth factor (EGF; Franks et al, 1988), decreased insulin-like growth factor 1 (IGF1)-binding protein (Pekonen et al, 1989; Suikkari et al, 1989) and increased free IGF1 which, along with insulin, stimulated the production of thecal androgens. All these modifications lead to an increased ovarian sensitivity to exogenous gonadotrophins. Furthermore, hyper-prolactinaemia (Yuen et al, 1979), which can of itself be associated with ovarian dystrophy and hyperthyroidism, can also lead to the occurrence of hyperstimulation by increasing ovarian sensitivity to human chorionic gonadotrophin (hCG; Morgan et al, 1983).

Treatment

Two conditions are most frequently associated with the development of hyperstimulation syndrome: the development of a multifollicular response to stimulation, with abnormally high plasma oestradiol and rapid luteinization following one or several injections of hCG. Although hMG is most often implicated, severe hyperstimulations have also been observed with more 'physiological' forms of stimulation such as clomiphene citrate (Morgan et al, 1983; Chow and Choo, 1984) LH releasing hormone (LHRH) pump (Lorcy et al, 1984) and pure FSH (Check et al, 1985). The introduction of LHRH agonists, which has certainly improved the pregnancy rate per cycle, does not seem to have reduced the risk of hyperstimulation and may even have increased it, especially related to PCO (Charbonnel et al, 1987; Salat-Baroux et al, 1988a). Recently Yeh et al (1989) have even reported a case of moderate hyperstimulation due to the flare-up effect of the agonist. It is rare for a spontaneous LH peak to cause hyperstimulation. More usually, hCG has been administered. Several risk factors need to be emphasized: doses of hCG ≥ 5000 IU intramuscularly, a short interval (24 h) between the last administration of hMG and that of hCG and, especially, repeated hCG injections in the luteal phase (Salat-Baroux et al, 1987).

Relationship to pregnancy

Our experience with in vitro fertilization without LHRH analogues showed a significant difference in the ongoing pregnancy rates obtained depending on whether the oestradiol level on the day of hCG administration was greater or less than 2500 pg/ml (5% of 34 cycles and 16% in 543 cycles respectively, $P < 0.05$) (Salat-Baroux et al, 1987). Several mechanisms could be envisaged, including poor oocyte quality with a reduced fertilization rate, poor endometrial quality (Forman et al, 1988), and a luteolytic effect of oestradiol. Our most recent data (Salat-Baroux et al, 1988b, 1990) suggest that when LHRH analogues are used, the high pregnancy rate still occurs in these conditions, even after fresh embryo replacement, possibly due to the more physiological rate of oestradiol to progesterone at the start of the luteal phase.

GENERAL COMPLICATIONS

Clinical description

The classification into six stages initially proposed by Rabau et al (1967) has been reduced by the WHO to three well-recognized degrees:

1. first degree (minor hyperstimulation)—increase in steroids and ovarian volume < 5 cm, accompanied by an increased chance of pregnancy;
2. second degree (moderate hyperstimulation)—presence of ovarian cysts, nausea, vomiting and abdominal distension;
3. third degree (severe hyperstimulation)—voluminous ovarian cysts, ascites, sometimes hydrothorax.

Even more severe complications can result, including hypovolaemic shock, renal insufficiency, acute respiratory distress (Zosmer et al, 1987) and even death.

Physiopathology

The underlying phenomenon is a massive passage of fluid and protein from the vascular space to the peritoneal and pleural cavities (Hanning et al, 1985). This leads to hypovolaemia with secondary increases in plasma renin activity, aldosterone and antidiuretic hormone (ADH) despite the low serum osmolality (Figure 1). These result in an antidiuretic effect, with sodium retention leading to oliguria, functional renal insufficiency and water retention, which aggravates the plasma extravasation and is a secondary source of haemodilution with hyponatraemia and hypo-osmolality. These latter can be accompanied by central nervous system problems: headaches, disorientation, confusion and, at worst, coma.

Hanning suggests that this plasma extravasation is only a rapid increase in the volume of peritoneal fluid which is normally observed in the second half of the cycle and is not related to rupture of ovarian follicles since it persists following extra-peritonization of the ovaries. A similar mechanism occurring over a longer period of time could also explain the characteristic effusions of Demons–Meigs syndrome. This association has already been suggested in the term 'acute Meigs syndrome' used by Neuwirth et al (1965) to describe hyperstimulation.

The origin of these different processes appears to be an ovarian hormonal factor which is hCG-dependent and seems to be responsible for increased capillary permeability on the peritoneal and pleural surfaces. This factor has not been definitely identified. It is known that it is not oestradiol and that prostaglandins and histamines are probably involved, since it is possible to inhibit hyperstimulation by indomethacin (Schenker and Polishuk, 1976) and antihistamines (Knox, 1974; Gergely et al, 1976). Antihistamines also increase the ovarian concentration of prostaglandin F (PGF; Pride et al, 1984). Recently, activation of the ovarian renin–angiotensin system (Fernandez et al, 1975) has been suggested by Navot et al (1987). He showed that in 21 women with clinical pictures of hyperstimulation caused by hMG there was a significant increase in plasma renin activity over that of controls. This was directly correlated with the severity of hyperstimulation and regressed in the absence of early pregnancy and persisted at high levels when pregnancy occurred. This ovarian renin–angiotensin system could play an important role in the onset of hyperstimulation syndrome by inducing the development of neovascularization and increasing capillary permeability.

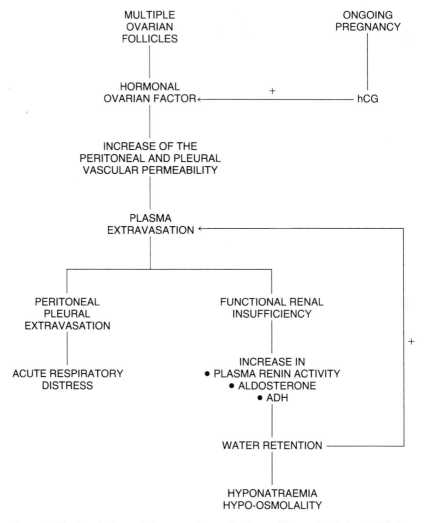

Figure 1. Physiopathology of the general complications of hyperstimulation. hCG, human chorionic gonadotrophin; ADH, antidiuretic hormone.

Other secondary physiological modifications have also been described. These include an increase of carcinoembryonic antigen (CA)-125 in hyperstimulation with exogenous gonadotrophins, although the levels are normal in patients who receive the same treatment without hyperstimulation (Jager et al, 1987). Transitory liver disturbances have also been described (Younis et al, 1988), which could constitute a marker for the severity of hyperstimulation.

LOCAL COMPLICATIONS

Several intermediary stages are possible, from simple ovarian cysts which persist in isolation after stimulation by hMG/hCG (as described by Tummon et al (1988) as an attenuated form of hyperstimulation) to true surgical complications occurring when polycystic ovaries are greatly increased in volume. These include rupture and torsion as causes of haemoperitoneum. Haemoperitoneum can also occur in relation to an associated extrauterine pregnancy.

THROMBOEMBOLIC COMPLICATIONS

Thromboembolic complications are rare but serious complications related to the initial haemoconcentration. Mozes et al (1965) reported two cases of arterial thrombosis following induction by hMG/hCG. One was a carotid thrombosis, which was fatal, and the other a femoral, necessitating amputation of the lower limb. Isolated coagulation disorders are more frequent. These include increased factor V, platelets, fibrinogen and thromboplastin formation.

TREATMENT

In all cases, the occurrence of clinical hyperstimulation necessitates discontinuation of stimulation. In mild and moderate forms this, associated with rest and possibly with cold packs on the abdomen, leads to spontaneous resolution over a variable period of time. However, in the severe forms hospitalization and often active treatment are necessary. This is both symptomatic, directed towards the consequences of hyperstimulation, and specific, against the mechanisms that produce and maintain the condition.

Symptomatic treatment

In the emergency situation, the risk of cardiovascular collapse must be prevented by the infusion of either dextran, fresh frozen plasma or human albumin, with monitoring of arterial pressure and central venous pressure. When effusions are present, either pleural or peritoneal, these should be aspirated, possibly using ultrasound monitoring. Thaler et al (1981) and

Borenstein et al (1989) report that evacuation of ascites leads to clear improvement of the clinical state and the biological parameters (renal function and haemoconcentration). When torsion or rupture of a cyst occurs or there is haemoperitoneum of extrauterine pregnancy, surgical intervention is necessary and, if possible, should be conservative.

When the situation is less urgent it is necessary to balance the efficacy and potential risks of several therapeutic modalities. Replacement of vascular fluid is useful to prevent haemoconcentration with associated thromboembolic complications and renal insufficiency, but could aggravate the water retention and the importance of the third sector and haemodilation. On the other hand, restriction of sodium and water and diuresis increase hypovolaemia and functional renal insufficiency. In the normal forms without renal insufficiency, typical management would include moderate sodium and water restriction, with simple replacement of water and electrolyte losses, sometimes associated with small doses of diuretics, particularly of the anti-aldosterone type. The question of whether to use anticoagulants is difficult because of the risks of intraperitoneal haemorrhage. Use in isocoagulant doses would seem indicated in purely biological disturbances of coagulation, while more potent anticoagulation should be reserved for obvious thromboembolic complications.

Specific treatment

Corticosteroids are a classic treatment for clinical hyperstimulation. The problems relate to knowing their efficacy in the absence of randomized studies, their tolerability with the risk of sodium and water retention, coagulation disturbances and the possible teratogenic risks. More recently, early aspiration of ovarian cysts by laparoscopy (Jahier et al, 1985) or transvaginally under ultrasound control (Dellenbach, personal communication) has been proposed to reduce the production of the ovarian factor responsible for the syndrome. However, because of the fragility of the cysts, this procedure is not devoid of the risk of haemorrhage and should be reserved for extremely severe cases. Other therapeutic modalities are not really compatible with ongoing pregnancy and should be reserved strictly for the forms of hyperstimulation not associated with pregnancy or with a very serious condition. In addition to interruption of pregnancy itself, both antihistamines (Pride et al, 1984; Kirshon et al, 1988) and antiprostaglandins (Shenker and Weinstein, 1978; Katz et al, 1984) are used, but their efficacy has been questioned (Borenstein et al, 1989).

PREVENTION

This must be a major preoccupation at all stages of ovarian stimulation.

Before start of treatment, identification of high-risk cases

The characteristic signs of polycystic ovaries should be carefully looked for.

These include long and irregular cycles, obesity, hirsutism, high baseline and stimulated LH, and increasing testosterone and δ-4-androstenedione. We have studied the pelvic ultrasound appearances before ovulation induction of 109 patients with non-obvious ovulatory problems prior to a cycle of in vitro fertilization (IVF; Tibi et al, 1989). The presence of ten follicles of more than 4–8 mm in at least one ovary gives a 75% probability of a polycystic response and a 42.8% chance of biological hyperstimulation (against 3.3 and 5.3% in the absence of these signs). These predictive criteria have a sensitivity of 50% and a specificity of 91.4%.

Choice of treatment

This is difficult, especially in cases of PCO. The most logical current solutions for simple stimulation would be clomiphene citrate and if this fails, pure FSH in small doses (Claman et al, 1986). For IVF the combination of the long period of desensitization with LHRH agonists and induction by FSH in small doses seems to be the best protocol (Salat-Baroux et al, 1988a), although even in these conditions there is still a risk of hyperstimulation.

Monitoring during treatment and the decision to trigger ovulation

Whenever gonadotrophins are used it is indispensable to use some form of monitoring in the last days of stimulation, by follicular ultrasound and rapid assays of plasma or urinary oestradiol. One should emphasize in these conditions that protocols of fixed ovulation stimulation run an avoidable potential risk of hyperstimulation, even when follicular aspiration is planned.

Blankenstein et al (1987) found that mild hyperstimulation at the time of hCG injection is characterized by the presence of eight or nine follicles, of which 68.7% are of intermediate size (9–15 mm diameter). Moderate to severe hyperstimulation is associated with 95% of preovulatory follicles less than 16 mm, of which 54.7% are <9 mm. In fact, isolated ultrasound examinations are insufficient to prevent the risk of severe hyperstimulation. The best parameter for monitoring remains plasma oestradiol (Hanning et al, 1983).

When excessive response to simple stimulation has been obtained (more than two or three mature follicles and > 500 pg/ml per mature follicle), hCG is usually not given to induce ovulation and patients are advised to avoid sexual intercourse. However, to avoid losing the benefit of the treated cycle, Hazout et al (1984) proposed aspirating the majority of the follicles on the 11th–12th day of the cycle and leaving just one or two intact. Belaisch-Allart et al (1988) induces ovulation with hCG and advises the patients to have sexual intercourse but aspirates all the follicles except one 35 h later and performs IVF with the oocytes obtained, followed by embryo cryopreservation. In the three reported cases, two pregnancies were obtained without complications. In the context of IVF, when the oestradiol is > 2500 pg/ml, caution is advised and it is suggested that ovulation should not be induced but LHRH agonist continued, to avoid a spontaneous peak of LH. We have tried to assess the possibility of inducing ovulation with hCG, aspirating all the follicles 36 h later, cryopreserving the embryos obtained with a view to later replacement, and continuing the administration of agonists until complete ovarian inactivity is obtained (Salat-Baroux et al, 1988b, 1990). Of 33 cases induced, with a mean oestradiol level of 3702 ± 885 pg/ml, 29 patients had secondary embryo replacement leading to eight pregnancies (24.2% per oocyte retrieval, 27.6% per replacement). However, 31% of pregnancies were obtained in 22 cases of biological hyperstimulation of a similar degree when fresh embryo transfer was performed. Interestingly, the only case of severe hyperstimulation obtained was in the first group.

Luteal phase support

Whenever there are patient risk factors, including polycystic type follicular response, abnormally high plasma oestradiol and/or number of oocytes obtained, or the ovaries are especially large and sensitive following aspiration, caution is advised before deciding to repeat the hCG injection in the luteal phase. It is better to avoid it and to use only progesterone in increasing doses.

In early pregnancy

This risk of hyperstimulation is increased by endogenous hCG secretion, which activates the phenomenon. Hormonal and ultrasound monitoring must be pursued.

CONCLUSION

Although the effects of the majority of ovulation-induction agents are incompletely understood and the physiopathology of severe ovarian hyperstimulation syndrome has not been completely worked out, the risk factors and the early mechanisms are known. These data suggest that an efficient policy for prevention while conserving the best success rate in the treatment of sterility is necessary.

SUMMARY

Clinical hyperstimulation is the most serious complication of ovulation induction, occurring in approximately 3% of cases (0.8% in the severe form). Paradoxically, it seems to be rare following in vitro fertilization, probably because all the follicles are aspirated. High-risk patients are those with polycystic ovarian disease, hyperprolactinaemia and hypothyroidism. All forms of ovulation induction have been implicated. Use of LHRH agonists have not reduced the incidence of hyperstimulation and they may even have increased it. An ongoing pregnancy seems to predispose to the occurrence of hyperstimulation, due to the secretion of hCG.

Clinically, three stages of hyperstimulation have been described by the WHO (mild, moderate and severe). The pathophysiology is not completely understood, although prostaglandins, histamines and, especially, the ovarian renin–angiotensin system may be involved. Local ovarian complications and thromboembolic complications have also occurred.

The treatment of severe hyperstimulation is both symptomatic (fluid replacement, aspiration of effusions, moderate sodium and water restriction, small doses of diuretics) and specific (corticosteroids, aspiration of ovarian cysts, even voluntary interruption of pregnancy in the most serious forms). If the hyperstimulation occurs in the absence of pregnancy, antihistamines or antiprostaglandins can be given.

Prevention is exceedingly important. This can be helped by recognition of polycystic ovarian disease and stimulation of these cases by clomiphene citrate or pure FSH associated, for use in in vitro fertilization, with prolonged desensitization using LHRH agonists. Daily ultrasound and hormonal monitoring of ovulation induction is required. When there is excessive response to stimulation, it is prudent not to induce ovulation with hCG or, alternatively, to aspirate all the follicles and freeze the embryos obtained without giving further injections of hCG in the luteal phase.

Clinical ovarian hyperstimulation is the classic form of iatrogenic disorder and is the most important complication of ovulation induction treatments, since it can be life-threatening in its most severe form. In this chapter we review current knowledge concerning the frequency, factors associated with its occurrence, clinical aspects, physiopathological mechanisms and, finally, the possibilities for treatment and prevention.

REFERENCES

Belaisch-Allart J, Belaisch J, Hazout A, Testart J & Frydman R (1988) Selective oocyte retrieval: a new approach to ovarian hyperstimulation. *Fertility and Sterility* **50:** 654–655.
Blankstein J, Shalev J, Saadon T et al (1987) Ovarian hyperstimulation syndrome: prediction by number and size of preovulatory ovarian follicles. *Fertility and Sterility* **47:** 597–602.
Borenstein R, Elhalah U, Lunenfeld B & Schwartz ZS (1989) Severe ovarian hyperstimulation syndrome: a reevaluated therapeutic approach. *Fertility and Sterility* **51:** 791–795.
Charbonnel B, Krempf M, Blanchard P, Dano F & Delage C (1987) Induction of ovulation in polycystic ovary syndrome with a combination of a luteinizing-releasing hormone analog and exogenous gonadotropins. *Fertility and Sterility* **47:** 920–924.
Check JH, Wu CH, Gocial B & Adelson HG (1985) Severe ovarian hyperstimulation syndrome from treatment with urinary follicle-stimulating hormone: two cases. *Fertility and Sterility* **43:** 317–319.
Chow KK & Choo HT (1984) Ovarian hyperstimulation syndrome with clomiphene citrate. Case report. *British Journal of Obstetrics and Gynaecology* **91:** 1051–1052.
Claman P, Seibel MM, McArdle C, Berger MJ & Taymor ML (1986) Comparison of intermediate-dose purified urinary follicle-stimulating hormone in patients with polycystic ovarian syndrome. *Fertility and Sterility* **46:** 518–522.
Fernandez LA, Tarlatzis BC, Rzasa PJ et al (1985) Renin-like activity in ovarian follicular fluid. *Fertility and Sterility* **44:** 219.
Forman R, Fries N, Testart J, Bellaisch-Allart J, Hazout A & Frydman R (1988) Evidence for an adverse effect of elevated serum estradiol concentrations on embryo implantation. *Fertility and Sterility* **49:** 118–122.

Franks S, Mason HD, Polson DW, Winston RML, Margara R & Reed MJ (1988) Mechanism and management of ovulatory failure in women with polycystic ovary syndrome. *Human Reproduction* **3**: 531–534.

Friedman CI, Schmidt GE, Chang FE & Kim MH (1984) Severe ovarian hyperstimulation following follicular aspiration. *American Journal of Obstetrics and Gynecology* **150**: 436–437.

Gergely RZ, Paldi E, Erlik Y & Makler A (1976) Treatment of ovarian hyperstimulation syndrome by antihistamine. *Obstetrics and Gynecology* **47**: 83–85.

Haning RV, Austin CW, Carlson IH, Kuzma DL, Shapiro SS & Zweibel WJ (1983) Plasma estradiol is superior to ultrasound and urinary estriol glucuronide as a predictor of ovarian hyperstimulation during induction of ovulation with menotropins. *Fertility and Sterility* **40**: 31–36.

Haning RV, Strawn EY & Nolten WE (1985) Pathophysiology of the ovarian hyperstimulation syndrome. *Obstetrics and Gynecology* **66**: 220–224.

Hazout A, Porchier J & Frydman R (1984) Une alternative à la réduction embryonnaire: la réduction folliculaire. *Gynécologie* **35**: 119.

Jager W, Diedrich K & Wildt L (1987) Elevated levels of CA-125 in serum of patients suffering from ovarian hyperstimulation syndrome. *Fertility and Sterility* **48**: 675–678.

Jahier J, Malbranche-Aupecle MH, Feldman JP et al (1985) L'hyperstimulation ovarienne: traitement des kystes volumineux par ponction percoelioscopique. *Revue Française de Gynécologie et Obstétrique* **80**: 109–111.

Katz Z, Lancet M, Borenstein R & Chemke J (1984) Absence teratogenicity of indomethacin in ovarian hyperstimulation syndrome. *International Journal of Fertility* **29**: 186–188.

Kirshon B, Doody MC, Cotton DB & Gibbons W (1988) Management of ovarian hyperstimulation syndrome with chlorpheniramine maleate, mannitol and invasive hemodynamic monitoring. *Obstetrics and Gynecology* **71**: 485–487.

Knox GE (1974) Antihistamine blockade of the ovarian hyperstimulation syndrome. *American Journal of Obstetrics and Gynecology* **118**: 992–993.

Lorcy Y, Bohec M & Allanic H (1984) Hyperstimulation ovarienne induite par l'administration pulsatile de gonadolibérine. *Presse Médicale* **42**: 300–302.

Lunenfeld B, Bloom S & Blankstein J (1986) Résultats de l'induction de l'ovulation par les ménotrophines chorioniques (HMG-HCG). In Dain (ed.) *Induction et stimulation de l'ovulation*, pp 155–162. Paris.

Morgan H, Paredes RA & Lachelin GCL (1983) Severe ovarian hyperstimulation after clomiphene citrate in a hypothyroid patient. Case report. *British Journal of Obstetrics and Gynaecology* **90**: 977–982.

Mozes M, Bogokowsky H, Antebi E et al (1965) Thromboembolic phenomena after ovarian stimulation with human gonadotrophins. *Lancet* **ii**: 1213–1214.

Navot D, Margalioth EJ, Laufer N et al (1987) Direct correlation between plasma renin activity and severity of the ovarian hyperstimulation syndrome. *Fertility and Sterility* **48**: 57–61.

Navot D, Relou A, Birkenfeld A, Rabinowitz R, Brzezinski A & Margaloth EJ (1988) Risk factors and prognostic variables in the ovarian hyperstimulation syndrome. *American Journal of Obstetrics and Gynecology* **159**: 210–215.

Neuwirth RS, Turksoy RN & van de Wilde RL (1965) Acute Meigs' syndrome secondary to ovarian stimulation with human menopausal gonadotropins. *American Journal of Obstetrics and Gynecology* **91**: 977–981.

Pekonen F, Laatikainen T, Buyalos R & Rutanen EM (1989) Decreased 34K insulin-like growth factor binding protein in polycystic ovarian disease. *Fertility and Sterility* **51**: 972–975.

Pride SM, Yuen BH & Moon YS (1984) Clinical, endocrinologic, and intraovarian prostaglandin F responses to H-1 receptor blockade in the ovarian hyperstimulation syndrome: studies in the rabbit model. *American Journal of Obstetrics and Gynecology* **148**: 670–674.

Rabau E, Serr DM, David A, Mashiach S & Lunenfeld B (1967) Human menopausal gonadotropins for anovulation and sterility. *American Journal of Obstetrics and Gynecology* **96**: 92–97.

Salat-Baroux J, Cornet D, Antoine JM, Alvarez S, Alfieri D & Bonnardot JP (1987) Un cas de stimulation, grave au cours d'une fécondation in vitro suivie de grossesse. *Gynécologie* **38**: 113–116.

Salat-Baroux J, Alvarez S, Antoine JM et al (1988a) Comparison between long and short protocols of LHRH agonist in the treatment of polycystic ovary disease by in vitro fertilization. *Human Reproduction* **3**: 535–539.

Salat-Baroux J, Alvarez S, Cornet D et al (1988b) Stratégie thérapeutique dans les hyper-stimulations biologiques au cours des fécondations in vitro. *Contraception Fertilité Sexualité* **16**: 589.

Salat-Baroux J, Alvarez S, Antoine JM et al (1990) Treatment of hyperstimulation during in vitro fertilization. *Human Reproduction* **5**: 36–39.

Schenker JG & Polishuk WZ (1976) The role of prostaglandins in ovarian hyperstimulation syndrome. *European Journal of Obstetrics, Gynecology and Reproductive Biology* **6**: 47–50.

Schenker G & Weinstein D (1978) Ovarian hyperstimulation syndrome: a current survey. *Fertility and Sterility* **30**: 255.

Suikkari AM, Ruutiainen K, Erkkola R & Seppala M (1989) Low levels of low molecular weight insulin-like growth factor-binding protein in patients with polycystic ovarian disease. *Human Reproduction* **4**: 136–139.

Thaler I, Yoffe N, Kaftory JK & Brandes JM (1981) Treatment of ovarian hyperstimulation syndrome: the physiologic basis for a modified approach. *Fertility and Sterility* **36**: 110–113.

Tibi C, Alvarez S, Cornet D, Antoine JM, Gomes AC & Salat-Baroux J (1989) Prédiction des hyperstimulations ovariennes. *Contraception Fertilité Sexualité* **17**: 751–752.

Tummon IS, Henig I, Radwanska E, Binor Z, Rawlins R & Dmowski WP (1988) Persistent ovarian cysts following administration of human menopausal and chorionic gonado-tropins: an attenuated form of ovarian hyperstimulation syndrome. *Fertility and Sterility* **49**: 244–248.

Yeh J, Barbieri RL & Ravnikar VA (1989) Ovarian hyperstimulation associated with the sole use of Leuprolide for ovarian suppression. *Journal of in Vitro Fertilization and Embryo Transfer* **6**: 261–262.

Younis JS, Zeevi D, Rabinowitz R, Laufer N & Shenker JG (1988) Transient liver function tests abnormalities in ovarian hyperstimulation syndrome. *Fertility and Sterility* **50**: 176–178.

Yuen BH, McComb P, Sy L, Lewis J & Cannon W (1979) Plasma prolactin, human chorionic gonadotropin, estradiol, testosterone, and progesterone in the ovarian hyperstimulation syndrome. *American Journal of Obstetrics and Gynecology* **133**: 316–320.

Zosmer A, Katz Z, Lancet M, Konichezky S & Schwartz-Shoham Z (1987) Adult respiratory distress syndrome complicating ovarian hyperstimulation syndrome. *Fertility and Sterility* **47**: 524–526.

14

Induction of ovulation—cost-effectiveness and future prospects

DAVID. T. BAIRD
WILLIAM L. LEDGER
ANNA F. GLASIER

In the last 30 years there have been spectacular advances in the treatment of anovulatory infertility. If the specific cause of the anovulation is diagnosed correctly and the appropriate treatment instigated, pregnancy rates approaching those described for normal fertile couples can be achieved. The object of any treatment of anovulatory infertility should be the birth of a single healthy baby at term. Unfortunately, this cannot always be achieved because one of the major side-effects of many methods of ovulation induction is the stimulation of the development of more than one ovulatory follicle. The deleterious effects of multiple pregnancies cannot be underestimated. There is a marked increase in the incidence of spontaneous abortion and preterm labour, which rise tenfold in twins as compared with singleton pregnancies. The perinatal mortality rate amongst preterm twins and triplets is very high, and even amongst the survivors there is an increased risk of serious handicap.

The risk of multiple births is not the only disadvantage associated with induction of ovulation. A few of the agents have recognizable side-effects which may be a hazard to mother and baby. These disadvantages must be considered when choosing treatment for a particular patient. Each couple should be carefully counselled about the risks and costs involved. Many infertile couples are so desperate to have a baby that they are unable to make a realistic assessment of the risk/benefit ratio. For example, when told of the risk of having triplets following treatment with gonadotrophins, many couples choose to ignore the obvious medical and social problems which inevitably accompanies their birth. In few other areas of medical practice is skilled counselling more important.

Another factor which has become increasingly important is the cost of treatment. Many of the drugs are extremely expensive, as are the sophisticated methods necessary to monitor the growth of the follicles. Although ovulation induction is highly successful, few couples realize that several courses of treatment may be necessary before pregnancy occurs. In many countries treatment of infertility is not available from a national health service or its cost is reimbursed only in part or not at all by private health

Baillière's Clinical Obstetrics and Gynaecology—
Vol. 4, No. 3, September 1990
ISBN 0–7020–1478–8

639

Table 1. Costs of treatment for ovulation induction.

Drug	Unit cost (£)	Dose and days of treatment	Cost of drugs (£)	Monitoring costs		Additional costs (£)	Total cost (£)	Pregnancy/cycle (%)
				Assays (£)	Scans (£)			
GnRH	0.5	15 µg/pulse every 90 min for 14 days	112	30	30	(pump) 30 (HCG) 5	207.00	25
Pergonal	10.24	2 ampoules for 10 days	205	55	30	(HCG) 5.00	295.00	5–30*
HCG	3.42	5000–10000 iu	3.42–6.84	—	—	—	—	—
Clomiphene	0.39	100 mg for 5 days	3.90	5	—	—	8.90	20
Tamoxifen	0.48	20 mg for 5 days	2.40	5	—	—	7.40	20
Dexamethasone	0.02	0.5 mg for 30 days	0.90	—	—	—	—	—
Metrodin	16.68	2 ampoules for 10 days	334	55	30	(HCG) 5.00	420.00	5–30*
Buserelin	0.42	600 µg for 20 days	50	15	—	—	—	—
Pergonal and buserelin			255	70	30	6.84	361.84	5
Bromocriptine	0.30	5 mg for 30 days	18	5	—	—	23	30

NB: Costs are given in pounds sterling. Monitoring costs are calculated at £5 per hormone assay and £10 per ultrasound scan.
* Pregnancy rate 5% for oligomenorrhoea, 30% for hypogonadotrophic hypogonadism.

insurance. Many couples have found the' selves bitter and disillusioned after years of unsuccessful and very expens 'e treatment. It is incumbent on the specialist to provide the couple with a realistic estimate of the likely success, side-effects and cost of any proposed treatment.

In this chapter we shall attempt to make an estimate of the cost/benefit ratio of the various forms of treatment of ovulation induction. We have assumed that investigations have been sufficiently detailed in order that the correct diagnosis can be made and that the only cause of infertility is the failure to ovulate. Clearly, if the male partner has suboptimal semen analysis or there is associated tubal disease, the pregnancy rate for any treatment will be lower, as will the cost/benefit ratio. We have taken the cost of drugs from *MIMS* in the UK in January 1990 (Table 1). The cost to hospitals or large institutions buying in bulk may be lower than this average, while the retail cost in pharmacies will be higher due to prescription costs etc. The actual cost of the drugs varies throughout European countries and the USA, but the relative costs remain fairly constant from country to country.

We have also made an attempt to price the cost of monitoring. It is appreciated that there may be large differences in the frequency of hormone and ultrasound measurements made, but the regimen on which we have based the costing is the minimum which we consider to be compatible with acceptable clinical practice.

HYPOGONADOTROPHIC HYPOGONADISM

This condition is characterized by low levels of oestradiol, as a consequence of the extremely low secretion of luteinizing hormone (LH) and follicle-stimulating hormone (FSH) (Yen, 1986). Because of the deficiency of gonadotrophins, these women are unresponsive to clomiphene and other anti-oestrogens. If the defect is hypothalamic, e.g. Kallman's syndrome or secondary amenorrhoea associated with weight loss or anorexia nervosa, it is possible to stimulate the anterior pituitary with gonadotrophin-releasing hormone (GnRH) administered in a pulsatile manner via a portable infusion pump (Leyendecker and Wildt, 1983). If there is pituitary disease it will be necessary to administer gonadotrophins.

Pulsatile GnRH

The treatment of choice in hypogonadotrophic women with an intact pituitary is pulsatile GnRH (Homburg et al, 1989). The advantage of this treatment is that it replaces the missing stimulation of the pituitary with GnRH. Because the feedback of ovarian steroids still occurs to regulate the secretion of FSH and LH by the anterior pituitary, the risk of multiple pregnancy is much reduced and minimal monitoring is necessary. Only a maximum of six hormone assays and three ultrasound scans are required to determine whether the treatment is effective.

It is, however, essential that the GnRH be administered in a series of pulses every 90 minutes day and night (Knobil, 1980). Continuous release of GnRH, such as could be achieved more conveniently by a biodegradable implant, rapidly leads to down-regulation of the anterior pituitary (Belchetz et al, 1978). Programmable pumps which are small enough to be worn continuously are available at a cost of £300–£500. The GnRH can be administered subcutaneously or intravenously via a fine disposable cannula (Archer, 1986). While the latter is more effective, it is also potentially more hazardous due to the risk of septicaemia. For this reason the infusion site is usually changed once or twice per week, adding to the cost and inconvenience of the procedure.

On average it may take 14 days treatment with GnRH to reach ovulation. Although theoretically it is possible to reduce the frequency of pulses to that found during the normal luteal phase (about every six hours), in practice the treatment is usually continued unaltered throughout the luteal phase. Alternatively, it is possible to induce ovulation with exogenous human chorionic gonadotrophin (HCG) when the leading follicle is > 18 mm. In this case it would be necessary to make daily ultrasound measurements around the time of expected ovulation and to give supplementary booster doses of HCG (1000 iu) every four days during the luteal phase. This second regimen involves the additional expense of frequent monitoring, but releases the pump during the luteal phase for other patients.

Treatment of suitable patients with pulsatile GnRH is highly effective, with a pregnancy rate of about 25% per cycle and a cumulative pregnancy rate approaching 90% (Mason et al, 1984; Santoro et al, 1986). It is safe and requires relatively little monitoring, but has the inconvenience of requiring the wearing a pump continuously, which is relatively expensive. The major cost is that of GnRH, so that the cost per cycle varies from £200 to £280 depending on which regimen is followed. Assuming an average of three treatment cycles per patient, the total cost per pregnancy is approximately £600, including a proportion of the capital cost of the pump.

Gonadotrophin treatment

If the anterior pituitary is missing or diseased, it will be necessary to stimulate the ovaries with gonadotrophins. It is not possible to use gonadotrophins prepared from animals due to the development of antibodies; the original material used by Carl Gemzell and his co-workers was extracted from human pituitaries (Gemzell et al, 1958). All preparations which are used currently are extracted from menopausal urine. The collection of urine from suitable subjects is time consuming and the extraction process cumbersome and, hence, human menopausal gonadotrophin (HMG) is extremely expensive. In recent years there has been an increased use of gonadotrophins for in vitro fertilization and other forms of assisted reproduction and there is therefore considerable impetus to develop an alternative source of FSH and LH by genetic engineering.

A major problem associated with the use of HMG is that the variability in response between patients is so great that it is necessary to adjust the dose in each treatment cycle from day to day. This involves frequent monitoring, with measurement of oestradiol in plasma or urine and ultrasound examination of the ovaries (Brown, 1986). We have assumed an average of 10 days treatment with two ampoules (150iu) or HMG per day. Including the cost of 5000iu HCG to induce ovulation and two further booster doses for luteal support, the total drug bill is £210 and the cost per cycle including monitoring about £300.

Gonadotrophin therapy in women with hypogonadotrophic hypogonadism is extremely effective and the pregnancy rate per cycle is about 30% (Oelsner et al, 1978; West and Baird, 1984). The major risks are hyperstimulation and multiple pregnancies. Severe hyperstimulation syndrome can be a life-threatening condition (Schenker and Weinstein, 1978) and, although its incidence can be reduced to less than 1% by careful monitoring and judicious withholding of the ovulatory dose of HCG when follicular development is excessive, this treatment should be supervised by those experienced in its use and with access to facilities for the management of acute emergencies. About 25% of pregnancies are multiple (Oelsner et al, 1978) and, although the majority are twins, even in experienced centres it has not been possible to avoid totally the occurrence of triplets or higher order births.

In summary, gonadotrophins given to women with hypogonadotrophic hypogonadism is probably the most effective treatment of infertile couples currently prescribed. However, it carries an appreciable risk of hyperstimulation and multiple pregnancy. Because frequent monitoring is required, it is inconvenient for the patient and relatively expensive, with a cost per treatment cycle of about £300 or £900 per baby.

OLIGOMENORRHOEA: NORMOGONADOTROPHIC ANOVULATION

Anti-oestrogens

Women with oligomenorrhoea and anovulation may have serum concentrations of gonadotrophins within the normal range or may have normal FSH levels with increased concentrations of LH, as in polycystic ovarian syndrome. In both cases serum oestradiol is usually within the range for the early to mid follicular phase of the cycle, and most of these women will respond to anti-oestrogens by increasing FSH and particularly LH, consequently stimulating follicle growth. Given orally and with an acceptable risk of multiple pregnancy, anti-oestrogens should be the drug of first choice for such women (Yen, 1980). Clomiphene citrate is the most widely used treatment, although other cheaper preparations such as tamoxifen are available (Klopper and Hall, 1971). As an absolute minimum, monitoring should aim to confirm that ovulation is indeed being induced successfully. In the absence of ovulation, the daily dose can be increased, in the case of clomiphene to 150–200 mg. If despite an increased dose follicular development occurs but without ovulation (i.e. a failure of positive feedback), HCG may be given in the presence of a preovulatory follicle but this significantly increases the cost of monitoring since ovulation will not occur if HCG is given too early or too late (Williams and Hodgen, 1980). Women with elevated serum concentrations of testosterone who fail to respond to high doses of clomiphene may ovulate if a small dose of dexamethasone is given daily in order to reduce the secretion of adrenal androgen which has a deleterious effect on developing follicles (Daly et al, 1984).

Anti-oestrogens are convenient to use as they are given orally without very intensive monitoring and are relatively cheap. Most women require treatment for several months, since the pregnancy rate per cycle is only about 20% (Hammond et al, 1983). Moreover, once pregnancy has been achieved there is still a 25% chance of spontaneous abortion and about 8% of pregnancies will be multiple (mainly twins). To date there is no evidence to suggest that pregnancies following clomiphene citrate have any additional risk of congenital malformation (Taubert and Kuhl, 1986).

In summary, anti-oestrogens are cheap, convenient and can be used with very little monitoring. The cost per cycle with a 20% chance of pregnancy is around £3.90, with an additional £5 for the cost of monitoring. The side-effects are minimal and the risks of both hyperstimulation and multiple pregnancy relatively small.

Gonadotrophins

Women with oligomenorrhoea who fail to respond to anti-oestrogens alone or in combination with HCG or dexamethasone may ovulate in response to gonadotrophins. The risks and costs of HMG (Pergonal, Serono Laboratories (UK) Ltd), have been discussed in the previous section. However, the pregnancy rate in this group of patients is significantly lower than in women with hypogonadotrophic hypogonadism. Therefore, more cycles of treatment are needed and some women may never conceive (Lunenfeld and Insler, 1978). For women with high levels of LH, 'pure' FSH (Metrodin, Serono Laboratories (UK) Ltd), was developed as a logical alternative approach (Claman and Seibel, 1986). The underlying concept was to administer only FSH, thereby correcting the LH:FSH ratio and avoiding giving yet more, possibly deleterious, LH. Unfortunately, there is no evidence to suggest that the incidence of either hyperstimulation or multiple pregnancy is reduced when compared with LH and FSH in combination. Moreover, the cost of drugs is higher—£334/cycle as compared with £205 for Pergonal—and there are no savings to be made on the monitoring costs of at least £85 per cycle.

Because women with oligomenorrhoea respond less consistently to gonadotrophin therapy than women with hypogonadotrophic hypogonadism, with the result that many more treatment cycles are abandoned, the cost, inconvenience, frustration and disappointment to the patients is increased. Down-regulation of endogenous pituitary gonadotrophin secretion with GnRH analogues administered both before and during gonadotrophin therapy (Chang et al, 1983) reduces the incidence of asynchronous follicle growth and premature LH surges and increases the chance of successful ovulation induction (Fleming et al, 1985; Fleming and Coutts, 1986). GnRH analogues are usually administered for 10–21 days before gonadotrophins are given and treatment continues during HMG therapy, so that a total of 20–31 days of administration at a total cost of £38–£57 is required. Costs also rise as a result of increased monitoring and prolonging the treatment, and the duration of the monitoring adds further inconvenience to the patient.

In summary, gonadotrophin therapy is expensive both in terms of the cost of the drugs and the requirements for intensive monitoring. GnRH analogues given in addition may reduce the number of cancelled cycles but are expensive. Whatever the regimen, the cost in terms of risk to the patient is high. Hyperstimulation can be fatal and multiple pregnancy a disaster. Many clinicians and most patients are unaware that the pregnancy rate achieved—perhaps because the women who are easy to treat have already conceived with anti-oestrogen therapy—is only around 5% per cycle.

HYPERPROLACTINAEMIC AMENORRHOEA

Of all disorders of ovulation, that associated with hyperprolactinaemia is the most amenable to treatment. Although the mechanisms by which increased circulating levels of prolactin inhibit ovulation remain unclear, the diagnosis is simple to make. Treatment is with a dopamine agonist such as bromocriptine which, acting like prolactin inhibitory factor (PIF), reduces pituitary prolactin secretion. Given orally at a dose of 5 mg/day for 30 days, the cost of the drug is £18 per cycle. In women with amenorrhoea or oligomenorrhoea the re-establishment of regular menstrual cycles is in itself enough to indicate ovulation and, with a pregnancy rate of 30% per cycle, many women conceive soon after starting treatment. Women with regular cycles who are not ovulating or who have luteal phase dysfunction in association with hyperprolactinaemia may need some monitoring to confirm regular ovulation. As multiple follicular development is not a consequence of dopamine agonist treatment, there is no risk of hyperstimulation and no increased incidence of multiple pregnancy, so monitoring can be minimal. To date there is no evidence that women conceiving on dopamine agonists have any increased risk of infants with congenital anomalies (Turkalj et al, 1982).

Unfortunately, some women are unable to tolerate the almost universal side-effect of nausea associated with dopamine agonist treatment and doses needed to achieve normoprolactinaemia are unattainable. New agonists (lisuride and pergolide) have become available (De Cecco et al, 1978; Franks et al, 1981) but in our hands results are disappointing as these drugs are seldom better tolerated. Women in whom ovulation cannot be induced with oral dopamine agonists can be successfully treated with surgery or radiotherapy, or ovulation can be induced with pulsatile GnRH or gonadotrophins in the presence of continued hyperprolactinaemia should the patient wish to avoid these more radical procedures (Grossman and Besser, 1985; Polson et al, 1986). Women with large pituitary tumours who respond to dopamine agonists with ovulation should be advised to defer pregnancy for some months as once treatment is stopped and with stimulation by high circulating levels of oestrogen, the tumour may expand significantly (Gemzell and Wang, 1979). Alternatively, in these women surgery may be the treatment of choice (Scanlon et al, 1985).

In summary, the treatment of anovulation in association with hyperprolactinaemia is effective, cheap and without major risks or side-effects.

FUTURE PROSPECTS

It is apparent from the previous sections that although the treatment of anovulatory infertility with the regimens currently available is highly successful in many cases, it is expensive, inconvenient and not without risk. The ideal of restoring the working of the hypothalamic–pituitary unit to normal cannot always be achieved conveniently, although treatment of hyperprolactinaemia with dopamine agonists approaches this ideal. Further developments in this field will depend on gaining a more comprehensive knowledge of the normal mechanisms controlling follicle growth and ovulation as well as of the pathophysiology of anovulatory states. In this section, we shall discuss what approaches are likely to lead to improvement in the treatment of different forms of anovulatory infertility.

Hypogonadotrophic hypogonadism

In the majority of women who present with secondary amenorrhoea associated with low levels of gonadotrophins, the origin is presumed to be hypothalamic. The absence of LH pulses reflects the inability of the hypothalamus to generate pulses of GnRH (Vaughan Williams et al, 1983). We know very little about the control of the activity of the GnRH 'pulse generator' in normal women and even less about the defects in women with 'hypothalamic' amenorrhoea (Marshall and Odell, 1989). Basic research in the rat has revealed that noradrenergic neurotransmitters are involved in normal control of GnRH neurones and that endogenous opioids may influence their activity (Meites et al, 1979; Rance et al, 1981). It has been shown in some women with hyperprolactinaemia that administration of the opioid antagonist naltrexone causes an immediate increase in the pulsatile release of LH (Quigley et al, 1980; Grossman et al, 1982). A preliminary report showed that the administration of naltrexone, a long-acting opioid antagonist, to women with secondary amenorrhoea resulted in restoration of ovarian cyclicity (Wildt and Leyendecker, 1987). These results suggest that in some women with hypothalamic amenorrhoea there is an increase in endogenous opioid tone which leads to inhibition of the activity of the GnRH neurones such as occurs during lactation (McNeilly, 1988). As more knowledge becomes available about the neurotransmitters involved in normal hypothalamic function it may be possible to give treatment with specific agonists or antagonists. It may even be possible to stimulate the neurones intermittently, such as has been done experimentally in rhesus monkeys with aspartate (Gay and Plant, 1987).

Another improvement in the treatment of women with hypogonadotrophic hypogonadism would be the development of a more convenient form of administering GnRH. At present it is necessary to use expensive pumps to deliver intermittent pulses, but it may be possible to devise an implant or long-acting depot which releases GnRH in a fluctuating manner. In certain types of amenorrhoea it may even be possible to prime the anterior pituitary by administration of continuous amounts of GnRH given at a dose below that which will induce desensitization of the anterior pituitary, as has been shown to be effective in anoestrus sheep (McLeod et al, 1982).

Mention has already been made of the fact that HMG is expensive, inconvenient to prepare and in limited supply. Moreover, as commercially available, each ampoule contains a fixed mixture of 75 iu of LH and FSH. 'Pure' FSH with minimal LH activity is also available (Metrodin), although it is also extracted from postmenopausal urine and is subject to the same disadvantages as HMG. The half-life of FSH extracted from urine is extremely long (about 48 hours) due to the fact that it is strongly glycosylated and acidic (Diczfalusy and Harlin, 1988). The fixed ratio of LH : FSH in Pergonal and the long half-life of FSH make it extremely difficult to adjust the dose from day to day.

In the normal cycle a single follicle is selected for ovulation each month by a process involving feedback between the ovary and the anterior pituitary (Baird, 1987). Once selected the dominant follicle suppresses the secretion of FSH to a level below that which is necessary to activate other antral follicles. In this way a single follicle is available for ovulation each month. LH is also necessary for normal growth of the follicle by stimulating the production of androgens from the theca layer which are then used as precursors for the synthesis of oestrogens by the granulosa cells. There is evidence, however, from experiments in sheep and from women with polycystic ovary syndrome that if the level of LH is raised above normal, the development of large preovulatory follicles is suppressed (Franks et al, 1983; Glasier et al, 1989a; Picton et al, 1990).

In view of these observations there would be considerable advantage in having available preparations of pure FSH and LH so that the amounts of each gonadotrophin could be varied to simulate the changes which occur during the normal ovarian cycle. Preliminary data have shown that it is possible to restrict the number of ovulatory follicles by progressively reducing the amount of FSH given after the threshold dose of HMG has been reached. The genes coding for the α and β subunits of LH and FSH have been cloned and transvected into ovarian cells of the Chinese hamster (Chappel, 1987). If the problems associated with controlling the degree of glycosylation can be overcome it should be possible to produce pure preparations of LH and FSH for clinical use.

Oligomenorrhoea

Another possible advance in treatment is the development of pure anti-oestrogens for the induction of ovulation in oligomenorrhoeic women. Clomiphene citrate is a mixture of two isomers of which only one (en) has anti-oestrogenic activity (Glasier et al, 1989). The zu isomer, which is a weak oestrogen, has an extremely long half-life and persists in the body for several weeks after ingestion. Even tamoxifen, which is a more potent anti-oestrogen than clomiphene, has agonist activity in women who are profoundly hypo-oestrogenic (Furr and Jordan, 1984).

It is thought that anti-oestrogens induce ovulation in women by virtue of antagonizing the negative feedback effect of endogenous oestrogens and causing an increase in the secretion of FSH (Adashi, 1986). The rise in LH which invariably accompanies administration of clomiphene citrate, and which may have a deleterious effect on follicular development, could be due to the oestrogenic zu isomer (Hsueh et al, 1978). A pure anti-oestrogen such as has been developed by ICI (ICI 164,384) may result in a preferential elevation of FSH by acting at the level of the pituitary (Wakeling and Bowler, 1988).

Another promising approach to increasing the concentration of FSH selectively in anovulatory women is by antagonizing inhibin. This glyco-protein is secreted by the granulosa cells of large antral follicles and suppresses the secretion of FSH from the anterior pituitary without affecting the levels of LH. In rats and sheep administration of antisera to inhibin results in a rise in the concentration of FSH and an increase in the number of preovulatory follicles (Rivier et al, 1986; Mann et al, 1989). In the future it may be possible to synthesize antagonists of inhibin which would be a powerful new class of compounds for use in the treatment of anovulatory infertility.

REFERENCES

Adashi EY (1986) Clomiphene citrate-induced ovulation. *Seminars in Reproductive Endocrinology* **4:** 255–276.

Archer DF (1986) Use of luteinizing hormone-releasing hormone for ovulation induction. *Seminars in Reproductive Endocrinology* **4:** 285–291.

Baird DT (1987) A model for follicular selection and ovulation: lessons from superovulation. *Journal of Steroid Biochemistry* **27:** 15–23.

Belchetz PE, Plant TM, Nakai Y, Keogh EJ & Knobil E (1978) Hypophyseal responses to continuous and intermittent delivery of hypothalamic gonadotropin releasing hormone (GnRH). *Science* **202:** 631–633.

Brown JB (1986) Gonadotropins. In Insler V & Lunenfeld B (eds) *Infertility: Male and Female*, pp 359–396. Edinburgh: Churchill Livingstone.

Chang RJ, Lauffer LR, Meldrum DR et al (1983) Steroid secretion in polycystic ovarian disease after ovarian suppression by a long-acting gonadotropin-releasing hormone agonist. *Journal of Clinical Endocrinology and Metabolism* **56:** 897–903.

Chappel S (1987) Factors that regulate follicle stimulating hormone biosynthesis and secretion. In Burger HG, de Kretser DM, Findlay JK & Igarashi M (eds) *Inhibin—Non-steroidal Regulation of Follicle Stimulating Hormone Secretion*, pp 1–15. New York: Raven Press.

Claman P & Seibel MM (1986) Purified human follicle-stimulating hormone for ovulation induction: a critical review. *Seminars in Reproductive Endocrinology* **4:** 277–283.

Daly DC, Walters CA, Soto-Albors C-E, Tohan N & Riddick DH (1984) A randomised study of dexamethasone in ovulation induction with clomiphene citrate. *Fertility and Sterility* **41:** 844–848.

De Cecco L, Foglia G, Ragni N, Rossato P & Venturini PL (1978) The effect of lisuride hydrogen maleate in the hyperprolactinaemia-amenorrhoea syndrome: clinical and hormonal responses. *Clinical Endocrinology* **9:** 491–498.

Diczfalusy E & Harlin J (1988) Clinical-pharmacological studies on human menopausal gonadotropin. *Human Reproduction* **3:** 21–27.

Fleming R & Coutts JRT (1986) Induction of multiple follicular growth in normal menstruating women with endogenous gonadotropin suppression. *Fertility and Sterility* **45:** 226–230.

Fleming R, Haxton MJ, Hamilton MPR et al (1985) Successful treatment of infertile women with oligomenorrhoea using a combination of an LHRH agonist and exogenous gonadotrophins. *British Journal of Obstetrics and Gynaecology* **92:** 369–373.

Franks S, Horrocks PM, Lynch SS, Butt WR & London DR (1981) Treatment of hyperprolactinaemia with pergolide mesylate: acute effects and preliminary evaluation of long-term treatment. *Lancet* **ii:** 659–661.

Franks S, Horrocks PM, Lynch SS, Butt WR & London DR (1983) Effectiveness of pergolide mesylate in long-term treatment of hyperprolactinaemia. *British Medical Journal* **286:** 1177–1179.

Furr BJ & Jordan VC (1984) The pharmacological and clinical uses of tamoxifen. *Pharmacology and Therapeutics* **25:** 127–205.

Gay VL & Plant TM (1987) N-Methyl-D-L aspartate elicits hypothalamic gonadotrophin releasing hormone release in prepubertal male rhesus monkeys (*Macaca mulatta*). *Endocrinology* **120:** 2289–2296.

Gemzell C & Wang CF (1979) Outcome of pregnancy in women with pituitary adenoma. *Fertility and Sterility* **31:** 363–372.

Gemzell CA, Diczfalusy E & Tillinger G (1958) Clinical effect of human pituitary follicle-stimulating hormone (FSH). *Journal of Clinical Endocrinology and Metabolism* **18:** 1333–1348.

Glasier AF, Baird DT & Hillier SG (1989a) FSH and the control of follicular growth. *Journal of Steroid Biochemistry* **32(1B):** 167–170.

Glasier AF, Irvine DS, Wickings EJ, Hillier SG & Baird DT (1989b) A comparison of the effects on follicular development between clomiphene citrate, its two separate isomers and spontaneous cycles. *Human Reproduction* **4:** 252–256.

Grossman A & Besser GM (1985) Prolactinomas. *British Medical Journal* **290:** 182–184.

Grossman A, Moult PJA, McIntyre H et al (1982) Opiate mediation of amenorrhoea in hyperprolactinaemia and in weight-loss related amenorrhoea. *Clinical Endocrinology* **17:** 379–388.

Hammond MG, Halme JK & Talbert LM (1983) Factors affecting the pregnancy rate in clomiphene citrate induction of ovulation. *Obstetrics and Gynecology* **62:** 196–202.

Homburg R, Eshel E, Armar NA et al (1989) One hundred pregnancies after treatment with pulsatile luteinising hormone releasing hormone to induce ovulation. *British Medical Journal* **298:** 809–812.

Hsueh AJW, Erickson GF & Yen SSC (1978) Sensitisation of pituitary cells to luteinising hormone releasing hormone by clomiphene citrate in vitro. *Nature* **273:** 57–59.

Klopper A & Hall M (1971) New synthetic agent for the induction of ovulation: preliminary trials in women. *British Medical Journal* **1:** 152–154.

Knobil E (1980) The neuroendocrine control of the menstrual cycle. *Recent Progress in Hormone Research* **36:** 53–88.

Leyendecker G & Wildt L (1983) Induction of ovulation and chronic-intermittent (pulsatile) administration of GnRH in hypothalamic amenorrhoea. *Journal of Reproduction and Fertility* **69:** 397–409.

Lunenfeld B & Insler V (1978) *Diagnosis and Treatment of Functional Infertility*, pp 61–89. Berlin: Grosse Verlag.

McLeod BJ, Haresign W & Lamming GE (1982) The induction of ovulation and luteal function in seasonally anoestrous ewes treated with small-dose multiple injections of GnRH. *Journal of Reproduction and Fertility* **65:** 215–221.

McNeilly AS (1988) Suckling and the control of gonadotropin secretion. In Knobil E & Neill J (eds) *The Physiology of Reproduction*, pp 2323–2349. New York: Raven Press.

Mann GE, Campbell BK, McNeilly AS & Baird DT (1989) Passively immunizing ewes against inhibin during the luteal phase of the oestrus cycle raises the plasma concentration of FSH. *Journal of Endocrinology* **123:** 383–391.

Marshall JC & Odell WD (1989) The menstrual cycle—hormonal regulation, mechanisms of anovulation, and responses of the reproductive tract to steroid hormones. In De Groot LJ (ed.) *Endocrinology*, vol. 2, pp 1940–1949. Philadelphia: WB Saunders.

Mason P, Adams J, Morris DV et al (1984) Induction of ovulation with pulsatile luteinising hormone releasing hormone. *British Medical Journal* **288:** 181–185.

Meites J, Bruni JF, Van Vugt DA & Smith AF (1979) Relation of endogenous opioid peptides and morphine to neuroendocrine functions. *Life Sciences* **24:** 1325–1336.

Oelsner G, Serr DM, Mashiach S, Blankstein J, Snyder M & Lunenfeld B (1978) The study of induction of ovulation with menotropins: analysis of results of 1897 treatment cycles. *Fertility and Sterility* **30:** 538–544.

Picton HM, Tsonis CG & McNeilly AS (1990) The antagonistic effect of exogenous LH pulses on FSH-stimulated preovulatory follicle growth in ewes chronically treated with GnRH agonist. *Journal of Endocrinology* (in press).

Polson DW, Sagle M, Mason HD, Adams J, Jacobs HS & Franks S (1986) Ovulation and normal luteal function during LHRH treatment of women with hyperprolactinaemic amenorrhoea. *Clinical Endocrinology* **24:** 531–537.

Quigley ME, Sheehan KL, Casper RF & Yen SSC (1980) Evidence for increased dopaminergic and opioid activity in patients with hypothalamic hypogonadotropic hypogonadism. *Journal of Clinical Endocrinology and Metabolism* **50:** 949–954.

Rance N, Wise PM, Selmanoff MK & Barraclough CA (1981) Catecholamine turnover rates in discrete hypothalamic areas and associated changes in median eminence luteinizing hormone-releasing hormone and serum gonadotropins on proestrus and diestrus Day 1. *Endocrinology* **108:** 1795–1802.

Rivier C, Rivier J & Vale W (1986) Inhibin-mediated feedback control of follicle-stimulating hormone secretion in the female rat. *Science* **234:** 205–208.

Santoro N, Wierman ME, Filicori M, Waldstreicher J & Crowley WF Jnr (1986) Intravenous administration of pulsatile gonadotrophin-releasing hormone in hypothalamic amenorrhoea: effects of dosage. *Journal of Clinical Endocrinology and Metabolism* **62:** 109–116.

Scanlon MF, Peters JR, Thomas JP et al (1985) Management of selected patients with hyperprolactinaemia by partial hypophysectomy. *British Medical Journal* **291:** 1547–1550.

Schenker JG & Weinstein D (1978) Ovarian hyperstimulation syndrome: a current survey. *Fertility and Sterility* **30:** 255–268.

Taubert HHD & Kuhl H (1986) Steroids and steroid like compounds. In Insler V & Lunenfeld B (eds) *Infertility: Male and Female*, pp 413–449. Edinburgh: Churchill Livingstone.

Turkalj I, Braun P & Kropp P (1982) Surveillance of bromocriptine in pregnancy. *Journal of the American Medical Association* **247:** 1589–1591.

Vaughan Williams CA, McNeilly AS & Baird DT (1983) The effects of chronic treatment with LHRH on gonadotrophin secretion and pituitary responsiveness to LHRH in women with secondary hypogonadism. *Clinical Endocrinology* **19:** 9–19.

Wakeling AE & Bowler J (1988) Biology and mode of action of pure antioestrogens. *Journal of Steroid Biochemistry* **30:** 141–147.

West CP & Baird DT (1984) Induction of ovulation with gonadotrophins—a ten year review. *Scottish Medical Journal* **29:** 212–217.

Wildt L & Leyendecker G (1987) Induction of ovulation by the chronic administration of naltrexone in hypothalamic amenorrhoea. *Journal of Clinical Endocrinology and Metabolism* **64:** 1334–1335.

Williams RF & Hodgen GD (1980) Disparate effects of human chorionic gonadotropin during the late follicular phase in monkeys: normal ovulation, follicular atresia, ovarian acyclicity, and hypersecretion of follicle-stimulating hormone. *Fertility and Sterility* **33:** 64–68.

Yen SSC (1980) The polycystic ovary syndrome. *Clinical Endocrinology* **12:** 177–208.

Yen SSC (1986) Chronic anovulation due to CNS–hypothalamic–pituitary dysfunction. In Yen SSC & Jaffe RB (eds) *Reproductive Endocrinology, Physiology, Pathophysiology and Clinical Management*, pp 500–545. Philadelphia: WB Saunders.

Index

Note: Page numbers of article titles are in **bold** type.